EADI Global Development Series

Series Editors
Isa Baud, University of Amsterdam, Amsterdam, The Netherlands
Andrew Mold, United Nations Economic Commission for Africa, Kigali,
Rwanda
Pedro Goulart, Instituto Superior de Ciências Sociais e Políticas,
University of Lisbon, Lisboa, Portugal

The **EADI Global Development book series** seeks to broaden our understanding of the processes that advance or impede human development, whether from a political, economic, sociological or anthropological perspective. Development Studies is a multi- and inter-disciplinary field of study. The European Association of Development Research and Training Institutes (EADI) reaches with over 120 development research institutes and regular conferences the most important institutes and researchers in this field.

The book series aims to better understand the interplay between social, economic, political, technological, ecological, cultural and gendered (inter-sectional) aspects of societal change at the local, national, regional and global levels. It focusses on the link between theory, policy and practice. New formats include: **"From past to present - and vice versa"** (development processes are not ahistorical); **"From theory to practice - and vice versa"** (dialogues between academics, policymakers and practitioners); and **"Development roundtable"** (a forum where major contributors engage in a debate about a specific topic. Original and thought-provoking perspectives based on evidence are encouraged).

The series editors invite proposals for manuscripts across all disciplines at bookproposals@eadi.org.

Anika Altaf · Dzodzi Tsikata ·
Gertrude Dzifa Torvikey · Marleen Dekker
Editors

EQUITY IN COVID-19

Mitigation and Policy Responses in Africa

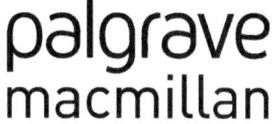

Editors
Anika Altaf
INCLUDE Knowledge Platform for
Inclusive Development Policies
African Studies Centre Leiden
Leiden, The Netherlands

Gertrude Dzifa Torvikey
Institute of Statistical, Social
and Economic Research (ISSER)
University of Ghana
Accra, Ghana

Dzodzi Tsikata
Department of Development Studies
SOAS, University of London
London, UK

INCLUDE Knowledge Platform for
Inclusive Development Policies
African Studies Centre Leiden
Leiden, The Netherlands

Marleen Dekker
African Studies Centre Leiden
Leiden, The Netherlands

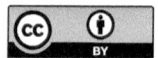

ISSN 2947-8529   ISSN 2947-8537   (electronic)
EADI Global Development Series
ISBN 978-3-031-58587-6   ISBN 978-3-031-58588-3   (eBook)
https://doi.org/10.1007/978-3-031-58588-3

This Palgrave Macmillan imprint is published by the registered company Springer Nature
Switzerland AG
The registered company address is: Gewerbestrasse 11, 6330 Cham, Switzerland

If disposing of this product, please recycle the paper.

Acknowledgements

We gratefully acknowledge the INCLUDE Knowledge Platform on Inclusive Development Policies for facilitating and funding the twelve country case studies of the *"Equity in COVID-19, Mitigation and Policy Responses in Africa"* research, as well as the synthesis study of the twelve case studies and for commissioning a paper on learning from past pandemic experiences such as Ebola.

We are grateful to all the authors of the country case studies who have carried out excellent research and shared important insights in the county case study chapters of this book.

Finally, we thank all reviewers for their helpful and constructive feedback of the country case studies and synthesis report, Désiré Assogbavi, Paul Litjens, Dennis Arends and Manon Heuvels.

CONTENTS

LIST OF CONTRIBUTORS

Anika Altaf INCLUDE Knowledge Platform for Inclusive Development Policies, African Studies Centre Leiden, Leiden, The Netherlands

Tesfaye C. Cholo Department of Development Economics, Ethiopian Civil Service University, Addis Ababa, Ethiopia

Angela Collet Centre for Democracy and Human Rights (CDD), Maputo, Mozambique

Akosua K. Darkwah Department of Sociology, University of Ghana, Accra, Ghana

Marleen Dekker African Studies Centre Leiden, Leiden, The Netherlands;
Institute of Statistical, Social and Economic Research (ISSER), University of Ghana, Accra, Ghana

Djénéba Diarra Groupe de Recherche en Économie Appliquée Et Théorique (GREAT), Bamako, Mali

Laura Ferguson Institute On Inequalities in Global Health, University of Southern California, Los Angeles, CA, USA

Majdi Hassen University of Tunis, ESSECT, Tunis, Tunisia

Rahmane Idrissa EPGA, Niamey, Niger

Chimere Iheonu Centre for the Study of the Economies of Africa (CSEA), Abuja, Nigeria

Ezra Ihezi Centre for the Study of the Economies of Africa (CSEA), Abuja, Nigeria

Tonny Kapsandui Reproductive, Maternal Child and Adolescent Health Programme, Amref Health Africa, Kampala, Uganda

Irene Kizito Corporate Programmes' Department, Amref Health Africa Headquarters, Nairobi, Kenya

Leonie Koumassa University of Princeton, Princeton, USA

Shiphrah Kuria Corporate Programmes' Department, Amref Health Africa Headquarters, Nairobi, Kenya

Miles Lambert-Peck Institute On Inequalities in Global Health, University of Southern California, Los Angeles, CA, USA

Mohamed Ali Marouani UMR Développement Et Sociétés, Université Paris 1 Panthéon-Sorbonne, Paris, France

Martin Luther Munu Department of International and European Law, Maastricht University, Maastricht, The Netherlands

Yannick Ngongang African School of Economics, IREEP, Abomey-Calavi, Benin

Adriano Nuvunga Centre for Democracy and Human Rights (CDD), Maputo, Mozambique

Thelma Obiakor Centre for the Study of the Economies of Africa (CSEA), Abuja, Nigeria

Thierry Ogoutchoro Innovation for Povercty Action, Washington DC, USA

Clara Osei-Boateng Independent Research Consultant, Cobquecura, Chile

Krishni Satchi Corporate Programmes' Department, Amref Health Africa Headquarters, Nairobi, Kenya

Dimas Sinoia Fórum de Monitoria Do Orçamento, Maputo, Mozambique

Kassa Teshager Department of Development Economics, Ethiopian Civil Service University, Addis Ababa, Ethiopia

Dorte Thorsen Institute of Development Studies, University of Sussex, Brighton, UK

Gertrude Dzifa Torvikey Institute of Statistical, Social and Economic Research (ISSER), University of Ghana, Accra, Ghana; Department of Development Studies, SOAS, University of London, London, United Kingdom

Ousmane Z. Traoré Department of Agricultural Economics and Consumer Science, Groupe de Recherche en Économie Appliquée Et Théorique (GREAT), Laval University, Québec, Canada

Dzodzi Tsikata Department of Development Studies, SOAS, University of London, London, UK; INCLUDE Knowledge Platform for Inclusive Development Policies, African Studies Centre Leiden, Leiden, The Netherlands

Zjos Vlaminck Cobquecura, Chile; Independent Governance and Social Development Expert, Accra, Ghana

Leonard Wantchekon African School of Economics, IREEP, Abomey-Calavi, Benin

Madeleine Wayack-Pambè Institut Supérieur Des Sciences de La Population, Université Joseph KI-ZERBO, Ouagadougou, Burkina Faso

Emilie Wojcieszynski School of Economics, Utrecht University, Utrecht, Nederland

LIST OF FIGURES

List of Tables

CHAPTER 1

Introduction

Anika Altaf, Dzodzi Tsikata, Gertrude Dzifa Torvikey, and Marleen Dekker

CONTEXTS MATTER: AFRICA'S EARLY COVID-19 RESPONSES

For Africa, the COVID-19 pandemic has compounded decades of cyclical socio-economic and health crises and changing policy frameworks and prescriptions. At the onset of the COVID-19 pandemic in the early 2020s, with growing global uncertainty and concern regarding the impact of COVID-19, many African governments acted quickly, both to prevent the spread of the virus and to mitigate its effects on their economies and citizens. They did this with various public

A. Altaf (✉) · D. Tsikata
INCLUDE Knowledge Platform for Inclusive Development Policies, African Studies Centre Leiden, Leiden, The Netherlands
e-mail: a.altaf@asc.leidenuniv.nl

D. Tsikata
e-mail: dt48@soas.ac.uk

G. D. Torvikey
Department of Development Studies, SOAS, University of London, London, United Kingdom
e-mail: torvikeydzifa@gmail.com

© The Author(s) 2024
A. Altaf et al. (eds.), *EQUITY IN COVID-19*, EADI Global Development Series, https://doi.org/10.1007/978-3-031-58588-3_1

1

health measures including (partial) lockdowns and mobilising health-care resources, support programmes for businesses and social protection measures for households and certain categories of workers (Rafalimanana and Sherif (2021), INCLUDE (2021). There were, however, significant variations in the severity and type of measures taken, as well as their accessibility and impacts (see, e.g., Konte et al., 2022). In the design and implementation of these measures, equity—the situation in which everyone is treated fairly according to their needs—was not a given. Therefore, important questions were raised about who was affected most by public health measures, who was benefiting from the support measures, and who was left unprotected. In Africa, COVID-19 was described as the inequality pandemic (Qureishi (2020), Berkhout et al. (2021), Gopalakr-ishnan et al (2021)) and the unequal impacts of the pandemic have been and continue to be documented. National level inequalities are part of a larger set of global inequalities and power dynamics that (re) surfaced during the pandemic, characterised by Antonio Guterres, UN Secretary General, quite early in the pandemic:

> COVID-19 has been likened to an x-ray, revealing fractures in the fragile skeleton of the societies we have built. It is exposing fallacies and false-hoods everywhere: The lie that free markets can deliver healthcare for all; The fiction that unpaid care work is not work; The delusion that we live in a post-racist world; The myth that we are all in the same boat. While we are all floating on the same sea, it's clear that some are in super yachts, while others are clinging to the drifting debris.
> –Antonio Guterres, UN Secretary General, 2020

The international development community responded to the pandemic by investing in strengthening country-level responses. In June 2021, G7 countries committed US$80 billion to support African countries to recover quickly from COVID-19. While this was a good example of

M. Dekker
Institute of Statistical, Social and Economic Research, University of Ghana, Accra, Ghana

African Studies Centre Leiden, University of Leiden, Leiden, The Netherlands

M. Dekker
e-mail: m.dekker@asc.leidenuniv.nl

solidarity, it fell far short of the demand for an effective and sustained anti-COVID-19 response. Reports of aid reduction decisions by certain bilateral donors, vaccine nationalism, point to the continuing economic and political inequalities and hierarchies in the global order (see also Sidibe (2022)) In the discussions about access to vaccines, Africa's aid dependence and the accompanying vulnerabilities, including the lack of policy autonomy, space to seize opportunities to build self-reliance and the compromised sustainability of innovations and inventions, have been topical.

Amidst this uncertainty in the early days of the pandemic in 2020, the knowledge platform on inclusive development policies (INCLUDE) initiated the research programme '*Equity in COVID-19*'. Focused on a critical examination of containment and mitigation responses to the pandemic and their impacts in 12 African countries, with special reference to marginalised, vulnerable and disadvantaged social groups, this project was one of several important efforts to respond to the imperative of research-based policy making, particularly on the issue of inequalities.

This edited volume presents the case studies that systematically reconstruct, document and analyse how national governments and other stakeholders have responded to the COVID-19 pandemic and if and to what extent governments have taken equity into account in COVID-19 policy responses. Based on a variety of empirical data and disciplinary perspectives, research teams from across the continent present evidence on the (non) inclusive nature of mitigation and policy responses. The book situates these findings on short-term interventions and impact in debates on the longer term implications of the COVID-19 on development on the continent.

This introduction to the edited volume provides a short description on the pandemics' trajectory in Africa, with a focus on the first wave in 2020, an elaboration of the research focus and approach, as well as a contextual description on the status of development in the country cases at the time the pandemic occurred.

Development of (the Narrative on) COVID-19 in Africa[1]

On 14 February 2020, the COVID-19 pandemic was confirmed to have spread to Africa, with the first case announced in Egypt (Egypt Today, 2020), followed by Nigeria at the end of February 2020 (BBC News, 2020). Within three months, the virus spread throughout the continent, with Lesotho being the last to report the first case on 13 May 2020.

With uncertainties about the transmission and mutation of the virus at the onset of the pandemic, and with reference to the generally weak health systems as well as the high number of people with underlying risks such as HIV and malnutrition, concerns on how the virus would affect Africa grew (WHO, 2020). In some circles, these concerns were expressed in dramatic scenarios and dystopian visions of extremely high death rates and total societal breakdown. One of the more dramatic expressions of concern was the often cited statement by Melinda Gates, co-chair of the Bill & Melinda Gates Foundation, in April 2020, that 'unless the world acts fast, dead bodies will litter the streets of Africa'(CNN Business, 2020). The United Nations Commission for Africa projected that without aid and intervention, up to 1.2 billion of the 1.6 billion Africans would be infected and between 300,000 and 3.3 million would die of COVID-19 (UNECA, 2020). A group of African scholars presented a more realistic projection of 150,078 deaths by May 2021 and between 16 and 26% of Africa's population infected within the first year of the pandemic (Cabore et al., 2020).

While there remain question marks about Africa's infection and mortality statistics because of the generally poor medical data collection and management systems, low diagnostic and testing capabilities and rates of testing and surveillance, there is evidence to suggest that infections and related mortality numbers have been relatively low. As of 3rd September 2021, COVID-19 infection and mortality rates were modest when compared with what countries in the Americas (84,498,889 cases), Europe (65,697,497 cases), South-East Asia (41,504,688 cases), Eastern Mediterranean (14,776,814 cases), Western Pacific (6,778,828 cases) had experienced. Africa recorded the lowest numbers of infections with 5,689,356 cases.

---

[1] Atuire and Rutazibwa (2021) provide a more detailed discussion on the discourse on COVID-19 in Africa.

Similarly, the impacts of COVID-19 on access to health in African countries have not been as devastating as earlier predicted. Data from the COVID-19 Household Monitoring Survey showed that in Ghana, Kenya, and Mali, for example, 90 per cent of survey respondents in June 2020 reported having been able to access health care while the figure for Nigeria was 66%. In Uganda, while many respondents accessed health facilities, those who reported that they could not do so cited lack of money or transportation challenges rather than reduced access due to COVID-19 infections.

The fears about infection rates soon gave way to the search for explanations for Africa's relatively lower numbers of infections and deaths. Explanations that have been offered include the high malaria drug intake (Ahmed, 2020), early precautions taken by countries, the demographic profile, intra-continental and community resource and information sharing, and the deployment of infrastructure inherited from Ebola containment measures at borders and health facilities (Maffioli, 2020; Kelly et al., 2020).[2]

Much more troubling for Africa have been the socio-economic impacts of COVID-19, such as the macro-economic contractions, livelihood disruptions, food insecurity, school closures, and growing inequality. The African Development Bank (2021) described the levels of contraction of economies in Africa, 2.1%, as a recession. Annual GDP growth declined sharply from impressive 2019 figures for many countries—Kenya (−0.3%), Mali (−1.6%), Mozambique (−1.3%), Nigeria (−1.8%), Rwanda (−3.4%) and Tunisia (−8.6) recorded negative growth in 2020. Tsikata and Torvikey (2022) provide a review of studies documenting the socio-economic impact.

RESEARCH FOCUS: THEMATIC APPROACH AND COUNTRIES

The Equity and COVID-19 programme was designed in the framework of INCLUDEs approach to inclusive development that posits that inclusive development is achieved when improvements are realised in the income and non-income dimensions of development and inequalities in these dimensions fall (Reinders et al, 2019). This approach emphasises dimensions of well-being beyond income and growth and a focus on the

---

[2] Other studies have documented the disconnect between Ebola and COVID-19 responses, see, for example, Konte et al. (2022) for Nigeria.

distribution of well-being in societies (Rauniyar & Kanbur, 2009) and advances equity as a lens to consider the redistribution of development gains. Equity has social and geographic dimensions. Social equity refers to inequalities in relation to vulnerable groups such as women, youth, the ultra-poor (the lowest 20% in the income distribution), disabled, and elderly. Spatial or geographical equity refers to regional differences, i.e. the extent to which there are differences in the distribution of well-being between neighbourhoods, urban and rural settings, or regions within a country (see also Awortwi & Dietz, 2019).

The 12 county case studies were guided by the following broad themes:

- Country socio-economic contexts that had a bearing on COVID-19 effects and responses.
- COVID-19 policy responses and measures in terms of their nature, purpose, who they are directed at, their inclusivity and effects on different socio-economic groups and geographies.
- The politics and implications of responses: including their origins and influences on measures; the role of state and non-state actors; the implications for structures and systems of power and governance and democratic consolidation; the implications for state citizen relations, trust, and civic space.
- Citizen responses to containment and mitigation measures—from compliance, protests to innovations and inventions.

The selection of counties for the case studies, Benin, Burkina Faso, Ethiopia, Ghana, Kenya, Mali, Mozambique, Niger, Nigeria, Rwanda, Tunisia, and Uganda, was guided by the representation of a variety of contexts and aimed at a continent-wide relevant analysis including regional variation, variation in population size and geography, political context with elections or upheaval and economic status.

The country studies researchers had the freedom to decide how to approach the study. Most of them were based on secondary sources and limited key informant interviews, with a few undertaking surveys to collect quantitative data (Nigeria, Tunisia, and Benin). There is therefore some variability in what information is available in each chapter. Moreover, the country case studies took place during the first year of the pandemic, capturing what took place in the first wave and parts of the second wave of the pandemic.

Contextualising the Country Case Studies at the Onset of the Pandemic

The responses of national governments and other stakeholders to the COVID-19 outbreak, as well as the impact of containment measures and other policy responses, have been shaped, in part, by pre-pandemic country socio-economic, geographical, and political contexts. This section briefly describes the variation in pre-pandemic country contexts for the cases included in this study. A more extensive discussion of context is provided by Tsikata and Torvikey (2022).

Geographical Contexts

The 12 case study countries are spread across Africa and have interesting similarities and differences. Half of the countries are in West Africa, four in East Africa, and one each in North Central and Southern Africa. There are several landlocked countries that are also vulnerable to severe episodes of drought (Burkina Faso, Ethiopia, Mali, and Niger).

Socio-economic Contexts

In terms of socio-economic contexts, eight of the study countries (Benin, Burkina Faso, Ethiopia, Mali, Mozambique, Rwanda, and Uganda) are both low income and LDCs,[3] while the other four (Ghana, Kenya, Nigeria, and Tunisia) are lower middle income. A common feature in the case studies is the composition of the economy in terms of economic sectors, with services sectors contributing the largest share of their GDP (Ghana, Kenya, Ethiopia, Nigeria, Rwanda, Tunisia, and Uganda). Even when it is not the most dominant, services are important for countries such as Mali and Niger. The size of the services sectors and their significance as a source of employment is a matter of concern because the services sectors in Africa are dominated by small precarious enterprises,

---

[3] LDC status denotes not just low per-capita income, but also significant social development deficits and environmental vulnerabilities.

which except for ICTs, were badly hit by the pandemic. Self-employment or informal employment is the dominant form of employment in the countries of study, except for Tunisia.

There were variations in income poverty levels, with national head-count levels before COVID-19 ranging from 15% for Tunisia, to 20–30% for Ethiopia, Ghana, Uganda, 31–40% for Benin, Kenya, Rwanda, between 41 and 50% for Burkina Faso, Mali, Niger, and Nigeria, and above 50% for Mozambique. Over the years, income inequalities in many African countries have become wider (see Tsikata & Torvikey, 2022).

Going by social development indicators, stunting in children under 5 years, is under 10% for Tunisia, under 20% for Ghana; between 20 and 29% for Burkina, Kenya, Mali, and Uganda; between 30 and 39% for Benin, Ethiopia, Nigeria, and Rwanda, and over 40% for Niger and Mozambique. Regarding literacy rates of persons 15 years and above, the countries with the lowest rates (between 30 and 39%) are Mali and Niger. Burkina Faso and Benin have between 40 and 49%, Nigeria, Ethiopia, and Mozambique have between 50 and 69%, while Ghana, Rwanda, Tunisia, Uganda, and Kenya have between 70 and 89%. The gender gap in literacy is up to 10% for Ghana, Kenya, and Rwanda; between 11 and 20% for Burkina Faso, Ethiopia, Mali, Niger, Nigeria, Tunisia, and Uganda; and above 20% for Benin and Mozambique. In terms of the pre-COVID-19 situation, reported cases of violence against women was under 10% for Burkina Faso, between 10 and 19% in Ethiopia, Mozambique, and Nigeria; between 20 and 29% in Ghana, Mali, Rwanda, and Uganda; and 40.7% in Kenya.

More generally, in terms of inequalities, all countries identified gender and rural–urban inequalities as important. In addition, Ethiopia, Ghana, Mozambique, and Nigeria identified geographical or regional inequalities.

Political Contexts

All the case study countries were identified as multi-party constitutional democracies with ruling and opposition parties. However, for many of the countries, COVID-19 represented a crisis within a crisis. Niger, Burkina Faso, and Mozambique were facing Islamic insurgencies of different degrees of severity, which had generated feelings of insecurity among the population. In the case of Burkina Faso, this had been compounded by the closure of 7.2% of health facilities in 2020 affecting 1.08 million people (OCHA, 2020). Ethiopia was on the brink of civil war and the decision to postpone elections to contain COVID-19 has deepened instability and tension in the country. Tunisia has been in the throes of political instability, unsettled since the Arab Spring. In Mali, a long-standing political crisis has resulted in coups d'état in August 2020 and May 2021. In Nigeria, the crisis has been manifested by a generalised breakdown of security, police/armed forces brutality, and mistrust of government, which at the height of COVID-19 boiled over into the End-SARS campaign. Kenya was facing a crisis of terror attacks and police brutality, while Rwanda's main political stressor was its closed political system, government intolerance of criticisms, and compliant CSOs. In Ghana, Uganda, Benin, and Niger, elections heightened political tensions, partisanship, and distrust for government, with citizens expressing suspicion of government intentions and about the seriousness of the pandemic in equal measure.

Pandemic Vulnerability

Since the outbreak of COVID-19, there have been efforts to classify countries according to their vulnerability to the pandemic.[4] The COVID-19 Community Vulnerability Index (CCVI) which measures the vulnerability context of countries using their age structure, epidemiological context, fragility, health system, population density, socio-economic structure and transportation and housing systems is one such effort. The index finds, based on all seven indicators, that of the country case studies covered in this book, Ghana is the least vulnerable while Ethiopia is the most vulnerable.[5] Other countries with high vulnerability scores are Niger, Mozambique, Mali, Burkina Faso, and Benin. An examination of each indicator separately shows that on age vulnerability (number of people aged 65 years and above), Ghana is the most vulnerable while Rwanda is the least vulnerable. On epidemiological vulnerability, Nigeria is the least vulnerable, while Kenya is the most vulnerable. On the fragility measure, which looks at civil unrest and food security, Ghana is the least vulnerable while Mali is the most vulnerable. With respect to health

---

[4] Similarly, there have been several initiatives to map sub-national differences in vulnerability to the pandemic, focusing on regional and demographic differences. For an example using the Oxford Policy Human Development Index (OPHI) in Nigeria, see Konte et al. (2022).

[5] Tunisia is missing from the CCVI.

systems vulnerability, Ethiopia is the most vulnerable while Uganda is the least vulnerable. Ghana is the least socio-economically vulnerable, while Niger is the most vulnerable. For transportation and housing, Ethiopia is the most vulnerable while Ghana is the least vulnerable. In terms of population density, Rwanda is the most vulnerable and Mozambique is the least vulnerable. It is instructive that the most vulnerable countries are all LDCS, and except for Mozambique, landlocked, and with high levels of social tension. While useful in flagging stressors that need attention, differences within countries are not reflected in the measurement. Thus, for example, Ghana's relatively high score on average conceals the regional, rural–urban, class, and gender differences in the vulnerability context (see also Konte et al., 2022 for an emphasis on regional differences in vulnerability based on a different index in Nigeria).

The country case studies in this volume document the economic factors that generate social issues in pandemic contexts, with agrarian and primary export commodity-dependent countries being exposed to global trade disruptions and countries with substantial informal economies seeing increased precariousness of work. Similarly, the effectiveness of national level responses was shaped by institutional capacities, the availability of timely data and existing targeting systems as well as the lack of or varying degree of involvement of citizens in formulating and shaping pandemic responses.

ORGANISATION OF THE BOOK

The book is organised in 12 country case study chapters, followed by a conclusion and reflection. The country case studies are organised in three broad regional sections covering West Africa (Benin, Burkina Faso, Ghana, Mali, Niger, and Nigeria), East and Southern Africa (Ethiopia, Kenya, Mozambique, Rwanda, Uganda), and North Africa (Tunisia).

REFERENCES

African Development Bank. (2021). African Economic Outlook 2021. AfDB
Ahmed, A. E. (2020) Incidence of coronavirus disease (COVID-19) and countries affected by malarial infections. Travel Medicine and Infectious Disease, Vol. 37, September–October 2020, 101693
Atuire, C. A., & Rutazibwa, O. U. (2021). An African reading of the COVID-19 pandemic and the stakes of decolonization. Yale University

Law School. https://law.yale.edu/sites/default/files/area/center/ghjp/doc uments/atuire_rutazibwa_commentary_v2.pdf

Awortwi, N., & Dietz, T. (2019). INCLUDE concept note for phase II (2019–2022).

BBC News. (2020, 28 February). *Nigeria confirms first coronavirus case.*

Berkhout, E., Galasso, N., & Lawson, M et al. (2021). The inequality virus: Bringing together a world torn apart by coronavirus through a fair, just, and sustainable economy. Oxfam briefing Paper.

Bolton, L., & Georgalakis, J. (2022). The socioeconomic impact of Covid-19 in low- and middle-income countries: A synthesis of learning from the Covid-19 Responses for Equity Programme. CORE_Synthesis_Report.pdf (ids.ac.uk).

Cabore, J. W., Karamagi, H. C., Kipruto, H., Asamani, J. A., Droti, B., Seydi, A. B. W., Titi-Ofei, R., Impouma, B., Yao, M., & Yoti, Z. (2020). The potential effects of widespread community transmission of SARS-CoV-2 infection in the world health organization African region: A predictive model. *BMJ Global Health, 5*(5), e002647.

CNN Business. (2020). Melinda Gates: COVID-19 will be horrible in the developing world. https://edition.cnn.com/videos/business/2020/04/10/melinda-gates-coronavirus.cnn-business

Gopalakrishnan, V., Wadhwa, D., Haddad, S., & Blake, P. (2021). 2021 year in review in 11 charts: The inequality pandemic. The World Bank: https://www.worldbank.org/en/news/feature/2021/12/20/year-2021-in-review-the-inequality-pandemic.

INCLUDE. (2021). COVID-19: Challenging inclusive development in Africa. https://includeplatform.net/inclusive-development-covid-19-pandemic/

Kelley, M., Ferrand, R. A., Muraya, K., Chigudu, S., Molyneux, S., Pai, M., & Barasa, E. (2020). An appeal for practical social justice in the COVID-19 global response in low-income and middle-income countries. *The Lancet Global Health, 8*(7), e888–e889.

Konte, M., Ndubuisi, G., & Okofor, A. (2023). The past and the present: The Nigerian Ebola experience and the Covid-19 Pandemic. INCLUDE. The-Past-and-the-Present-The-Nigerian-Ebola-experience-and-the-Covid-19-Pandemic.pdf (includeplatform.net)

Maffioli, E. M. (2020). How is the world responding to the novel coronavirus disease (COVID- 19) compared with the 2014 West African Ebola Epidemic? The importance of china as a player in the global economy. *American Journal of Tropical Medicine and Hygiene, 102*(5), 924–925. https://doi.org/10.4269/ajtmh.20-0135

Qureishi, Z. (2020). *Tackling the inequality pandemic: Is there a cure?* Brookings Institution.

Rafalimanana, H., Sherif, M. (2021). Social policy and social protection measures to build Africa better post-COVID-19. UNDESA. https://www.un.org/development/desa/dspd/wp-content/uploads/sites/22/2021/03/PB_93.pdf

Rauniyar, G., & Kanbur, R. (2009). Conceptualizing inclusive development: With applications to rural infrastructure and development assistance. Asian Development Bank.

Reinders, S., Dekker, M. Kesteren, F. van, & Oudenhuisen, L. (2019). Synthesis report Inclusive Development in Africa. INCLUDE synthesis report series. https://includeplatform.net/downloads/synthesis-report-inclusivedevelopment-in-africa/

Sidibé, M. (2022) Vaccine inequity: Ensuring Africa is not left out. Africa in Focus. Brookings Institution.

Egypt Today. (2020, 14 February). Egypt announces first Coronavirus infection. Egypt Today.

Tsikata, D., & Torvikey, D. (2022). COVID-19 in Africa, A synthesis of 12 country studies. INCLUDE. https://includeplatform.net/wp-content/uploads/2022/06/COVID-19-Synthesis-Report.pdf

UNECA. (2020). Economic effects of the COVID-19 on Africa. UNECA.

WHO. (2020). Coronavirus (COVID-19) | WHO | Regional Office for Africa.

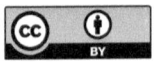

PART I

West Africa

CHAPTER 2

Benin

Leonard Wantchekon, Leonie Koumassa, Thierry Ogoutchoro,
and Yannick Ngongang

INTRODUCTION

In Benin, the first case of the Covid-19 virus was detected on March 16, 2020. Benin's statistical service, Institut National de la Statistique et de l'Analyse Economique (INSAE), estimates the population of Benin at 11,884,127 in 2019. Benin has the characteristic of a very young population. Almost 65% of its population is under 25 years. In 2019, the population under 25 reached 7,628,592 people. More than half (55.2%) of the population lives in rural areas, with Cotonou and Abomey-Calavi accommodating most of the urban population. Taking advantage

L. Wantchekon
University of Princeton, Princeton, USA

L. Koumassa (✉) · Y. Ngongang
African School of Economics, IREEP, Abomey-Calavi, Benin
e-mail: lbonou@africanschoolofeconomics.com

Y. Ngongang
e-mail: yngongang@africanschoolofeconomics.com

T. Ogoutchoro
Innovation for Povercty Action, Washington DC, USA

of its political stability, Benin has continuously recorded an increase in its Human Development Index (HDI) over the past thirty years, which rose from 0.348 in 1990 to 0.531 in 2019 which is an increase of 0.182 points. This increase is the result of the progress made by the country on three dimensions namely, health, education, and livings standards. Indeed, between 1990 and 2019, Benin experienced successive gains in the life expectancy at birth of its citizens. An average of 0.3 years per year increase is recorded yearly but with a period of stagnation between 1996 and 2000. The country also generally recorded an improvement in its Gross National Income per capita (GNI/inhabitant) over the period, which rose from USD 1431 in 1990 to USD 2217.57 US PPP in 2019. Table 2.1 presents a selection of comparative macroeconomic and demographic statistics in 2018 (unless otherwise indicated) for Benin and some of its West African counterparts.

The Covid-19 health crisis occurred when the country's economy had seen a significant boost. Benin's economic growth remains robust and is estimated at 6.7% in 2019. The growth rate has been consistent over the past two decades (World Bank, 2020). The growth figures are partly due to the increase in public investments, which rose from 21% of GDP in 2016 to 29.6% in 2019. On the supply side, the growth is attributable to the performance of the agricultural sector, particularly in the cotton production sector, which is a major cash crop in the country. Cotton production rose from 269,222 tons in 2016 to 726,831 tons in 2019. Other sectors of the economy, including construction, public

Table 2.1 Comparative macroeconomic and demographic statistics for 2018

Indicator	Benin	Senegal	Ghana	Nigeria	Ivory Coast
GDP per capita (US$)	1 234.9	1550	1920	2240	1880
GDP growth (annual%)	6.7	6.7	7.6	2.3	7.0
Population growth (annual%)	2.71	2.39	2.17	2.43	1.84
Life expectancy at birth (years) (men/women)	63.0/66.2	60/64.3	64.5/69.6	52.8/55	57.8/60.2
Primary school enrolment rate (% net)	96.4	72.3	85.1	64.1	83.8
Mortality rate before five years (per 1000 births	96	49.1	35.2	124	108

Source FMI, CIA World Factbooks et UNICEF

works, agro-industry, and the Port of Cotonou, have contributed significantly to the positive growth figures. Inflation in Benin has remained low at an estimated rate of −0.1% in 2019 and below the WAEMU limit of 3%. The CFA franc, pegged to the euro, appreciated against the dollar over 2017–2019 (AFDB, 2020).

Benin's economy is dominated by the services sector comprising banking, transport, telecommunications, public administration, and other trade sectors. The country's economic boost is also driven by the dynamism of trade with Nigeria, which averaged 48.9% of nominal GDP between 2013 and 2019. The share of the agricultural sector, composed mainly of cotton, cashew, and pineapple cultivation, represented on average of 26.9% between 2013 and 2018. The manufacturing sector, comprised mainly of energy and construction, accounted for 15.9% of GDP during the same period, while taxes and duties contributed 8.2% of nominal GDP over the same period (INSAE, 2020). Table 2.2 shows the sectoral contribution to GDP trend from 2013 to 2019.

The country's budget deficit, financed by loans and grants, narrowed to 2.5% of GDP in 2019. The current account deficit, which improved due to improvement in cotton production, is mainly financed by official loans (33%), private loans (27%), and foreign direct investment (19%) (AFDB, 2020). Benin's foreign exchange reserve fell to 20.93 million USD in 2018 (or 0.07 months of import). Public debt was estimated at 54% of the GDP in 2019. The country issued an Eurobond of 500 million Euros (5.2% of GDP) in March 2019; however, its risk of debt distress is considered moderate. Benin is rated B + by the Standard and Poor's Agency regarding its debt and financial position. However, 40% of

Table 2.2 Sectoral contribution to GDP growth (2013–2019) in percentage

	2013	2014	2015	2016	2017	2018 (Est)	2019 (Prev)
Primary sector	1.6	2.2	0.0	2.4	2.1	2.1	1.5
Secondary sector	0.9	0.6	2.0	0.1	0.1	0.7	2.0
Tertiary sector	4.4	2.5	0.0	0.9	2.7	2.8	2.5
Taxes and duties net of subsidies	0.2	1.1	-0.2	-0.1	0.8	1.1	0.9
GDP	7.2	6.4	1.8	3.3	5.7	6.7	6.9

Source INSAE (2020)

the Beninese population is rated poor, reflecting the inequality and non-inclusiveness inherent in the country's impressive growth figures (AFDB, 2020). The structural inequalities also show in the differential ways social groups access information, basic services, health care, and means of livelihood. This study seeks to analyse how different socioeconomic groups are differently affected by the Covid-19 pandemic and how various mitigation measures designed to target these multiple groups affected them differently.

METHODOLOGY

The study used multiple approaches for data and information gathering. These include key informant interviews, phone surveys, and media reports. Individuals and companies were the units of analysis for the study. In addition, state and non-state actors who coordinated and worked in the management of Covid-19 were also interviewed. Besides that, the research team also interviewed the leaders of various workers organisations and trade unions to have a broader view of the implication of the pandemic on their sectors of work and members.

In the context of the pandemic, the study's primary concern was not to reach all actors but to investigate those most impacted by the pandemic. Thus, teachers, students, hospitality sector workers, transporters, agricultural producers, merchants, artists, and marginalised people in the Social Promotion Centres (CPCs) were involved. The representatives of the organisations gave the list of their members which was used for the study.

The study also includes formal and informal enterprises. Formal companies were sampled from a list of formal enterprises (INSAE, 2017). Regarding informal enterprises, this group comprises only artisans whose lists and contacts were obtained from the artisans' association of each commune. Data were mainly collected using the phone survey method.

The study covered Benin's four territorial departments namely Atlantic, Littoral, Borgou, and Atacora. The study systematically considered the Atlantic and Littoral departments, which were the epicentres of Covid-19 in Benin. These locations are crucial because most cross-border transactions happen in these two departments. Furthermore, to see the differential effects of the pandemic on the various regions, two departments in the north namely Borgou and Atacora were also sampled. A rural and an urban commune in each of these departments were selected to account for locational differences. The seven communes chosen for the study were Cotonou, Abomey-Calavi, Toffo, Parakou, Kalalé, Natitingou, and Cobly.

SAMPLE SIZE AND SAMPLING STRATEGIES

The target of this study include nine categories of individuals who are transporters (zem,[1] city cab, and minibus), agricultural producers, the marginalised people in CPCs,[2] traders, students, secondary school teachers, pharmacists, artists, and restaurant and eatery place operators. Since a sampling database was not at our disposal, we obtained the lists of participants from the diverse associations to which these individuals belong. The list for vulnerable people such as people with disabilities, older people, poor people, and orphans were obtained from Social Promotion Centers (CPS) in each of the municipalities covered by the study. All these lists together helped us define a database with different essential characteristics of these targets which have been used as a sampling base. Once the sampling frame was available, the strategy adopted was to determine the total sample size and distribute it among the different communes.

The sample size calculation was performed using the formulas below.

$$n_1 = \left(z^2 \frac{P(1-P)}{e^2} \right)$$

With "z" the confidence level of the estimates, "p" the proportion of individuals who have undergone, in one way or another, directly or indirectly, the influence of the "Cordon Sanitaire" on their activities, "e" the marginal error term and "n_1" the initial sample size. For the calculation of the initial size of the sample, we chose a confidence level of 95%, with a margin error of 3% and a proportion of $p = 0.5$.

Furthermore, since the population size was not infinite, an adjustment was made to account for this size using the formula:

$$n_2 = \frac{n_1 N}{N + n_1}$$

---

[1] Commercial motorbike operators.

[2] Social promotion centres.

With "N", the size of the population of actors identified based on the exploratory phases and "n_2", the modified sample size.

Finally, an adjustment is made for the expected response rate through the relationship, where the expected response rate provides the final sample size for the study. As a result of these various calculation procedures, the sample size selected for the study was 1200.

After collecting the data, we got a sample size of 1067 individuals corresponding to a non-response rate of 11–08%.

At the enterprise level, the sampling base was the list of formal enterprises (INSAE, 2017). The enterprises used for the sampling are those operating in the sectors probably most affected by Covid-19, such as accommodation and food services, arts and recreation services, wholesale and retail trade, pharmaceutical services, beverage manufacturing, food manufacturing, real estate activities, office services activities, human health activities, and social action, specialised scientific and technical support activities. The total number of enterprises working in these sectors for the seven communes was 1624. The same sampling method was used to determine the size of 101 enterprises to be surveyed.

The sampling of informal enterprises follows the same process described for individual actors. Applying the same methodology, we obtained a sample size of 200 artisans distributed among the different communes. After the phone data collection, 113 individuals and 217 enterprises were surveyed in the formal and informal sectors.

COVID-19 RESPONSE MEASURES

Following the record of the 1st case of Covid-19 infection in Benin on March 16, 2020, the number of contaminations exceeded 1000 infections by June 24, 2020. The first case of death linked to Covid-19 was recorded on April 6, 2020. On January 4, 2021, the country recorded 75 active cases for 3,304 confirmed cases, including 3,185 cured and 44 deaths. It should be noted that the relative spread of Covid-19 was triggered by its trivialisation and the vulgarisation because of false information spread. Thus, some believe that the Covid-19 virus is a divine punishment in response to the multiple injustices, atrocities, and wickedness that people on earth generally commit. Others believed that this health crisis was God's will for mankind. Others still link this pandemic to fate, believing that those who die from it can do nothing to prevent it. Another category of people confused the coronavirus disease with ordinary flu that can be treated with usual herbal remedies.

However, the state took pragmatic measures to curb the infections with a US $ 320,338,983 national prevention plan. Following the confirmation of this first case, the government and its partners set a plan to fight against the pandemic. It also worked on proposing mitigation strategies to limit the effects of this pandemic on the socioeconomic activities of the populations. The public health measures included cordon sanitaire imposed on April 14, 2020, which restricted the movement of populations in Cotonou, Abomey-Calavi, Allada, Ouidah, Tori, Zè, Sèmè-Podji, Porto-Novo, Akpro-Missérété, and Adjarra. In addition, the public gathering was restricted to fifty people while there was a total ban on funerals, parties, and concerts. Furthermore, rotational and remote work arrangements were enforced across the country. In addition, social distancing measures were instituted together with promoting hygienic practices such as hand washing, sanitiser use, and nose mask-wearing.

The state used many media channels to disseminate Covid-19 information. Access to Covid-19 information was determined by channels through which information was disseminated. Among the surveyed population, more than 74% of people received Covid-19 information through radio, 72% through television, and 53% through social networks (Fig. 2.1).

We also assessed people's perception of the risk of contamination since this determines their risk-taking behaviour. Since the advent of Covid-19, the perception of some Beninese on the risk of contamination has seemed the same during the lockdown,[3] and the post-lockdown. More specifically, about 32% of people said that the risk of contamination was "high" during the lockdown compared to 33% of respondents during the post-lockdown (Fig. 2.2).

The research team also assessed the risk exposure of the surveyed population generally in the social life compared to the risk during working periods. Among the working population, more than 36% felt that they were exposed to the risk of contamination of Covid-19. However, only 28% of individuals in social life asserted that the risk of exposure was high

---

[3] The lockdown in the Benin context refers to what the government called "Cordon Sanitaire". This has forbidden people from moving from the areas most infected by the pandemic (15 communes in the South) to other areas of the country to limit the spread.

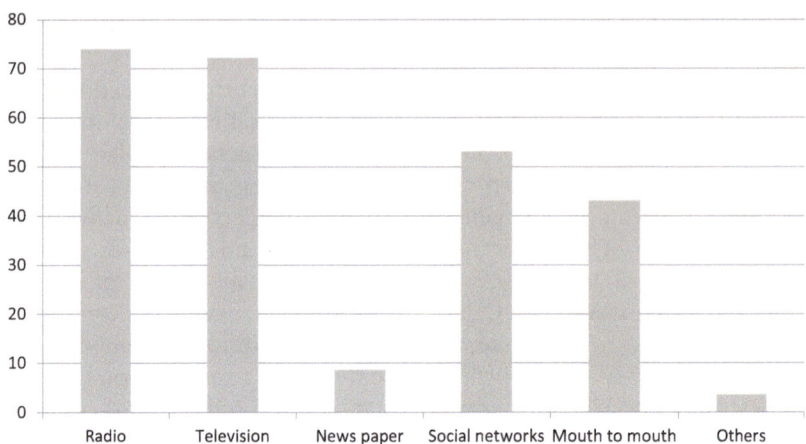

Fig. 2.1 Information channel of the surveyed population (*Source* ASE data collection, December 2020)

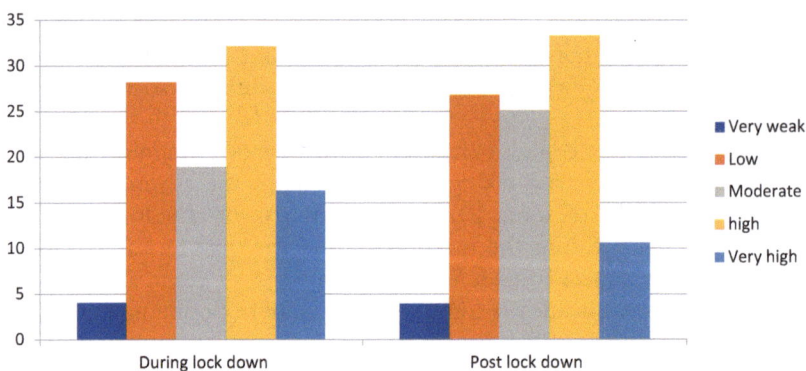

Fig. 2.2 Contamination risks of the surveyed population (*Source* ASE data collection, December 2020)

(Fig. 2.3). This means that people felt they could be exposed to the virus through their work rather than through their social activities.

Among socioeconomic groups surveyed, **91.41%** of teachers and **89%** of traders think their economic activities expose them to the virus. However, more traders (**84%**) and interurban taxis (**80.36%**) operators

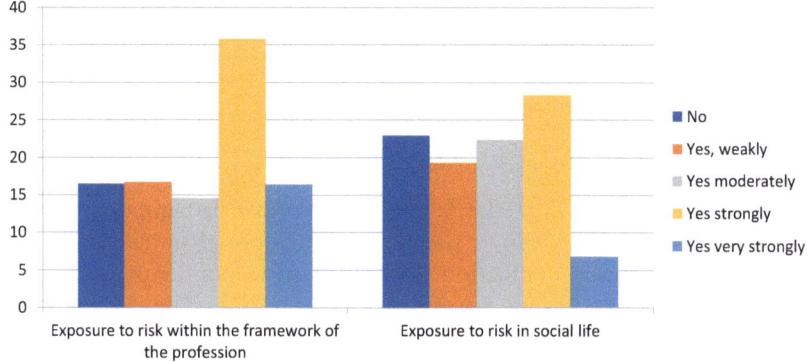

Fig. 2.3 Risk exposure in social life and employment (*Source* ASE data collection, December 2020)

thought that they were more exposed to the virus through their social life (Table 2.3).

Due to the high level of access to Covid-19 information, we found that there was high compliance with the protocols and measures. Compliance to facial mask-wearing (99%) was the highest while the weres are hand washing (92%), reduction in participation in public events (92%), social distancing (92%), and restriction on movement (90%) among others. As

Table 2.3 Risk exposure by socioeconomic groups

Categories	Exposure to risk in professional life (%)	Exposure to risk in social life (%)
Zem	85.56	83.33
City taxi/minibus	80.00	72.00
Interurban taxi	85.71	80.36
Artist	86.11	73.61
Teacher	91.41	79.19
Trader	89.00	84.00
Bartender/restorer	83.84	73.74
Student	75.93	74.53
Agricultural producer	76.22	73.61
Overall	**83.46**	**77.15**

Source ASE data collection, December 2020

the next section will show, compliance also came with consequences and this will have implications for economic activities and income losses.

Impacts of Response Measures on Sectors and Social Groups

It is abundantly clear that the Covid-19 measures had impacts on the population. Figure 2.4 shows the type of measure that had the most impact on the survey population. Over 70% of respondents mentioned *cordon sanitaire* as having adverse effect on them. The rest include measures that ban large gatherings and those that enforced closures of places such as closure of schools, places of worship, and ban on large gatherings (Fig. 2.4).

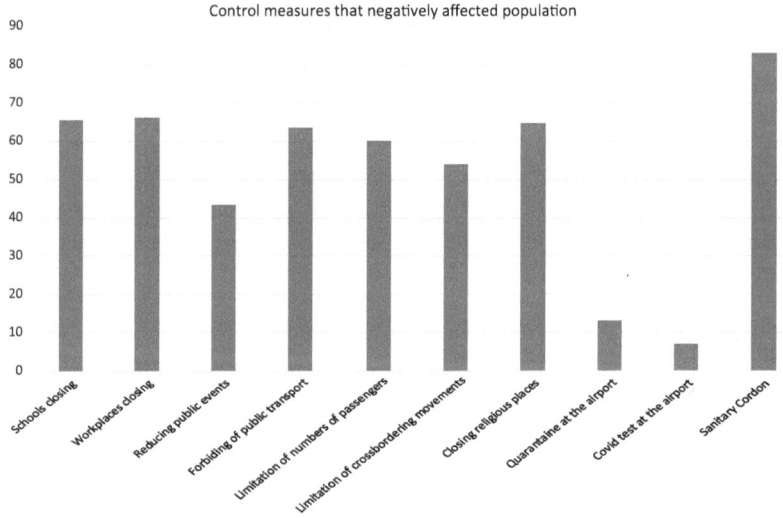

Fig. 2.4 Impacts of control measures on population (*Source* ASE data collection, December 2020

DIFFERENTIAL IMPACTS OF COVID-19 ON SOCIAL GROUPS AND SECTORS

The measures instituted by the Beninese State affected social groups differently. In Benin, the government did not prohibit access to markets for goods and services to fight Covid-19. That is shown by the proportion of individuals (64.48%) who declared they had no difficulty accessing markets. However, some Covid-19 related measures prevented a significant proportion of people from accessing markets. A total of 21.65% of the survey participants believed they did not have access to some local markets in their municipalities, 4.69% could not access the stores; 2.25% could not access supermarkets, and 1.31% believed they could not access international markets.

The leading cause of non-accessibility to markets for goods and services was the closure of specific shops. More than half (51.48%) of respondents attributed the inaccessibility of markets to the physical closures of those spaces. Also, 40.66% of respondents blamed the implementation of the safety measures in fighting against Covid-19 for constraining their access to markets. The rest of the reasons included travel restrictions (26.89%) and quarantining (3.93%).

THE DIFFERENTIAL IMPACT OF COVID-19 ON THE EMPLOYMENT OF SOCIOECONOMIC GROUPS

Since the cordon sanitaire was mentioned as the measure with the most adverse effects on the population, we examined how its impacts were felt by different sectors. The ordinal logistic regression shows the effect of lockdown on the activity level of some socioeconomic groups. Table 2.4 reveals the impact of the lockdown on the level of activity. Almost all the socioeconomic groups, except agricultural producers, have completely stopped their activity during the lockdown.

Table 2.5 presents the Average Adjusted Predictions (AAP) for diverse activity groups. Looking at the results of this table, teachers (59.2% of probability) were more likely to have their activity completely stopped during the lockdown. There are followed by students (47%), bartenders(42.3%), and artists (41.9%). The result reflects the nature of the pandemic response which included closure of schools and places of entertainment.

Table 2.4 Activity level of various socioeconomic groups

Activity level	
Zem	(ref)
City taxi/minibus	−1.123**
Interurban taxi	−1.067***
Artist	−1.352***
Teacher	−2.054***
Trader	−0.742**
Bartender/Restaurant worker	−1.369***
Student	−1.560***
Agricultural producer	0.577*
Unemployed, retired	−0.103
Constant 1	**−1.681***
Constant 2	**0.166**
Constant 3	**0.966***
Constant 4	**3.410***
N	**956**
* p < 0.05, ** p < 0.01, *** p < 0.001	

Source ASE data collection, December 2020

Table 2.5 Average adjusted predictions for the level of activity of socioeconomic groups

Main activity	Average adjusted predictions for the level of activity				
	Complete cessation	Significant drop	Moderate drop	Activity unchanged	Increase of activities
Zem	0.157	0.384	0.183	0.244	0.032
City taxi/minibus	0.364	0.420	0.106	0.099	0.011
Inter-cities	0.351	0.423	0.110	0.105	0.011
Artist	0.419	0.402	0.090	0.081	0.008
Teacher	0.592	0.310	0.051	0.042	0.004
Trader	0.281	0.431	0.134	0.138	0.015
Bartender/Restorer	0.423	0.400	0.089	0.080	0.008
Student	0.470	0.379	0.077	0.067	0.007
Agricultural producer	0.095	0.304	0.197	0.348	0.056

Source ASE Data Collection, December 2020

We also found that agricultural producers had a higher probability (5.6%) of seeing their level of activity increase during the lockdown. In contrast, a lower chance (0.4%) is observed at the teachers' level. Agricultural production was considered an essential activity during the period and therefore had little restrictions compared to other non-agricultural sectors.

The activities of the various socioeconomic groups evolved with the intensity of the measures and the pandemic. Overall, 36.72% of respondents reported that their economic activity levels dropped during the lockdown against 19.04% during the post-lockdown period. The effect was highest among city taxi drivers (60%). In general, 35.77% stopped their economic activities altogether during and after confinement. High school teachers (63.64%) had the highest economic activity decline rate due to school closures.

Effects of Changes in the Level of Economic Activities

Changes in activity level during or after confinement have essential consequences for workers' employability. While 33.47% temporarily stopped their activities during confinement, only 6.07% of the same was reported post-lockdown. Also, most of those who have kept their activities have experienced significant reductions in working hours or wages.

Thus, 29.08% had a moderate decrease in working hours or wages during and after confinement. Tables 2.6, 2.7, 2.8, 2.9, and 2.10 show the results on implications of Covid-19 on employment conditions.

The Covid-19 pandemic has negatively impacted the conditions of employability at the level of socioeconomic groups. About 43% of the individuals interviewed saw their wages reduced. For the few of these workers who continue to receive their regular wages without reduction, nearly 5% maintain that their salaries came late.

Among other difficulties, among the Zem operators surveyed, some said they had not experienced problems in developing their activity while others evoked the lack of customers since people were afraid to go out. This fear has also caused a considerable decrease in the number of passengers among city taxi drivers due to restrictions on movement.

Artists raised difficulties related to the pandemic, such as reduction in assets and especially the prevention of honouring their social contributions as members of their associations. Teachers said that although they

Table 2.6 Consequences in Activities Level Changes During the Lockdown

Sectors/ social groups	During lockdown					
	Permanent loss of my job (%)	A pause of my job/ technical leave (%)	A moderate reduction in working hours and wages (%)	I continued / I continue to work normally (%)	Increase in working hours/ overtime (%)	Increase in salary/ income (%)
Zem	5.56	12.22	35.56	27.78	10.00	1.11
City taxi/ minibus	4.00	48.00	32.00	12.00	0.00	0.00
Interurban taxi	8.93	33.93	39.29	10.71	3.57	1.79
Artist	9.72	44.44	33.33	5.56	2.78	0.00
Teacher	3.54	60.61	13.64	15.15	0.51	0.51
Trader	7.00	27.00	31.00	20.00	2.00	1.00
Bartender/ Restorer	8.08	35.35	37.37	9.09	0.00	2.02
Student	2.47	31.48	26.54	11.11	0.00	0.62
Agricultural producer	2.08	8.33	37.50	41.67	2.78	0.00
Overall	**5.02**	**33.47**	**29.08**	**18.41**	**2.09**	**0.73**

Source ASE Data Collection, December 2020

did not have so much financial difficulties, they were nevertheless exposed to psychosocial risks at work attributed to the fear of being contaminated in school.

The Covid-19 health crisis has relatively impacted employment. In general, 11.40% of respondents were dismissed from work during the period. The rate of dismissals was high people in the hospitality industry (32.32%), city taxi/minibus drivers(24%), agricultural producers(15.97%), and traders (13%). Zem operators (6.67%) and teachers(6.57%) had the least dismissals because of the high rate of layoffs among workers in bars or restaurants (32.32%).

In terms of location, the communes of the *cordon sanitaire* such as Cotonou and Abomey-Calavi have experienced more layoffs in companies due to the coronavirus pandemic. More than half of the individuals surveyed who declared having seen the companies in which they work to carry out redundancies were in the municipalities of Abomey-Calavi

Table 2.7 Consequences in activities level change during post-lockdown

	Post-lockdown					
	Permanent loss of my job (%)	Temporary stoppage of my job/ technical leave (%)	A moderate reduction in working hours and wages (%)	I continued/I continue to work normally (%)	Increase in working hours/ overtime (%)	Increase in salary/ income (%)
Zem	4.44	5.56	30.00	51.11	3.33	0.00
City taxi/ minibus	4.00	16.00	40.00	24.00	16.00	0.00
Interurban taxi	1.79	8.93	50.00	26.79	7.14	3.57
Artist	2.78	16.67	48.61	30.56	0.00	0.00
Teacher	0.51	2.02	10.61	60.61	18.69	0.51
Trader	9.00	5.00	27.00	44.00	5.00	0.00
Bartender/ Restorer	3.03	5.05	40.40	40.40	2.02	2.02
Student	2.47	7.41	16.67	44.44	6.17	0.62
Agricultural producer	2.78	4.17	15.97	64.58	6.25	0.69
Overall	**3.24**	**6.07**	**24.90**	**48.01**	**7.74**	**0.73**

Source ASE Data Collection, December 2020

Table 2.8 Covid-19 and employability difficulties on sectors

Social groups	Decrease in salary (%)	The total cessation of salary (%)	Late wages (%)	Other difficulties (%)
Zem	68.42	3.51	0.00	33.33
City taxi/ minibus	72.73	0.00	0.00	36.36
Inter-cities taxis	57.14	0.00	7.14	35.71
Artists	46.43	3.57	3.57	50.00
Teachers	19.30	1.75	17.54	66.67
Traders	47.06	1.96	0.00	58.82
Bartender/ Restorer	60.87	0.00	13.04	39.13
Students	18.03	0.00	3.28	81.97
Agricultural producers	36.84	0.88	0.88	65.79
Overall	**42.29**	**1.32**	**4.85**	**57.05**

Source ASE Data Collection, December 2020

Table 2.9 Effect of Covid-19 on the income of socioeconomic groups

The proportion of income decreasing	
Zem	(ref)
City taxi/minibus	0.677
Interurban taxi	0.592
Artist	1.234***
Teacher	−0.887**
Trader	0.252
Bartender/Restorer	1.251***
Student	−0.154
Agricultural producer	0.266
Public	
Constant1	**−1.958***
Constant2	**0.015**
Constant3	**1.656***
R-squared	
N	779

*$p< 0.05$, **$p< 0.01$, ***$p< 0.001$
Source ASE data collection, December 2020

Table 2.10 Average adjusted predictions (AAP) on revenue decreasing

Main activity	Average adjusted predictions (aap)			
	Less_than_25%	From_25_to_50%	From_50_and_75%	From_75_and_100%
Artists	0.044	0.207	0.379	0.370
Bartenders/restaurant workers	0.041	0.197	0.375	0.387

Source ASE data collection, December 2020

(28.69%) and Cotonou (22.95%). Moreover, this phenomenon has also been more frequent during the period of the *cordon sanitaire* in the commune of Natitingou, where 20.49% reported layoffs. The tourist status of the city could explain this last observation. In reality, tourism drives economic activities in Natitingou. Since travel was almost restricted, especially for foreign visitors, the economic actors who previously lived off this have almost closed or at least have had a consideration reduction in workforced. As a result, even though, Natitingou was not part of the *cordon sanitaire* area, it was significantly affected by the effects of the pandemic response measures. The lowest employee layoff was reported at Cobly, which recorded 2.46%.

DIFFERENTIAL IMPACT OF COVID-19 ON THE INCOME OF SOCIOECONOMIC GROUPS

In this section, an ordinal logistic regression has been run to show how Covid-19 has impacted diverse socioeconomic groups regarding their income. In Table 2.9, only the categories of bartenders and artists have seen their revenue significantly decrease during the *cordon sanitaire* period.

To get a tangible feel of how significant and essential these differences are, we computed the Average Adjusted Predictions (AAP) for these categories of economic groups. Looking at the results, among the bartender/restaurant workers and the artists, more than three quarters (37.0% versus 38.7%) were likely to have their income decreased with a proportion of more than 75%(Table 2.10).

The model shows that bartender/restaurant workers and artists have a higher probability (76.2% versus 74.9%) of having their income decrease with the proportion decreasing more than 50%.

Consistent with the earlier results, the marginal effects (Table 2.11) show that, on average, bartenders/restaurant workers were 24.4 percentage points more likely than Zem operators to say their income decreased in proportion more than 75%, and about 20.2 percentage points less likely to say their income decreases in a proportion from 25 to 50%.

Artists are 22.8% points more likely than Zem to say their income decreases in proportion more than 75%, and about 19.2% points less likely to say their income decreases in a proportion from 25 to 50%. Table 2.12 shows the income-level variation in the context of the pandemic among the surveyed population with interurban taxi operators, artists, and restaurant workers having major declines in income which is linked to restrictions on movement and ban on large gatherings.

Table 2.13 shows the percentage of surveyed populations that experienced an increase, decrease, or stability of revenue during and after Cordon sanitaire containment measures. In all, 81.63% have seen their income decline during the main phase of the *cordon sanitaire* and the figure fell to 69% and 56% after applying the mitigation measures to the

Table 2.11 Marginal effect of income decrease by socioeconomic groups

The marginal effect of income decrease

	Less than 25%	From 25 to 50%	From 50 to 75%	From 75 to 100%
City taxi / minibus	−0.060	−0.091	0.058	0.093
Interurban taxi	−0.059	−0.090	0.058	0.092
Artists	−0.097	**−0.192**	0.062	**0.228**
Teacher	0.056	0.040	−0.054	−0.042
Trader	−0.041	−0.056	0.042	0.055
Bartender/ Restorer	−0.100	**−0.202**	0.058	**0.244**
Student	−0.015	−0.017	0.015	0.016
Agricultural producer	−0.031	−0.039	0.032	0.039
Unemployed, retired	−0.037	−0.048	0.038	0.047

Source ASE data collection, December 2020

Table 2.12 Income level variation in Covid-19 context

	Revenue proportion diminution			
	Less than 25%	Between 25 and 50%	Between 50 and 75%	More than 75%
Zem	13.43	44.78	38.81	2.99
City taxi/ minibus	15.79	31.58	36.84	15.79
Interurban taxi	12.77	40.43	25.53	21.28
Artist	8.47	22.03	49.15	20.34
Teacher	35.14	40.54	22.97	1.35
Trader	15.12	40.70	34.88	9.30
Bartender/ Restaurant workers	7.69	38.46	35.90	17.95
Student	20.18	45.61	27.19	7.02
Agricultural producer	21.30	41.67	27.78	9.26
Overall	**17.43**	**39.91**	**32.11**	**10.55**

Source ASE data collection, December 2020

Table 2.13 Impact of control and mitigation measures on revenue

	During "Cordon Sanitaire"	After removing cordon sanitaire	Once mitigation actions are applied
Increase of revenue	1.41	9.28	6.09
Decreasing of revenue	81.63	68.88	56.23
Stable revenue	16.96	21.84	37.68
Total	100	100	100

Source ASE data collection, December 2020

population. That shows that the mitigation measures had positive impacts on the population.

Covid-19 and Food Price Variability

Most individuals surveyed believed that there was an increase in the prices of certain than during the pandemic compared to pre-Covid-19 prices. For example, from the analysis of Table 2.14, more than 95% of respondents reported an increase in the prices of maize, sorghum or millet, rice, and gari.[4] beans, pepper, peanut oil, and palm oil. In the post-confinement period, an average of 85% of participants still believed that the price of these products remained high compared to the pre-Covid-19 period.

The increase in staple food items coupled with declines in economic activities, income, and job losses have implications for households' food security.

The Covid-19 pandemic has also impacted the cost of sanitary products, including soap, bleach, ointment, detergent, and hydroalcoholic gel, which increased compared to pre-pandemic times. This was confirmed by 96% of the people surveyed during the lockdown and 76% at the end of the lockdown period confirmed this information (Table 2.15).

Similarly, more than 93% of the respondents confirmed an increase in the cost of essential pharmaceutical products like paracetamol, amoxicillin, and chloroquine during the confinement. This same proportion is about

---

[4] During the lockdown, local food was made of ground cassava, dried and roasted.

Table 2.14 Covid-19 impacts on cost of food and essential goods

Some foodstuffs	During lockdown (%)		Post-lockdown (%)	
	Price increase	Price drop	Price increase	Price drop
Maize	96.06	3.94	83.86	16.14
Sorghum/Millet	97.42	2.58	82.50	17.50
Rice	98.43	1.57	83.27	16.73
Gari	97.42	2.58	89.98	10.02
Bean	98.06	1.94	87.06	12.94
Pepper	92.97	7.03	80.17	19.83
Peanut oil	99.28	0.72	86.12	13.88
Palm oil	95.95	4.05	89.80	10.20

Source ASE data collection, December 2020

Table 2.15 Hygienic products price variability during Covid-19

Hygienic products	During lockdown		Post-lockdown	
	Price increase	Price drop	Price increase	Price drop
Soap	92.19	7.81	72.00	28.00
Bleach	94.91	5.09	77.11	22.89
Ointment	99.09	0.91	75.73	24.27
Detergent	95.83	4.17	81.74	18.26
Hydroalcoholic gel	97.70	2.30	75.00	25.00

Source ASE data collection, December 2020

75% during the post-lockdown period. The implication is that, access to this item would be difficult for poorer households.

Perhaps, one of the high cost elements associated with Covid-19 was transportation. More than 95% of survey participants reported an increase in transport fares during confinement against 77.51% during the post-confinement period.

Covid-19 Impact Mitigation Measures

The government and other non-state actors instituted measures to improve health care resources, communication, and information dissemination by the media. The plan to mitigate the effects caused by Covid-19 was based on three dimensions, namely, **63.380 billion FCFA** financial support for businesses, **4.98 billion FCFA** financial support for artisans and small traders, and 5.76 billion FCFA water and electricity supply subsidies for all citizens. Besides the actions taken by the Benin government, the partners have worked to set up some specific measures for specific groups. Table 2.16 contains those measures. They targeted pregnant women, people with HIV, older people, and rural populations. In addition, Social Promotion Centres, which usually help people in need, the partners have increased their contribution to vulnerable groups. Those groups typically depend on other people that support them, and as activities have ceased, it increases the dependence on vulnerable people. Social Promotion Centers have then switched their intervention plan and devoted more financial resources to their target groups such as orphans, people with disabilities, older people, and poor households. The state actors have promoted three main types of mitigation actions. First, there is financial support for businesses, artisans and small traders, and household electricity and water bill subsidies. Besides those measures to mitigate Social Promotion Centers have undertaken the impact of the pandemic, specific mitigation measures, and the reorganisation on public service delivery among others.

Mitigation Actions Received
by Socioeconomic Groups

Although mitigation actions were put in place, the analysis of the surveyed population shows that only a tiny proportion of the population actually accessed them (Table 2.17). Except for water and electricity subsidies which were universally applied, the access options for other social support schemes was not accessible to everyone. In addition, the total amount devoted could not cover the target population. As a result, decision-makers had proposed a second round of registration to obtain mitigation measures, which were implemented when the data collection was completed.

Regarding support, 66% of the surveyed population did not receive tangible support, while 31% received facial masks, and 16% and 10% received washing hands kits and alcohol solutions respectively. The donations were from social support centres and some international partners. In addition, the survey population proposed several social actions and programmes to mitigate the impacts of Covid-19. In all, support for economic activities topped with 40.58%, followed by unemployment support (31.49%), ease of remote administrative procedures (24.09%),

Table 2.16 Mitigation measures promoted government and its partners[5]

Type of measures	Intended beneficiaries	Conditions of access	Excluded categories not likely to benefit
Social protection 1-Subsidy for facial masks	General public	1- None[6]	1- None
2-Sanitary lockdown	General public	None	2- Population outside the 15 communes are not involved in the location
Income support 1-Subsidy to artisans and carriers	1- Artisans and carriers	1- Fill online and on paper to deposit	1- all over categories except the artisans and porters has excluded
2- Taxes exemption for enterprises	2- Businesses	2- Formal enterprises to be registered and request the aid	2- Informal enterprises
3- Electricity and water free of charge for households for three months	3- Households	3- None	3- None
Access to services 1- Online service for taxes payment	1- the general public	1- none	1- None
2- Online service for judicial record acquisition	2- the general public	2- none	2- None
Regulations/advisories Advertising campaigns to sensitise the population through television, radio, and social media about Covid-19 and ways to fight against the disease	General public	None	None
Business Stimulus Taxes exemption for enterprises	Businesses	Formal enterprises to be registered and request the aid	Informal enterprises

[5] https://sgg.gouv.bj/cm/2020-06-10/.

[6] Facial masks are available at drug stores. Initially, it was sold at 500FCFA. However, the government makes it available at 200FCFA everywhere, even in rural areas. Additionally, facial masks made of local fabrics are also available.

Table 2.17 Mitigation actions received by specific socioeconomic groups

Mitigation action received	None	From my employer	From an organisation	Yes, from a state institution	From a private institution	From colleagues	From friends and family	Others	Total
Unemployed	93.33	0	6.67	0	0	0	0	0	100
Zem	100	0	0	0	0	0	0	0	100
Taxi ville/ minibus	96	0	0	4	0	0	0	0	100
Taxi interurban	87.5	3.57	0	7.14	0	0	0	1.79	100
Artists	98.61	0	0	1.39	0	0	0	0	100
Teachers	80.81	1.52	0.51	14.65	1.01	0	0	1.52	100
Merchant	98	0	0	1	1	0	0	0	100
Restaurant	96.97	0	0	3.03	0	0	0	0	100
Student	91.36	0.62	0.62	3.7	0.62	0.62	1.85	0.62	100
Agricultural Producer	96.53	0	0.69	0.69	1.39	0	0.69	0	100
Pharmacist	96.67	0	0	0	3.33	0	0	0	100
Retired	100	0	0	0	0	0	0	0	100
Others	83.33	6.06	3.03	7.58	0	0	0	0	100
Total	92.13	0.94	0.56	4.78	0.66	0.09	0.37	0.47	100

Source ASE data collection, December 2020

deadline waivers for statutory payments (21.37%), and others such as subsidies, food aid, and increased sensitisation among others which constituted 39.64% (ASE Data Collection, December 2020).

MAIN SUPPORTS DESIRED BY SOCIOECONOMIC GROUPS UNDEREMPLOYMENT

Following the measures to fight Covid-19, several measures to mitigate the adverse effects have also been initiated and implemented by the government. These include, among others, nationally applied water and electricity subsidies, financial assistance provided to specific individuals belonging to certain socioeconomic groups such as artisans and transporters, and tax exemption for formal businesses. However, the appropriateness of the measures targeting the groups must be examined. The data shows a disjuncture between what the groups wanted and what was provided. It emerged that, first and foremost, many survey participants (62%) wanted financial support (62%) from the government to mitigate the pandemic effects. Others include the provision of health kits (9.93%) or adaptive training (7.87%). Interestingly, many individuals did not desire support measures such as Covid-19 advisories, food supply, electricity and water subsidies, and exemption from taxes or levies.

However, location-based differences existed in the support measures desired by the survey population. From the results of Fig. 2.5, we essentially note that in the *cordon sanitaire* areas of Cotonou and Abomey-Calavi, socioeconomic groups mainly saw their activity cease during the lockdown. Since the most affected were teachers and students, they preferred water and electricity subsidies, training, supply of health kits, and Covid-19 advisories. However, in the area outside the *cordon sanitaire* areas such as Cobly, Toffo, Natitingou, Parakou, and Kalalé, financial aid and food supply were the most desired support measures. In this area, merchants, bartenders or restaurant owners, artists, and taximen constitute the target socioeconomic groups of the study. These groups had a significant drop in their level of their economic activities (Fig. 2.5).

COVID-19, CITIZENSHIP AND GOVERNANCE

Most Benin citizens were not involved in the Covid-19 management decision-making processes. We found that 19 per cent of the surveyed population engaged in taking actions related to control measures.

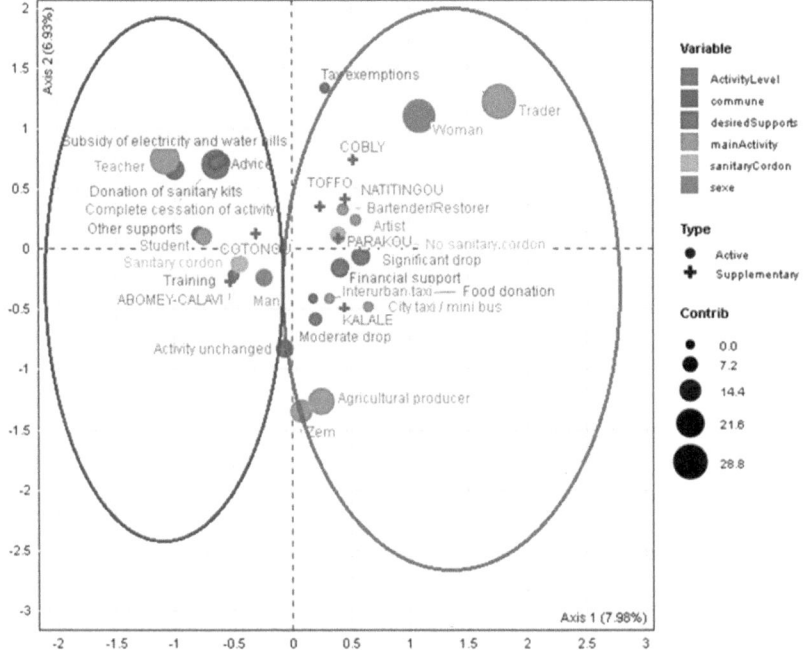

Fig. 2.5 Differences economic activities in and outside *cordon sanitaire* areas (*Source* ASE data collection, December 2020)

However, participation in the public protest was not substantial. Only a few respondents participated in Covid-19 management decisions. Nineteen per cent reported being part of control measure decisions, 8.15% in *cordon sanitaire* decision making, and 6.94% in mitigation measure decision making (ASE Data Collection, December 2020).

CONCLUSION AND RECOMMENDATIONS

Like all countries, Benin has been affected by the health crisis, weakening its reformed economy. Benin has opted for a *cordon sanitaire* to curb the spread of the pandemic to counter the negative impacts on the economy. The *cordon sanitaire* measure seems to be preferable and, at the same time, the most appropriate to avoid spreading the virus in the Beninese context. Benin is a small country with a large informal economy where a general lockdown would create more than considerable damage at the socioeconomic level. Therefore, the country instituted measures to mitigate the economic impacts of the pandemic. Our findings show that most of the various socioeconomic actors would primarily like financial support from the government in terms of mitigation measures. In addition, others would have liked support measures such as the supply of health kits or adaptive training. These individuals less desired supportive measures were counselling, food supply, subsidies for electricity and water bills, and exemption from taxes or levies. In light of this, the response put in place by the government by providing financial assistance to certain key socioeconomic actors aligns to meet the most pressing needs of these various actors.

The financial assistance measure also targeted stakeholders affected by the pandemic in their daily activities, such as stylists, hairdressers, transporters, restaurant workers, and artists. However, the available amount to assist the population was insufficient to cover most targeted group. Only 1–14% of the targeted people received such support. Therefore, although most socioeconomic actors desired an accurate mitigation measure, it has also been a potential source of inequality since many did not receive them despite high compliance with Covid-19 response measures.

Regarding the stakeholder's decision-making implication, only 19% of the actors' lead representatives were informed about the control measures decisions taken for their groups' categories. The proportion of group actors involved in the mitigation measures decisions is even fewer. The relevance of the measures taken by the government is well established for companies and socioeconomic groups. However, they did not seem to have experienced in practice the involvement of local authorities in managing the crisis. They were also observed disparities in the allocation of grants.

In summary, the governments' methods and actions for fighting the Covid-19 crisis agree with the population's expectations. However, there were some shortcomings in terms of participation and the distribution of resources.

In light of the study's findings, here are three main recommendations:

- Continuous awareness creation on safety measures and the risk of contamination.

- Increase efforts to subsidise agricultural producers to reduce the inflation in the prices of food products induced by the pandemic.
- Strengthen financial aid programmes for different socioeconomic groups in the different locations to relaunch their activities.

REFERENCES

AFDB. (2020). African Economic Outlook 2000.

INSAE (2017) Synthèse des analyses sur l'état et la structure de la population. Institut National de la Statistique et de l'Analyse Économique (INSAE).

INSAE. (2020). Note sur la pauvreté en 2019. INSAE—juillet 2020. https://docplayer.fr/191936953-Note-sur-la-pauvrete-en-2019-insae-juillet2020.html

USEFUL LINKS

Benin responds to covid-19: "Cordon Sanitaire" without generalized containment or lockdown? /https://www.gouv.bj/actualites/categorie/coronavirus--covid-19

"Gouvernement de la République du Benin" COVID-19 web page https://www.gouv.bj/actualites/categorie/coronavirus%2D%2Dcovid-19-/

https://www.worldbank.org/en/country/benin/overview

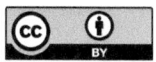

CHAPTER 3

Burkina Faso

Madeleine Wayack-Pambè, Dorte Thorsen, and Akosua K. Darkwah

INTRODUCTION

The first cases of Covid-19 infections were confirmed in Burkina Faso on 9 March 2020, amidst complex socioeconomic and political perturbations. Burkina Faso's social and political context has been particularly marked by instability since 2011. A significant factor producing instability was the fall of Blaise Compaoré's regime in October 2014, compounded by a security and humanitarian crisis that began in 2015 and clashes between ethnic groups. The Burkinabe state, particularly its army, has

M. Wayack-Pambè (✉)
Institut Supérieur Des Sciences de La Population, Université Joseph KI-ZERBO, Ouagadougou, Burkina Faso
e-mail: madeleine.wayackpambe@ujkz.bf

D. Thorsen
Institute of Development Studies, University of Sussex, Brighton, UK
e-mail: d.thorsen@ids.ac.uk

A. K. Darkwah
Department of Sociology, University of Ghana, Accra, Ghana
e-mail: adarkwah@ug.edu.gh

© The Author(s) 2024
A. Altaf et al. (eds.), *EQUITY IN COVID-19*, EADI Global Development Series, https://doi.org/10.1007/978-3-031-58588-3_3

been weakened considerably at the state level by these crises, encouraging the emergence of multiple groups exercising violence. Among these are ethnic self-defence militias known as "Kolgowéogo", Islamist armed groups claiming to be jihad, and groups of brigands (Kane, 2019). The 2019 report from the Legatum Institute, which analyses a country's potential to move from poverty to prosperity in an inclusive manner, gave Burkina Faso scores of 63.14% for safety and security, 60.68% for individual freedom and 44.12% for governance. These different scores placed Burkina Faso 117th, 58th and 108th, respectively compared to other countries.

Regarding corruption, Burkina Faso was ranked 85th out of 180 countries in 2019 by Transparency International, scoring 40%. Twenty-eight per cent of the Burkinabè population believed that corruption had increased in 2019 and 16% of the users of public services reported paying a bribe in 2019. In addition, Amnesty International (2019) states that human rights violations have increased in Burkina Faso. The country amended its Penal Code in June 2019 by adopting Law No. 044–2019/AN. This law defines what constitutes offences, but critics consider the definitions excessively broad and note that they could be used to repress human rights defenders, journalists and bloggers and restrict access to information.

The pandemic has thus added further strain to the country's resources, with two-fifths of the population (40%) living in poverty. Burkina Faso is classified as a lower-income country with an HDI of 0.434, according to the 2018 Human Development Report (UNDP, 2019). The value of the Gini Index was 35.3% in 2014[1] Furthermore, in 2018, the country's real GDP was 5,264.9 billion CFA francs [8.03 billion euros, much of which derived from the services sector (46%), despite this sector comprising only 17.7% of the working population (MINEFID, 2019). The relative contribution of other sectors to the GDP amounted to 21% for the industry sector, 20% for agriculture and 13% for tax revenues. Poverty affects around two-fifths of the Burkinabe population, or 40.1%, according to the latest household surveys (INSD, 2015a). It is higher in rural areas (47.5%) than in urban areas (13.7%). Only 25.5% of households had access to electricity in 2014, 9.3% in rural areas and 62.4% in urban areas (INSD, 2015b).

---

[1] https://donnees.banquemondiale.org/indicator/si.pov.gini?locations=bf

In terms of employment, while 63.4% of the population was actively employed in 2014, women's employment rate was lower (54.6.%) than that of men (73.3%)(INSD, 2015c. Significantly, 84% of the jobs are precarious. In 2018, the industry sector created the most employment (31.1%), followed by agriculture (29.9%), trade (21.3%) and services (17.7%).

Access to basic education has improved in Burkina Faso to the point of being almost universal, including in rural areas. For primary school (grade1-6), the gross admission rate was 104.8% in the 2017–2018 school year (INSD, 2019a). The enrolment rate was around 90.7%, with perfect parity between girls and boys, i.e. 90.9% and 90.6%, respectively. However, gender and locational inequalities increase as one progresses through the school system. For example, in 2015–16, there were 513 students in tertiary education per 100,000 inhabitants and disaggregation of the data revealed that only 330 students were female (Wayack-Pambè, 2020).

Burkina Faso's health indicators relating to access to the public health system show that in 2018 health centres had an average action radius of 5.9 km, a distance that tends towards the international standard of less than 5 km (Ministère de la santé, 2019). The average population within a Centre for Health and Social Promotion's (CSPS) catchment area was 9645 persons. Coverage for health professionals within the public health system was one doctor per 12,000 inhabitants despite the international standards recommending one doctor per 10,000 inhabitants; one nurse per 2419 inhabitants against standards recommending one nurse per 3000 inhabitants, and one midwife per 5510 inhabitants compared with standards recommending one midwife per 5000 inhabitants.

Maternal and infant mortality indicators remain high. In 2018, the maternal mortality rate was 320 deaths per 100,000 women, and the child mortality rate was 94 deaths per 1000 live births. The analysis of infant mortality rates according to children's place of residence shows that in 2010 infant mortality was lower in urban areas (46 pro mille) than in rural areas (82 pro mille). Children living in the poorest households were the most affected (95 pro mille) by mortality compared to those living in the wealthiest households (45 pro mille) (Ministère de l'économie et des finances, 2012). HIV-AIDS prevalence rate changed from 1% in 2010 (EDS-BF 2010) to 0.80% in 2018 (Présidence du Faso, 2019). Severe malaria remains the leading cause of death in medical centres and hospitals. In 2015, malaria accounted for 23.9% of the causes of death, followed by severe acute malnutrition (6.2%) and infections in newborn babies (5.2%) (Ministère de la santé, 2017).

The rate of access to drinking water in Burkina Faso was 75.4% in 2019, with disparities between rural (68.4%) areas and urban areas (92.9%) (Ministère de l'eau et de l'assainissement, 2020). However, it should be noted that in the Burkinabè context, the mere availability of a water source is insufficient to give an idea of the population's actual access to water. Access to water sources must be coupled with service quality criteria that consider the flow and continuity of supply. Discontinuity of service increases the risk of pathogen contamination of the water, as well as the difficulty of collecting water. Women and children usually carry out this chore, and the consequences of poor access to water (including time consumption) severely limit women's economic empowerment (Dos Santos and Wayack-Pambè, 2016).

In terms of sanitation, the proportion of households with improved toilets (VIP latrine, EcoSan, manual flush toilet, mechanical flush toilet) remained very low, with only 8.1% of the population having improved toilets in 2014 to 4.7% in 2009. In 2016, 40.4% of households had access to electricity,[2] 27.7% in rural areas and 75.3% in urban areas. Only 9.2% of female-headed households had access to electricity compared to 42.6% of male-headed households (MINEFID, 2017). Indicators on access to ICT show significant differences by gender and area of residence. A survey of access to ICTs among the population aged 15 years or older indicated that in 2014, 64.3% of Burkinabè owned a mobile phone, of which 51.7% were women and 79.4% men (INSD-EMC-TICs, 2015). The proportions according to the place of residence were 87% of the urban population had a mobile phone compared to 55.8% of the rural population.

Burkinabè societies are generally marked by unequal gender relations that expect women to be submissive to men. This is reflected in women's possibilities for exercising agency, i.e. having the power to decide for themselves. For example, in 2010, only 20% of women reported being able to make informed decisions for themselves regarding sexual relations, contraceptive use and reproductive health care (Ministère de l'économie et des Finances, 2012). Similarly, only 12% of women reported having participated in all three types of important decisions in their household at the same time: those related to their health, those related to major

---

[2] Access to electricity refers to the possession of grid electricity from the Société Nationale burkinabè d'électricité (SONABEL), solar energy and generators.

household purchases and those related to family visits. In addition, the proportion of women who had experienced domestic violence in the year preceding the survey was 9.3% in 2010, according to the same report.

The chapter analyses the inclusiveness of the public health strategies adopted and the measures taken to combat the Covid-19 pandemic in Burkina Faso. More specifically, it examines whether and how the different stakeholders were involved in defining and implementing the proposed responses and the multidimensional aspects of the consequences of these responses on the different groups of vulnerable populations. The study adopted an intersectional feminist approach allowing us, beyond gender, to take into account various groups of marginalised populations, such as the elderly, people living with a disability, street children, rural populations, the prison population or socio-economically disadvantaged populations through a feminist intersectional theoretical lens.

Methodology

The analysis is based on a Covid-19-focused review of the online press, government policy documents and reports published online by state and non-state actors. Several documentary sources were mobilised for the analyses presented in this study. These include existing national programme and policy documents, activity reports or study reports produced by ministries, documents and reports produced by the government, associations or other civil society actors reporting on actions taken on the pandemic, web pages of national and international institutions and online press articles. The information gathered from programme and policy documents, reports and institutional websites was used firstly to present an overview of the political, economic and social context in which Burkina Faso found itself at the time of the emergence of the Covid-19 pandemic on its territory. They also served to clarify the existing mechanisms for caring for vulnerable population groups and their potential for inclusion.

The data used to analyse the management of the pandemic derived mainly from the online private news outlets and a government information site. For the national press, the vast majority of the articles were identified on the site lefaso.net, the leading online news organ in Burkina Faso, and on Burkina24. Lefaso.net is a popular site serving as a relay for information from the various sectors of the country's political, social and economic life. It publishes articles written by academics, activists and other members of civil society residing in Burkina Faso or outside the country. Lefaso.net provides regular reports on the activities of the state, NGO associations, universities and educational centres. The Information Service of the Government of Burkina Faso (SIG) publishes press releases and reports on government action.

The information was collected from 9 March, the start date of the pandemic, to 30 September 2020. The research was carried out on the lefaso.net site and the GIS, in the files that each of these sites devoted to the Covid-19 pandemic, compiling all the information held by the site on the subject. For the other sites, the search was carried out on their search engines using the word "covid". A first selection was made by selecting any article or document containing Covid-19 in the title. A second selection was made by reading the first few lines, which made it possible to either classify the document in one of the predefined headings according to the search questions or to eliminate it based on keywords. A total of 859 articles from the lefaso.net site and 285 articles from the GIS were selected for content analysis. Finally, some information was supplemented by articles from the international online press dealing with the same subject or allowing for a more in-depth analysis.

Situating Covid-19 in Burkina Faso's Security Crisis

A recent report published the 13 March 2020 by the Office for the Coordination of Humanitarian Affairs (OCHA) indicates that 5.3 million people are affected by the security crisis in Burkina Faso and that 2.2 million need humanitarian aid assistance. Table 3.1 summarises the needs of those estimated to be in need of humanitarian assistance, as well as the type of need. Of the 579,000 people identified as in need, the majority are women (52%) or children (59%). There is also a substantial proportion of people with disabilities (1.2%). The assistance and protections needed include shelter and essential household items (EHI), education and food security. Concerning the latter, the nutritional situation of the population, already fragile due to the chronic drought and climatic hazards, is also exacerbated by the current humanitarian crisis. It is estimated that 954,000 people need nutritional assistance.

Table 3.1 Assistance and protection needs in the population most affected by the security crisis

Assistance/protection area	Population (No of persons)	Women (per cent)	Children (per cent)	Persons living with disability (per cent)
Humanitarian assistance	2.2 million			
• Shelter and essential household items	579,000	52	59	1.2
Water, Hygiene and Sanitation assistance	1.9 million	52	59	1.2
Education assistance	544,000	52	100	1.0
Food security	1.5 million	52	59	1.2
• Nutritional assistance	954,000	52	59	1.2
Security	948,000	52	59	1.2
• Gender-based violence protection	240,000	100	–	1.2

Source OCHA (2020)

Covid-19 Responses in Burkina Faso

On 9 March 2020, Burkina Faso confirmed its first cases of Covid-19, with the number of daily cases fluctuating between 0 and 50 cases per day between March and September 2020 and a peak of 193 on 12 September 2020, which is explained by a massive screening of students from the Ecole Nationale d'Administration (ENA) in military training in Bobo Dioulasso (Fig. 3.1).

Available statistics on the Covid-19 pandemic in Burkina Faso, therefore, indicate very low levels of pandemic-related lethality and mortality compared to other countries or regions of the world. However, extensive responses to the Covid-19 pandemic were taken in Burkina Faso. In the early stages of the outbreak, these responses were primarily aimed at curbing the spread of the disease and mitigating measures' impact on the population's living conditions. These responses focused on four aspects. The first two, health measures and those specific to the education sector, were primarily aimed at preventing the spread of the epidemic in the

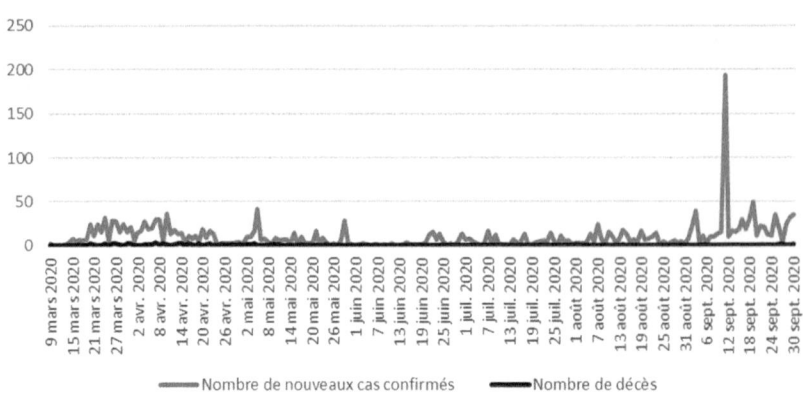

Fig. 3.1 Trends in confirmed cases and deaths related to Covid-19 in Burkina Faso (9 March–30 September 2020). *Source* Data on Covid-19 in Burkina Faso (INSD, 2020)

country. These were complemented by measures to mitigate the socioeconomic consequences of the proposed responses, as well as actions to ensure trust and reassurance of good governance of the pandemic by the government. Almost all of the measures were government-initiated but with diversified sources of funding.

Health Sector Measures

One of the initial health measures taken to manage the Covid-19 outbreak when the first cases appeared in Burkina Faso in March 2020 was the requisitioning of a hospital centre (in Tengandogo, a suburb of Ouagadougou) to receive and care for Covid-19 patients only. Screening units and tracing of contact cases were also set up. The dissemination of awareness-raising messages accompanied these measures on preventive measures through the media and a tour by the Minister of Health to raise awareness of the disease.[3] In May, they were supplemented by a digital system for monitoring and detecting cases suspected of having contracted Covid-19 with support from the World Health Organization (WHO),

---

[3] https://lefaso.net/spip.php?article95463;   https://www.sig.gov.bf/actualites/details?tx_news_pi1%5Baction%5D=detail&tx_news_pi1%5Bcontroller%5D=News&tx_news_pi1%5Bnews%5D=291&cHash=bc6791311989b21980dfc333e4fa33dd.

UNICEF and Terre des Hommes (TdH). Measures with a narrower remit included training of health sector actors in communication and community engagement to disseminate knowledge about the risks associated with the disease. In line with scientific developments at the international level, two clinical trials were initiated by the Ministry of Scientific Research, one on chloroquine and the other on a plant-based drug, Apirivine.[4]

Public Health Responses

During his first message to the nation on the Covid-19 pandemic, President Roch Marc Christian Kaboré announced several movement-related restrictions. He announced a ban on gatherings of more than fifty people, and imposition of curfew hour from 5 am to 7 pm throughout the country, starting from 21 March 2020.[5] The local authorities in affected cities subsequently issued by-laws ordering the closure of establishments likely to gather large numbers of people, such as markets, restaurants and entertainment venues, and later, places of worship.[6] The government also decreed the closure of all schools throughout the country in a communiqué dated 14 March.[7] The number of people permitted at family celebrations (weddings, funerals, etc.) was restricted to forty, with a procession ban. Visits to patients in hospitals and to prisoners were also

[4] https://www.sig.gov.bf/actualites/details?tx_news_pi1%5Baction%5D=detail&tx_news_pi1%5Bcontroller%5D=News&tx_news_pi1%5Bnews%5D=314&cHash=952f6d59c976703e5a84b57196d567c0.
https://www.sig.gov.bf/actualites/details?tx_news_pi1%5Baction%5D=detail&tx_news_pi1%5Bcontroller%5D=News&tx_news_pi1%5Bnews%5D=321&cHash=3afafb7827ed0f0ccc79af298dbb081a

[5] https://www.sig.gov.bf/fileadmin/user_upload/Decret_PRES_n__2020-0215_port ant_instauration_d_un_couvre-feu_page-0001.jpg;
https://www.sig.gov.bf/actualites/details?tx_news_pi1%5Baction%5D=detail&tx_news_pi1%5Bcontroller%5D=News&tx_news_pi1%5Bnews%5D=343&cHash=23ae834476018d450670743e46af594a

[6] https://www.sig.gov.bf/actualites/details?tx_news_pi1%5Baction%5D=detail&tx_news_pi1%5Bcontroller%5D=News&tx_news_pi1%5Bnews%5D=304&cHash=80c05b937c04a13681e163e0130beabe

[7] https://lefaso.net/spip.php?article95470
https://www.sig.gov.bf/fileadmin/user_upload/Communique_Gouvernement_Fermet ure_anticipee_Etalissements_d_enseignement_scolaire_universitaire_Burkina_Faso-page-001_1_.jpg

banned[8] and a thousand prisoners had their sentences commuted.[9] Large-scale administrative operations such as voter registration[10] and issuing of national identity cards were also interrupted.[11]

The second type of measure to contain the epidemic involved the reduction of the daily and spatial mobility of individuals. This materialised through the closure of all land and air borders, and the introduction of a night curfew[12] in cities affected by the pandemic.[13] These cities were quarantined and the movement of people to other locations was strictly forbidden.[14] Police controls were introduced at the exit points of the cities. Finally, all spaces and structures open to the public were required to implement a protocol of measures to prevent the spread of the virus, essentially providing hand-washing facilities and hydroalcoholic gel to users, and making compulsory the wearing of face masks within the premises.[15] The latter measure was made compulsory in all public places at the end of April 2020.[16]

One month after school closures, the Ministry of National Education, Literacy and Promotion of National Languages (MENAPLN) presented

[8] https://www.sig.gov.bf/actualites/details?tx_news_pi1%5Baction%5D=detail&tx_news_pi1%5Bcontroller%5D=News&tx_news_pi1%5Bnews%5D=299&cHash=6e869ea5f430d7669e593bdbeff624eb

[9] https://www.sig.gov.bf/actualites/details?tx_news_pi1%5Baction%5D=detail&tx_news_pi1%5Bcontroller%5D=News&tx_news_pi1%5Bnews%5D=316&cHash=92425765829c9f1f26d5cf3268cfeef0

[10] Burkina Faso held presidential elections on 22 November 2020.

[11] https://www.sig.gov.bf/actualites/details?tx_news_pi1%5Baction%5D=detail&tx_news_pi1%5Bcontroller%5D=News&tx_news_pi1%5Bnews%5D=303&cHash=2753b6a72cdadd2624a5be84a41583b3

[12] https://www.sig.gov.bf/actualites/details?tx_news_pi1%5Baction%5D=detail&tx_news_pi1%5Bcontroller%5D=News&tx_news_pi1%5Bnews%5D=320&cHash=f99b9bb926490f1c777c5643529af8f4

[13] https://www.sig.gov.bf/actualites/details?tx_news_pi1%5Baction%5D=detail&tx_news_pi1%5Bcontroller%5D=News&tx_news_pi1%5Bnews%5D=303&cHash=2753b6a72cdadd2624a5be84a41583b3

[14] https://www.sig.gov.bf/actualites/details?tx_news_pi1%5Baction%5D=detail&tx_news_pi1%5Bcontroller%5D=News&tx_news_pi1%5Bnews%5D=344&cHash=014aa58d0816d403d37d59f354758c25

[15] https://www.sig.gov.bf/actualites/details?tx_news_pi1%5Baction%5D=detail&tx_news_pi1%5Bcontroller%5D=News&tx_news_pi1%5Bnews%5D=303&cHash=2753b6a72cdadd2624a5be84a41583b3

[16] https://lefaso.net/spip.php?article96248

a response plan for educational continuity in the context of the pandemic, which included e-learning resources, promotion of hygiene in schools and sensitisation of learners and teachers among others.

RESPONSES TO MITIGATE THE ECONOMIC IMPACTS OF THE PANDEMIC

The government was faced with the question of how to mitigate the impact of the measures taken to contain the spread of Covid-19 on the population as soon as they were implemented. Questions were also raised by civil society as to the need for these nationwide measures given the realities of the country, particularly regarding measures that had an impact on the population's income. As a result, the government announced a series of measures to mitigate the consequences two weeks after issuing decrees that limited the mobility and activities of the population.

The mitigation measures mainly concerned actors in the economic sector, people working in markets and categories of people identified as vulnerable. Concerning economic sector actors, a battery of fiscal measures were taken in their favour, consisting of a waiver by the state of the collection of various taxes, deferral or exemption from payment and suspension or remission of penalties, to secure the country's supply of consumer goods and pharmaceutical products. In compensation, after consultation with traders, the Ministry of Trade secured stocks of consumer goods[17] (sugar, milk, rice, oil, soap, etc.) to guarantee the availability of stocks and reinforce the mechanisms for combating clandestine storage and price controls throughout the country.[18] Moreover, the government took over the operating costs of the traders working in markets. The latter has thus benefited from a suspension of rents and fees and an exemption from security fees.

The rest of the population enjoyed means-based subsidies aimed to ensure access to basic services, such as water and electricity.[19] For the poorest households, a three-month exemption from payment of water

---

[17] https://lefaso.net/spip.php?article42392

[18] https://www.burkina24.com/2020/03/21/covid-19-au-burkina-le-gouvernement-prend-des-mesures-pour-faire-face-A-limpact-economique/

[19] https://www.sig.gov.bf/actualites/details?tx_news_pi1%5Baction%5D=detail&tx_news_pi1%5Bcontroller%5D=News&tx_news_pi1%5Bnews%5D=318&cHash=7885bfed1 6f9887c68b530207ee4d310

and electricity bills was introduced, while other households benefited from a 50% rebate on electricity. Free water supply was introduced at standpipes in cities,[20] prompting the Ministry of Water and Sanitation to declare during a meeting with the media that the rural population had not been forgotten. However, according to the Ministry, the modalities for implementing mitigation measures for water supply in rural areas within the framework of the Covid-19 pandemic were under consideration. The location-specific management of rural water supply made the operationalisation of responses complex.[21]

Food was distributed to vulnerable populations—female heads of households, people living with disability and elderly people—in all the communes of Ouagadougou and the surrounding rural communes by the Ministry in charge of social action. These operations were to mark the beginning of a phase of support for vulnerable people through food distribution in the thirteen Burkina Faso regions.[22] Cash transfers of 20,000 CFA francs [30 euros] per month for three months were sent directly to 43,000 people affected by Covid-19 and identified through the *Burkina-Naong-Sa Ya* social safety nets programme.[23]

Finally, as a gesture of national solidarity, the government took other symbolic measures, such as the renunciation of salaries of members of the government: six months for the President of the Republic, four months

---

[20] https://www.sig.gov.bf/actualites/details?tx_news_pi1%5Baction%5D=detail&tx_news_pi1%5Bcontroller%5D=News&tx_news_pi1%5Bnews%5D=325&cHash=81bbed89c9298ac6404c58dbd7dc3c2b

[21] https://www.sidwaya.info/blog/2020/06/07/coronathon-plus-de-450-millions-F-cfa-collectes/

[22] https://www.sig.gov.bf/actualites/details?tx_news_pi1%5Baction%5D=detail&tx_news_pi1%5Bcontroller%5D=News&tx_news_pi1%5Bnews%5D=365&cHash=b45002b28c8ad81712569e3fa3499db9

[23] The "Social Safety Nets" are instruments of social Protection. They are defined as non-contributory transfer programmes that target poor or vulnerable populations in one way or another. They aim to stimulate—directly or through a substitution effect—household consumption of basic commodities and essential services. These programmes target poor and vulnerable people who are unable to meet their own basic needs or who are at risk of falling into poverty as a result of exogenous shocks or socioeconomic problems such as age, illness or disability. The Social Safety Nets "Burkina-Naong-Sa Ya" project in Burkina Faso is supported by the World Bank and aims to reduce chronic poverty and malnutrition. The project has a targeting strategy that allows the selection of beneficiaries according to defined criteria, followed by their registration and the attribution of a unique identifier. (Burkina Faso-Filets sociaux, 2011).

for the Prime Minister, two months for ministers of state and one month for other members of the government to contribute to the financing of Covid-19 prevention and mitigation measures.[24]

Innovations Arising from the Pandemic and Involvement of the Scientific Community

Scientific research in Burkina Faso, whether academic or industrial, is typically allocated very few financial resources. In the context of Covid-19, some studies were initiated by Burkinabè researchers. A study funded by the World Bank delivered its results on the impact of Covid-19 in artisanal mining communities in July 2020.[25] The aim was to examine how Covid-19 related restrictions affect children's and their families economic and social lives. In September 2020, the National Institute of Public Health presented a multidisciplinary research project on Covid-19 involving Burkinabè, French and Canadian researchers.[26] This project aims to generate epidemiological and socio-anthropological knowledge to assist the country in responding to the pandemic. Technological initiatives to help improve the management of the pandemic in the health system have also been developed. These include *Mondjossi*, a platform for connecting users with the medical profession,[27] ePresc (https://epresc. care/) is a web/mobile application dedicated to the digital management of patient's medical information throughout their lives and throughout their care,[28] Moreover, DMS is a pharmacy management software that facilitates data traceability.[29] Other innovations included a proposal for constructing a prefabricated hospital, a pedal-powered hand-washing system and software for distance learning (easyschool).

[24] https://www.sig.gov.bf/actualites/details?tx_news_pi1%5Baction%5D=detail&tx_news_pi1%5Bcontroller%5D=News&tx_news_pi1%5Bnews%5D=341&cHash=66cfb52c9af3f6c1447f5aaad715fa25

[25] https://lefaso.net/spip.php?article99154

[26] https://lefaso.net/spip.php?article99538

[27] https://lefaso.net/spip.php?article95805

[28] https://lefaso.net/spip.php?article95811

[29] https://lefaso.net/spip.php?article96384

Inclusiveness of Strategies
and Policy Responses: An Analysis

In Burkina Faso, as in the rest of the world, Covid-19 mortality is higher among men than women (Wayack-Pambè, Lankoandé & Kouanda, 2020). However, numerous studies show that poor and female populations are the most negatively impacted by epidemics, particularly regarding the social consequences and responses to them. The consideration of these populations has not been explicitly expressed or anticipated in the Covid-19 response documents developed by the government of Burkina Faso. As a result, an inclusive dimension is almost totally absent in the strategies and responses to mitigate the consequences of the Covid-19 pandemic. The inclusiveness of the government's strategies and responses to Covid-19 can only be seen in specific measures aimed at limiting the immediate socioeconomic effects of the preventive responses to the pandemic. The specific needs of populations traditionally discriminated against, for example, in terms of schooling, were not taken into account in the MENAPLN response plan. Hence the measures proposed for educational continuity were likely to increase educational inequalities. However, while the government's overall pandemic response plan did not initially target specific vulnerable groups, it was adapted over time in response to feedback from the population, opposition political parties, civil society organisations and donations from various contributors.

The temporary closure of schools will likely lead the most vulnerable children to drop out of school or not be enrolled. Given the conditions prior to the onset of the pandemic, it is conceivable that the solutions issued by the MENAPLN to limit the consequences of school closures were unable to curb the increase in pre-existing educational disparities between the advantaged and disadvantaged population groups, i.e. between urban and rural areas, between wealthy and poor households and between male and female children. Firstly, concerning children living in rural areas and those living in economically disadvantaged households, the virtual absence of electricity supply in rural areas, and to a lesser extent in peripheral urban areas, has de facto excluded children in these areas from the educational continuity offered by MENAPLN. As for the teaching offered by radio, even if the experiments on a small scale indicate that it is a medium that favours distance learning, it would have been necessary for every Burkinabe child attending school to have a personal radio to follow the lessons. Moreover, the proportion of the population with a

3 BURKINA FASO 57

computer or mobile phone and the proportion with access to the internet suggest that only a tiny minority of children have been able to access online teaching resources.

For girls, gender relations in society that assign them to caregiving roles increase the educational inequalities generated by school closures (Bandiera et al., 2020; Burzynska & Contreras, 2020). School closure thus has long-term deleterious effects on girls. Once out of school, they are more likely to stay out. School closures increase in this practice in contexts where early marriage is widespread. In Burkina Faso, for example, an increase in early marriage is feared due to the Covid-19 school closures. Indeed, 51.3% of the female population aged 20–24 declared in 2014 that they had married before 18, compared to 1.6% of the young men in the same age group (INSD, 2019b). Burkina Faso is thus among the countries in the world where the prevalence of early marriage is high. These rates are even higher in rural areas, where 62.9% of young women had married before the age of 18 compared to 2.2% of young men. In urban areas, 19.9% of women were in this situation, and no men were affected. Prevalence levels of early marriage were also high in the East and the Sahel regions, where the median age at marriage for girls was 16. These regions were already experiencing school closures due to attacks by armed groups. In 2015, nearly seven out of ten girls (65.2%) aged 20–24 years reported having been married before 18 in the Eastern region, whereas the phenomenon was almost non-existent among young men. In the Sahel region, eight out of ten girls (76.6%) in the same age group reported the same situation, compared to only one out of ten boys (10.4%) in the same age group.[30]

Another consequence of school closures is increasing the demand for girls for domestic and reproductive work. As a result, they have to substitute for adult women in tasks and activities related to this area. Girls are thus more unable than boys to become involved in a pedagogical continuity at a distance.

While the state's assumption of financial responsibility for water and electricity bills as part of a desire to minimise the economic inequalities generated by the pandemic, it did not take into account the specific needs of women and the accentuation of unequal situations between men and

---

[30] It should be noted that although the gender comparison shows a substantial difference to the detriment of girls, the proportion of boys married before they reach the age of majority is ten times higher than at national level in these regions.

women generated by the pandemic. The Covid-19 pandemic appeared in Burkina Faso during the dry season, when water is scarce, including in standpipes—moreover, introducing free water only concerned women in urban areas, while women in rural areas get their water mainly from rivers, wells or boreholes. However, even in urban areas, where water collection remains a predominantly female chore (Dos Santos & Wayack Pambè, 2016), this measure has not been inclusive, as it has not reduced the drudgery of waiting at the water point. This is all the more so as March, April and May are the hottest months and those with very low flows in the standpipes.

One of the significant shortcomings of the Covid-19 response plan,[31] as well as the strategies and measures put in place to deal with the pandemic is that they incorporate very little of the social dimensions of the security situation related to Jihadist insurgents. Thus the response plan does not consider the prolonged closure of various administrative services, schools and health centres in the regions most affected by the crisis or the displacement of people caused by the crisis.

Finally, the increase in domestic violence was very quickly identified as a "pandemic within the pandemic" because it affects all countries affected by Covid-19. This violence, which mainly affects women and girls, was denounced by the UN Secretary-General, who called on all states to take appropriate measures to end it. Nevertheless, the issue of gender-based violence has not been raised in Burkina Faso in any governmental or social forum. Therefore, it is difficult to know whether this is due to a lack of manifestation of the phenomenon in the Burkinabè context or whether it has simply been forgotten. Nevertheless, it should be noted that domestic or child abuse rates are low in Burkina Faso (Ministry of Economy and Finance, 2012; ISSP, 2018; Wayack Pambè et al., 2014).

It is difficult to determine the origin of the responses to the Covid-19 pandemic in Burkina Faso. However, the measures taken by the government can be read in the light of the social, political and economic situation prior to the pandemic, as well as the debates and developments at the regional and international levels.

---

[31] https://www.sig.gov.bf/actualites/details?tx_news_pi1%5Baction%5D=detail&tx_news_pi1%5Bcontroller%5D=News&tx_news_pi1%5Bnews%5D=387&cHash=301e88e8e56744ce646fe7771909a69e

Regarding the social, political and economic climate at a domestic level, the first measures were perceived by certain sections of the population as a willingness on the part of the government to take advantage of the health crisis to tackle internal difficulties. Thus, the closure of schools from 16 to 31 March and a ban on gatherings of more than fifty people were decreed on 14 March 2020, just two days before a protest march and the start of strike action among primary and secondary school teachers. In addition, a strike call for 16–20 March 2020[32] was issued by the Union of Trade Union Action (UAS) against the application of the Single Tax on Salaries and Wages (IUTS) to the bonuses and allowances of public employees. The closure of educational institutions during the weekend on a Saturday evening, with immediate effect on the following Monday, was therefore interpreted as a means of silencing the social movements being prepared in the country. This suspicion was reinforced by the fact that the government vacillated a great deal before closing places of worship and markets. Nevertheless, here, too, the government was accused of being afraid that it would have to confront specific religious and traditional communities resisting the preventive measure.

The temporal nature of decisions also led people to question the independence of the government in decision-making, as well as the legitimacy of the measures taken and their appropriateness to the country's situation. The decisions announced by the government were thus often welcomed and perceived as "following in the footsteps" of what was done in developed countries, particularly in France, without taking into account national realities. Indeed, the closure of schools was decreed on 14 March, two days after the same measure was decided in France. Similarly, the introduction of measures to limit the mobility of individuals, taken on 20 March, took place four days after confinement was imposed throughout France.

The desire to set up clinical trials[33] on Chloroquine and Apivirine (a remedy derived from local plants) stemmed both from the desire to position oneself internationally in the debate on the effect of chloroquine, and from the desire of African countries to contribute to the fight against the pandemic. Furthermore, a proven effect of chloroquine or Apirivine would have provided African states with a low-cost treatment

[32] https://lefaso.net/spip.php?article95232
[33] https://lefaso.net/spip.php?article95769

for the disease. However, the official launch of these clinical trials by the Ministry of Research has been followed by slow implementation. In the case of Apivirine, the first protocol was rejected by the Health Research Ethics Committee (HREC).[34] It was only in December 2020 that the first results of Apivirine were delivered, prompting challenges from some researchers and medical practitioners.[35]

Governance, Power Relations and Contestations of Covid-19 Responses

As a result of the various corruption cases involving the political elite that have been reported in the press for more than a decade, civil society and the population, in general, show a lack of confidence in the government's management of public assets. This situation has prompted the government to communicate very early on the management of the pandemic in an effort to be transparent and to give an image of good governance. Nevertheless, all the initiatives taken by the government remained marred by suspicion among the population. Some of the public image restoring programmes include daily Covid-19 briefings which were reduced gradually to weekly and monthly updates. The national Covid-19 coordinator Prof. Martial Ouédraogo was sacked after the poor handling of the death of the first patient. Covid-19 updates were broadcast on various media outlets in the country.

The government also held stakeholder consultations with political parties, market women and transport associations to improve the management of the pandemic. To resume economic activities, consultations were held with the actors of the various economic sectors, in particular, the urban passenger transport sector and the interurban, peri-urban and rural passenger transport sectors. These meetings led to the signing of protocols of an agreement to organise the resumption of activities in these sectors.[36] After the closure of the Ouagadougou central market, Rood-Wooko, the medium and small markets and the itinerant markets

[34] https://lefaso.net/spip.php?article96914; https://lefaso.net/spip.php?article95769

[35] https://lefaso.net/spip.php?article101643;   https://lefaso.net/spip.php?article10 1684

[36] https://www.sig.gov.bf/actualites/details?tx_news_pi1%5Baction%5D=detail&tx_news_pi1%5Bcontroller%5D=News&tx_news_pi1%5Bnews%5D=379&cHash=15f2c7fc2 690c1a262542c52a2926d33

also closed on 26 March 2020.[37] At the insistence of the population, the Ouagadougou city council initiated consultation with actors of the informal economy and the associations of market traders on 1 April 2020.[38] The consultation aimed to propose ways and means of reopening commercial infrastructures in the capital. These exchanges led to the establishment of a memorandum of understanding between the two parties for the strict observance of preventive measures to curb the pandemic and subsequently to the reopening of the prominent market in Ouagadougou on 20 April 2020.[39] However, a few days after the reopening of the market, the clauses of the protocol relating to the preventive measures were not respected.[40]

At the same time, a national committee for the crisis management of the pandemic was created, made up of government representatives, technical and financial partners working in the health sector, representatives of private health structures and civil society.[41] The High Council for Social Dialogue also initiated a framework bringing together members of the government, employers and workers to encourage joint reflection on the socioeconomic consequences of the pandemic and the development of palliative measures acceptable to the population.[42]

The various initiatives undertaken by the public authorities to demonstrate their good management of the pandemic have not always succeeded in restoring a climate of trust between the government and the population. One of the reasons for this is probably the fact that very few Burkinabès have been infected with Covid-19, and the pandemic's health effects were imperceptible to most of the population. The confusion surrounding the management of the first Covid-19 death in Burkina Faso (also the first recorded death of Covid-19 in sub-Saharan Africa) sowed

---

https://www.sig.gov.bf/actualites/details?tx_news_pi1%5Baction%5D=detail&tx_news_pi1%5Bcontroller%5D=News&tx_news_pi1%5Bnews%5D=378&cHash=6c3f9d394ec6b29df2a4d9aef505bfb0

[37] https://lefaso.net/spip.php?article96282

[38] https://lefaso.net/spip.php?article95976

[39] https://lefaso.net/spip.php?article96310

[40] https://lefaso.net/spip.php?article96419

[41] https://lefaso.net/spip.php?article96784

[42] https://lefaso.net/spip.php?article97107

doubt about the natural causes of this death[43]and contributed to the scepticism among ordinary people regarding the existence of the disease. Moreover, the first people to be affected, and whose contamination was widely publicised, were members of the government[44] and people from wealthy social classes. The measures implemented were therefore felt to subject most of the population to resolving a problem that only affected the elite. Meanwhile, the consequences of these measures affected the majority but not the elite. Despite the authorities' attempts to establish participation in the politics surrounding Covid-19 management through consultations with actors in the informal sector, the popular demonstrations by market traders forced the authorities to reopen earlier than planned.[45]

Similarly, mass demonstrations by members of an association of Muslim practitioners demanding the reopening of mosques[46] forced the government to authorise the immediate reopening of places of worship for all other religious denominations.[47] On the strength of this victory, the population subsequently demonstrated to demand the lifting of the curfew,[48] leading the government to capitulate again, thus removing any pretence of consensus in Covid-19 politics.

As is becoming increasingly clear, the management of the pandemic in Burkina Faso took place in a context of permanent contestation of public authority as well as under pressure from civil society, opposition political parties and various professional bodies to encourage the government to take appropriate measures to contain the pandemic and limit its adverse effects on the population.

Thus, the closure of the borders to the transport of people following the example of countries such as France and the USA, as well as the prohibition of large gatherings in all public places, was demanded as early as 17

---

[43] https://lefaso.net/spip.php?article96634

[44] https://lefaso.net/spip.php?article95632

[45] https://www.burkina24.com/2020/04/28/covid-19-au-burkina-faso-des-commer cants-reclament-louverture-du-marche-de-dassasgho/;   https://www.burkina24.com/2020/04/28/covid-19-au-burkina-faso-les-commercants-de-nabi-yaar-manifestent-pour-la-reouverture-du-marche/; https://lefaso.net/spip.php?article96460

[46] https://lefaso.net/spip.php?article96582

[47] https://lefaso.net/spip.php?article96585

[48] https://lefaso.net/spip.php?article97148

March by an opposition party, the UPC,[49] and the doctors' union.[50] The latter also called for subsidies and price controls on pharmaceutical products needed to fight the pandemic, such as hydroalcoholic gels and masks. At the same time, the government was also questioned the measures taken[51] to mitigate the effects of the measures to combat the pandemic on the population, particularly the most disadvantaged and those directly affected by these measures.[52]

Long before this turned into mood swings leading to the lifting of preventive measures, voices were raised to challenge almost every action or intervention of the government in its disease management.[53] These challenges came from ordinary citizens through social networks and in comments in the online press, political parties, trade unions or civil society, challenging the power of control. These non-governmental actors not only analysed the situation but also criticised the government's approach by making counter-proposals. These stances have contributed to increasing the fragility of the government's pandemic management. Thus, in the face of the preventive measures enacted by the government, the leader of the opposition as well as legal actors[54] denounced severe violations of individual freedom. Nevertheless, they have also made it possible to direct the state's actions more specifically towards the population's needs.

The socioeconomic measures subsequently introduced to mitigate the consequences of the response to the pandemic were deemed unsuitable by trade unions and civil society organisations. The Syndicat National des artistes musiciens du Burkina (SYNAMUB) denounced the clannish management of funds allocated to cultural and tourist actors. The Coalition Against the High Cost of Living (CCVC), a civil society organisation, described the management of the pandemic in Burkina Faso as "haphazard" and made up of "trial and error", intending to organise the plundering of the country's wealth.[55] Another party, Soleil d'Avenir,

---

[49] Union pour le Progrès et le Changement.

[50] https://lefaso.net/spip.php?article95542; https://lefaso.net/spip.php?article95539

[51] https://lefaso.net/spip.php?article95798

[52] https://lefaso.net/spip.php?article95806

[53] https://lefaso.net/spip.php?article96020

[54] https://lefaso.net/spip.php?article96555

[55] https://lefaso.net/spip.php?article96528

questioned the government on the disastrous results of its pandemic management.[56]

CONCLUSION AND RECOMMENDATIONS

Like the rest of the world's leaders, the Burkinabè government was caught off guard by the arrival of the Covid-19 pandemic in the country. Coinciding with a deleterious social, economic, political and security context, the emergence of the pandemic made it imperative for the government to show that it was capable of meeting this new health challenge while continuing to take on its pre-existing ones. This was all the more important as the disease appeared only a few months before the presidential elections due to take place on 22 November 2020.

The first measures taken by the Burkinabe government to counter Covid-19 did not target vulnerable population groups. However, government actions gradually became more inclusive as they were readjusted progressively under pressure from social movements and criticism from trade unions, political parties and the general population of the pandemic management and its lack of inclusiveness. This social pressure has thus contributed to reorienting the government towards more participatory management of the pandemic, through the multiplication of consultations with various actors. Also, the measures taken to mitigate the social and economic consequences of the response to the disease on the population have ultimately made it possible to include different categories of vulnerable populations, such as pregnant women, children who have been orphaned and are living on the street, prisoners and the elderly and poor female heads of household.

However, the specific needs of women and girls related to the higher impact of health crises on them due to unequal gender relations in societies were not taken into account in this reorientation of government action on the pandemic. Thus, issues such as the exacerbation of domestic violence during the confinement or closure of places of commerce and entertainment, the overload of domestic work due to preventive measures and school closures, as well as the potential increase in the de-schooling of girls, with the corollary of early marriage, do not appear in the interventions and actions taken in Burkina Faso to respond to the Covid-19

---

[56] https://lefaso.net/spip.php?article95876

pandemic. This is because the street and social networks were the main channels used by the population to express their concerns and disagreement with the government's response to the pandemic. However, these two spaces are still used less by women in Burkina Faso than men. On the one hand, they are not very present in corporate organisations or do not occupy a position that allows them to highlight the specificity of their situations, and on the other hand, their access to new information technologies and social networks remains low. The fact that the disease affects fewer women has probably contributed to the invisibility of women in political action against Covid-19 in Burkina Faso. Ultimately, the structuring of social and spatial inequalities in Burkina Faso, as well as the experiences of other epidemics that have impacted the West African subregion, suggest that females, especially girls, as well as rural populations will bear the brunt of the pandemic, mainly as a result of measures taken to contain it.

However, the interventions and actions taken in Burkina Faso to respond to the pandemic suffer from many shortcomings that give the impression of a lack of control over its management. First, they lack clarity regarding their adequacy and continuity with existing development programmes, particularly those stemming from the National Economic and Social Development Plan. Furthermore, as they have not been adopted in a participatory approach, they suffer from a lack of inclusiveness. Thus, neither the specific needs of the populations defined as vulnerable in the national development programme nor those of the populations particularly affected by the security crisis are reflected in the responses and measures proposed by the government to deal with the pandemic.

Ultimately, while, as in almost all sub-Saharan African countries, the Covid-19 disease has had little effect on Burkina Faso in terms of health, the Burkinabè population suffered the social and economic costs of the pandemic in the long term. The pandemic responses constitute risk factors for increasing the vulnerability of already disadvantaged populations, particularly girls and women. The effects resulted from the ad hoc manner in which responses were implemented, while the consequences of the measures taken to contain the pandemic have a potentially long-term impact on populations (Bandiera et al., 2020; Burzynska & Contreras, 2020).

In our recommendations and flowing from the analysis, Burkina Faso needs to democratise its decision-making spaces to make them more inclusive. Again, in times of crisis, the state must communicate clearly about programmes and their sustainability and continuity plans. It is also crucial for the state to own its plans and programmes, which must be fashioned to suit the various contexts in the country. Finally, vulnerable social groups such as women, people living with disability, youth, children, the aged and the extremely poor must be prioritised adequately in the implementation of social protection programmes.

References

Bandiera, O, Buehren, N., Goldstein, M., Rasul, I., Smurra A. (2020). Do school closures during an epidemic have persistent effects? Evidence from Sierra Leone in the Time of Ebola

Burzynska, K. & Contreras, G. (2020). Lancet. Gendered effects of school closures during the COVID-19 pandemic. *The Lancet, 395*(10242), 1968. https://doi.org/10.1016/S0140-6736(20)31377-5.

Dos Santos, S., & Pambè, M. W. (2016). Les Objectifs du Millénaire pour le développement, l'accès à l'eau et les rapports de genre. *Mondes En Développement, 2*, 63–78.

Burkina Faso. (2011). *Filets sociaux*. Ouagadougou.

Burkina Faso. (2012). *Politique nationale de protection sociale 2013–2022*. Ouagadougou.

Burkina Faso. (2016). *Plan national de développement économique et social 2016–2020*. Ouagadougou.

INSD. (2015a). *Enquête multisectorielle continue (EMC) 2014: Accès aux technologies de l'information et de la communication*. Ouagadougou.

INSD. (2015b). *Enquête multisectorielle continue (EMC) 2014:* Alphabétisation et scolarisation. Ouagadougou.

INSD. (2015c). *Enquête multisectorielle continue (EMC) 2014: Emploi et chômage*. Ouagadougou.

INSD (2015d). *Enquête multisectorielle continue (EMC) 2014:* Habitat, assainissement Et accès à l'eau potable. Ouagadougou.

INSD. (2015e). *Enquête multisectorielle continue (EMC) 2014:* Profil de pauvreté et d'inégalités. Ouagadougou.

INSD. (2019). *Annuaire statistique 2018*. Ouagadougou.

INSD. (2019). *Mutilations Génitales Féminines & Mariage d'Enfants : Rapport thématique basé sur l'EDS 2010 et l'EMC-MDS 2015*. Ouagadougou.

Institute, L. (2019). *Legatum prosperity index 2019*. United Kingdom.

ISCOM. (2019). *Etude sur l'expansion et les usages des TIC au Burkina Faso en 2018*. Ouagadougou.

Kane. (2019, 5 Juin). Au Burkina Faso, l'affaiblissement de l'État fait le lit du terrorisme. *The conversation*.

MINEFID. (2019). Annuaire statistique de l'économie et des finances 2018. Ouagadougou.

Ministère de l'économie et des finances. (2012). *Enquête Démographique et de Santé et à Indicateurs Multiples (EDSBF-MICS IV) 2010*. Ouagadougou.

Ministère de l'économie, des finances et du développement (2017) *Tableau de bord social du Burkina Faso*.

Ministère de la santé. (2017). *Profil sanitaire complet du Burkina Faso: Module 1, Situation socio-sanitaire du Burkina Faso et mise en œuvre des ODD*.

Ministère de l'économie, des finances et du développement. (2019). Annuaire statistique de l'économie et des finances 2018. Ouagadougou.

Ministère de la santé. (2019). *Annuaire statistique 2018*.

OCHA. (2020). Aperçu des besoins humanitaires Burkina Faso. OCHA

PNUD. (2019) *Rapport sur le développement humain 2019 Au-delà des revenus, des moyennes et du temps présent : les inégalités de développement humain au XXIe siècle, Burkina Faso*.

Présidence du Faso. (2019). *Rapport d'activité sur la Riposte au sida au Burkina Faso*.

RFI. (25 août 2015). Burkina Faso: une brigade de gendarmerie attaquée à Oursi. www.rfi.fr. https://www.rfi.fr/fr/afrique/20150825-burkina-faso-att aque-oursi-gendarme-blessure-grave

Savadogo, M. (5 Septembre 2019). Comment s'explique la prolifération des groupes extrémistes au Burkina Faso? *The conversation*. https://theconversat ion.com/comment-sexplique-la-proliferation-des-groupes-extremistes-au-bur kina-faso-122566

Wayack-Pambè, M. (2020). Inégalité entre les sexes en matière d'éducation au Burkina Faso: évolutions actuelles à partir des statistiques scolaires 1936–2019. Les presses Africaines, p. 153.

Wayack-Pambè, M., Lankoandé, B., & Kouanda, S., (5 Juin, 2020). Comment la jeunesse de sa population peut expliquer le faible nombre de morts de Covid 19 en Afrique? *The conversation*.https://theconversation.com/com ment la-jeunesse-de-sa-population-peut-expliquer-le-faible-nombre-de-morts-du-covid-19-en-afrique-sexplique-la-proliferation-des-groupes-extremistes-au-burkina-faso-139832

Wayack-Pambè, M., Gnoumou, B., & Kaboré, I. (2014). Relationship between women's socioeconomic status and empowerment in Burkina Faso: A focus on participation in decision-making and experience of domestic violence. *African Population Studies, 28*, 1146–1156.

WEBSITES

https://databank.worldbank.org/source/africa-development-indicators/Type/
TABLE/preview/on
https://data.worldbank.org/indicator/SL.EMP.VULN.ZS
https://donnees.banquemondiale.org/indicateur/SI.POV.DDAY?locations=
1W&start=1981&end=2015&view=chart
https://donnees.banquemondiale.org/indicateur/SI.POV.GINI?locations=BF
https://data.worldbank.org/indicator/SG.DMK.SRCR.FN.ZS?most_recent_
value_desc=true
https://data.worldbank.org/indicator/FX.OWN.TOTL.FE.ZS
https://afrobarometer.org/fr/results?field_country_tid=462&page=1
https://www.transparency.org/en/countries/burkina-faso
https://www.amnesty.org/fr/countries/africa/burkina-faso/
https://www.leconomistedufaso.bf/2015/06/15/tourisme-317-milliards-pour-
le-secteur/
https://www.humanitarianresponse.info/en/op%C3%A9rations/burkina-faso/
document/burkina-faso-aper%C3%A7u-des-besoins-humanitaires-hno-2020
https://donnees.banquemondiale.org/indicateur/SI.POV.GINI?locations=BF
https://www.hrw.org/fr/report/2020/05/26/leur-combat-contre-leduca
tion/attaques-comises-par-des-groupes-armes-contre-des
https://www.humanitarianresponse.info/en/opper   centC3per   centA9rations/
burkina-faso/document/burkina-faso-aperper   centC3per   centA7u-des-
besoins-humanitaires-hno-2020

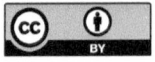

CHAPTER 4

Ghana

Clara Osei-Boateng and Zjos Vlaminck

INTRODUCTION

Ghana announced its first cases of Covid-19 on March 12, 2020. The country's experience with Covid-19 occurred when it was preparing for the eighth Presidential and Parliamentary elections since the commencement of the Fourth Republic Constitution in 1992. The December 2020 elections passed with some constatations that led to violence and court actions. However, there was a consensus among political actors and civil society organisations that Ghana's electoral management systems are adequate (CDD-Ghana, 2016), although mistrust of the electoral management body has plummeted since 2012 (Afrobarometer Surveys, 2016–2020); and electoral choices of the majority of Ghanaians are issue-based (Harding, 2015; Lindberg & Morrison, 2008). In addition, Ghana's voter turnout has been relatively high, averaging 71% between 1992 and 2016 (Afram & Tsekpo, 2017).

C. Osei-Boateng
Independent Research Consultant, Cobquecura, Chile

Z. Vlaminck (✉)
Independent Governance and Social Development Expert, Accra, Ghana
e-mail: zjos.vlaminck@gmail.com

© The Author(s) 2024
A. Altaf et al. (eds.), *EQUITY IN COVID-19*, EADI Global
Development Series, https://doi.org/10.1007/978-3-031-58588-3_4

Two political parties, namely the National Democratic Congress (NDC), a centre-left social democratic party and the New Patriotic Party (NPP), a centre-right and liberal, conservative political party, have dominated the political scene since the return to constitutional rule in 1992. Patronage politics and hyper-partisan competition between the two dominant parties means that access to services and resources is sometimes politically determined rather than based on technical or developmental considerations. As a result, the state tends to systematically redistribute resources towards members of the government, the ruling party, and influential leaders while weakening the political and economic bases of (real or perceived) members of the political opposition.

This structure also affects Ghana's decentralisation governance system, embedded in the 1992 Constitution and the Local Government Act (Act 462) of 1993. Under Ghana's decentralisation system, legislation, policies, and guidelines determine the relationships between central- and local government entities. The central government maintains the policy-making role and a vertical relationship with local government institutions. The sub-national governments (Metropolitan, Municipal, and District Assemblies (MMDAs)) act as implementing entities and have primary responsibility for planning, financing, and delivering services to local people. However, the central government retains most of the spending power and determines where developmental programmes are situated. The Municipal governments remain poorly equipped in budget planning, preparation, execution, and accounting, with many demonstrating weak compliance with regulatory frameworks, including procurement and contract management (World Bank, 2018).

In terms of Ghana's economic standing, while the country achieved Millennium Development Goal 1 by halving poverty ahead of the 2015 deadline, inequality continued to increase, and since 2012, the reduction in poverty rates has stagnated (GSS, 2018). In 2016/17, nearly a quarter (23.4%) of the Ghanaian population was classified as poor persons, with as many as 2.4 million Ghanaians (8.2%) considered extremely poor (GSS, 2018). Despite improvements in both income and non-income dimensions of development, inequality has been rising, a situation that speaks to Ghana's growth rate not being inclusive (Oduro et al., 2018). Ghana's Gini coefficient increased consistently between 1991 and 2016, from 38.4 to 43.5 (although there was a drop of 0.4 points between 2005 (42.8) and 2012 (42.4)) (World Bank, 2020).[1] However, Ghana has a relatively low Gini coefficient compared with other sub-Sahara African countries. The alarming issue with Ghana is that it is one of the few countries on the continent where income inequality has systematically increased over the last three decades (UNDP, 2017).

It has been argued that the following six factors have driven Ghana's growing inequality. These are jobless export-driven growth with low job creation and world market price vulnerabilities, poor public financial management fraught with corruption, significant regional and rural–urban disparities, unequal access to and quality of public services; gender inequality; and political capture and corruption (UNDP, 2017; Oduro et al., 2018). In addition, before Covid-19, Ghana was already under high debt, which has implications for spending and the reach of support programmes.

This chapter analysed the impact of Covid-19 responses of state and non-state actors on the well-being of Ghana's poor and vulnerable, which is analysed through four dimensions of well-being, namely material well-being operationalised as work and income as well as access to essential services (notably education, water, and electricity), relational well-being operationalised as social relations and social capital, subjective well-being operationalised as the subjective evaluation of the quality of life (prior and post-Covid-19) and collective well-being operationalised as political empowerment.

METHODOLOGY

The research was conducted in line with existing Covid-19 restrictions and protocols. The research team analysed vital government policies, presidential speeches, reports from CSOs, NGOs and development partners, and media output on response to the Covid-19 crisis. In addition, literature review of existing studies and surveys on the impact of COVID-19 in Ghana was conducted. The secondary data was then complemented with key stakeholder interviews with government officials at national and district levels, NGOs, development partners, local Civil Society Organisations (CSOs), trade unions, and workers associations. Lastly, to understand the impact on the well-being of the poor,

---

[1] https://data.worldbank.org/indicator/si.pov.gini?locations=gh

the research team conducted focus group discussions and interviews with head porters (*Kayayei*) in Accra, residents of Chorkor and market women in Bolgatanga. The research consisted of the following phases (a) socioeconomic and political context analysis, (b) mapping of Covid-19 mitigation responses by state and non-state actors, (c) identification of specific vulnerable groups for in-depth case studies of social and spatial equity issues, namely head porters (*Kayayei*), residents of Chorkor, market women/cross-border traders in Bolgatanga, and (d) equity assessment which interrogated how the identified policies/programmes have affected the well-being of the identified vulnerable groups in the short term. Moreover, it also examined how the identified policies/programmes have affected work and income, access to basic services and political empowerment of the poor and vulnerable in the longer term.

Theoretical and Analytical Framework

There has been a rise in scholarship and policy attention on inclusive development and the importance of addressing poverty and inequality (see e.g., Piketty, 2014; Bourguignon, 2015; OECD, 2014). However, the concept of equity in secular philosophy dates to ancient Greece with Plato, who pointed out the dangers of inequality for political stability (Attinc et al., 2006, p.76). Since the 1970s, the focus was shifted from looking at final welfare to creating equality in liberties (Rawls), opportunities (Roemer, Dworkin), and capabilities (Sen) (Attinc et al., 2006, p. 77). In a nutshell, social equity based on Rawls, Sen, Dworkin, and Roemer's theories roughly entails an equal starting point or equal set of opportunities or capabilities. However, creating a level playing field or equal opportunities still does not always result in more equal societies. Firstly, by taking the gaze away from the result, equality of opportunity theories has been used to justify inequality, as it is argued that existing inequality results from differences in individual effort or merit or lack thereof (Natasnon, 2016). Secondly, when translated into policies, focusing on equality of opportunities often implies creating "universal" basic services such as public healthcare or free basic education. Although egalitarian in theory, such programmes often overlook structural inequalities that discriminate against certain people from accessing these public goods. In the context of Covid-19 and related policy responses, such "egalitarian" approaches have been widely adopted, excluding certain groups of citizens.

We have re-centred the result in the analysis to explain the extent to which the Covid-19 policies have taken equity into account. More precisely, rather than only looking at the design of policies, which in theory could seem egalitarian, we will focus on their impact on the well-being of the poorest and most vulnerable. Our conceptualisation of well-being is drawn from McGregor and Pouw (2017, pp. 1134–5), who portray well-being as a multidimensional concept consisting of material well-being (e.g., income, housing), relational well-being (e.g., social relationships), and subjective well-being (or a person's evaluation of the quality of life). This allows the research team to analyse the impact of Covid-19 and related state and non-state responses on (1) income and other material sources of well-being such as housing and access to basic services (e.g., water); (2) social support networks and safety nets as well as associations and organisations of the (working) poor; (3) the individual perceptions of the impact on well-being and; and lastly (4) the collective well-being of the vulnerable groups we have identified (Fig. 4.1).

To understand why certain groups of people are more vulnerable to the current crisis and their differentiated nature of resilience, the research

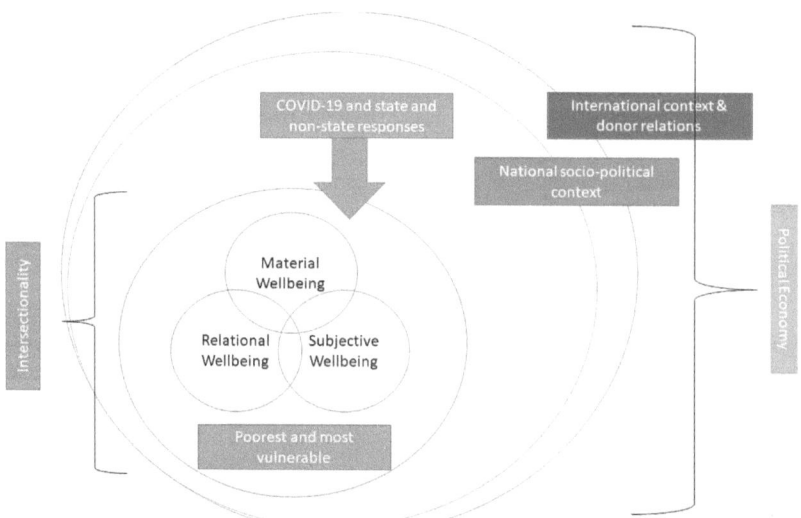

Fig. 4.1 Analytical framework. *Source* Developed by authors based on McGregor and Pouw (2017)

team adopted an intersectionality lens in the analysis. The intersections of existing economic, political, and social inequalities allow the research team to understand why specific groups of people are especially vulnerable to the Covid-19 health and related socioeconomic crises (Chaplin et al., 2019).

Mapping Ghana's Mitigation Measures and Policy Responses

It is important to note that Ghana's Ministry of Health (MoH) started public health promotion exercises before the first case of Covid-19 was recorded in the country. In its Press Release on January 31, 2020, six weeks prior to Ghana recording its first case, the Ministry of Health (MOH) advised the public to observe the following measures regular washing of hands with soap and water.

(i) Use alcohol hand rub when available.
(ii) Avoid touching of nose, eyes, and ears when one encounters a sick person or potentially infected surfaces; and
(iii) Seek immediate treatment if the symptom is suspected, among others ((MoH, 2020).

On March 12, 2020, Ghana recorded its first two cases of COVID-19. Public health, health sector, and socioeconomic responses were announced and implemented in a swift response. As a result, the responses were graduated and eased with increase and decrease in cases.

Public Health Responses

Restriction on movement and social distancing was the first public health response to contain the virus following the confirmation of the two cases of Covid-19. Accordingly, all public gatherings, including conferences, workshops, funerals, festivals, political rallies, sports, and church/mosque activities, were banned. These were announced at the President's Covid-19 status update briefing on March 15, 2020. Others include school closures, work from home and rotational work regimes, decongestion of markets, travel restrictions on inbound passengers to Ghana, and their attendant quarantining orders.

Restrictions on the number of passengers in public transport were coordinated by the Ministry of Transport in collaboration with private and public transport unions and operators to ensure enhanced hygienic conditions in all commercial vehicles and terminals, and transport unions agreed to reduce the number of passengers per commercial vehicle to allow for social distancing. Bonful et al. (2020) found that the majority (80%) of lorry stations in Accra had at least one Veronica Bucket with flowing water and soap, but the number of washing places at each station was inadequate.

Similarly, the Ministry of Local Government and Rural Development (MoLGRD) worked with the MMDAs to ensure enhanced hygiene conditions in the country's markets. As a result, some marketplaces in urban areas were sanitised, but the government did not provide WASH materials on a structural basis (Amankwaah & Ampratwum, 2020).

The Imposition on Restrictions Act (Act 1012) was passed by Parliament on March 21, 2020, under a certificate of urgency. The Minority in Parliament critiqued it for giving too much power to the executive. The MPs argued that the Act could be used to encroach on the freedoms of citizens. The Act gives legal backing for imposing restrictions on persons in the event of a disaster, emergency, or similar circumstances, for public safety and protection with no specific mention of Covid-19. The President cited that the Bill was consistent with Sect. 169 of the Public Health Act, 2012 (Act 851), but critics have argued that the Constitution and other Acts (e.g., Public Health Act, Immigration Act and National Disaster Management Act) have adequate provisions to cover such situations and therefore a new law was not necessary. Indeed, these existing laws had guided Act 1012 (FAAPA, 2020).

In his third National Address on March 28, 2020, the President of Ghana announced a partial lockdown of the Greater Accra Metropolitan Area, including Kasoa in the Central Region and Greater Kumasi Metropolitan Area, effective March 30, 2020, to contain the spread of the virus. Travel between regions was banned to prevent the virus' importation from affected regions. The lockdown was introduced when the country recorded 141 cases with five (5) fatalities and evidence of community spread. Security agencies were deployed to strategic locations within Accra, Kumasi, and Kasoa to ensure compliance. There were reports of the use of force which in some cases led to abuse of civilians. For instance, about 171 *Kayayei* disguised as cargo travelling from Accra to northern Ghana were intercepted and returned to Accra (CNR, 2020).

The lockdown ended three weeks after the imposition as the government reiterated that the decision was supported by science. However, this was received with mixed reactions. Civil society and professional groups, including the Ghana Medical Association, reacted in shock to the President's decision noting the rise in cases from 141 to 1024. In addition, there was evidence of community spread as 82% of 1024 cases had no travel history and, therefore, the belief that easing the lockdown could spark further spread. In a study conducted by the CSO Platform on SDGs (August 2020), most respondents reported that the government's restrictions were adequate to contain the spread of the virus and should not have been relaxed.

On the other hand, the restrictions were lifted with excitement by vulnerable groups, including people living in slums, head porters (*Kayayei*), and small- and medium-scale business owners. The Trade Union Congress and persons in academia called the decision progressive, highlighting the dire consequences of a prolonged lockdown on the economy and vulnerable people, including informal sector workers who survive on daily earnings.[2] The ease of restrictions on movement and social and economic activities continued amidst public anxiety. By September 2020, all restrictions had ended except for partial closure of schools, closure of land borders and social centres such as nightclubs and beaches.

Contrary to suggestions that the relaxation of the restrictions was going to cause hikes in cases, Ghana continued to record high recoveries and lower new cases. By November 4, 2020, Ghana had less than 1200 active cases, dropping further to less than 900 in December, creating a false sense that the pandemic was nearly over (see Fig. 4.2).

With the sharp rise in new infections since late December 2020, the government re-introduced some measures, as shown in Table 4.1. The second wave of the virus appears more deadly, with over 80 fatalities in January 2021 alone and more severely ill persons, which could have a detrimental effect on Ghana's already vulnerable health system. By January 31, 2021, the country's active cases stood at 5515, with a total case count of 67,782 and 424 deaths since March 2020 (GHS, 2021).

Awareness of the measures has been relatively high. For example, an online survey conducted by Lamptey et al. (2020) to assess the public

---

[2] Interview with TUC representative and UNIWA representative.

Daily new confirmed COVID-19 cases

Shown is the rolling 7-day average. The number of confirmed cases is lower than the number of actual cases; the main reason for that is limited testing.

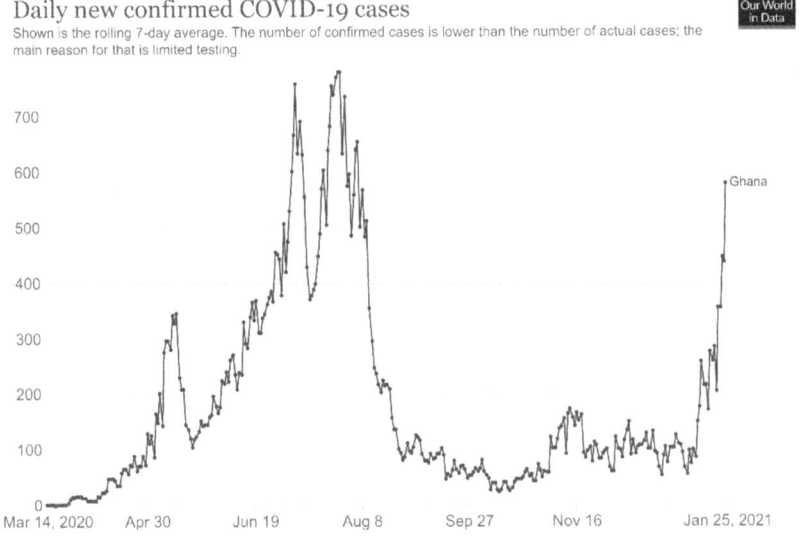

Source: Johns Hopkins University CSSE COVID-19 Data – Last updated 26 January, 09:02 (London time)

CC BY

Fig. 4.2 Daily new Covid-19 cases in Ghana. *Source* Our World in Data, 2020

knowledge, risk perception and preparedness to respond to the pandemic in the early stage of the outbreak in Ghana found that 62.7% had "good" knowledge about the outbreak. Saba et al. (2020) have equally found that the knowledge and preparedness were high in the Northern Region of Ghana, although differences existed between awareness levels in rural and urban areas.

HEALTH SECTOR RESPONSES

In collaboration with other government departments (e.g., Customs and Immigration), the Ghana Health Service (GHS) trained and provided resources (e.g., thermometers) to screen travellers at the ports of entry.[3] Travellers who recorded temperatures of more than 37 degrees Celsius were further screened. Before the closure of all borders, all international

---

[3] Initially, only the country's 13 ports of entry, one by air, two by seaport and ten by ground, were operated by Port health authorities, but 31 more (making 44) were later identified and secured with interventions.

Table 4.1 COVID-19 protocol ease timelines

Date	Easing of restriction	Effective date	Case count
May 31	Religious activities (churches and mosque) to resume for an hour of service with not more than 100 congregants under strict Covid-19 protocols	June 6, 2020	8070 cases and 36 deaths
	Final year University and other tertiary education students to report back to complete academic year. University lectures are to take place with half class sizes	June 15, 2020	
	Final year senior high school (SHS3) students, together with SHS 2 Gold Track students, were to go back to school. A maximum of 25 students for the SHS	June 22, 2020	
	Final year junior high school students were to report back to school. JHS class size is limited to 30 students	June 29, 2020	
	Private burials to continue with up to 100 in attendance	Immediate	
	Restaurants providing seated services, could operate under appropriate social distancing arrangements and hygiene protocols	Immediate	
	Individual, non-contact sports, conferences, workshops, weddings, and political activities, except rallies, can now occur, but with limited numbers not exceeding one hundred persons present, with the appropriate social distancing and hygiene protocols	Immediate	
	Exemptions marketplaces, workplaces, public transport, and constitutional and statutory bodies such as the Electoral Commission, the National Commission for Civic Education and the National Identification Authority from the restrictions		
July 27	Restriction of a number of worshippers eased, and hours of worship extended to two	August 1 2020	32,437 cases and 168 deaths
August 30	Kotoka International Airport opens to international flights	September 1 2020	44,205 and 276 deaths

(continued)

Table 4.1 (continued)

Date	Easing of restriction	Effective date	Case count
January 3 2021	Re-opening of all schools	January 9 2021	55,220 cases (879 active cases) and 336 deaths
January 31 2021	Re-introduction of ban on funerals, parties, theatrical gatherings, weddings, and concerts. Beaches, nightclubs, cinemas, pubs, and land borders remain closed		67,010 (5358 active cases) 416 deaths

Sources National addresses by the President, 1–3

travellers were put under mandatory quarantine and tested at a cost to the taxpayer, which enabled early detection, isolation, and treatment of cases. The GHS Helplines required citizens who showed symptoms to call and be picked up by an ambulance to be transported to Isolation Centres for screening. While this process was smooth initially, it became fraught with challenges as the number of cases surged over time. There were instances where patients transported themselves using modes that violated the Covid-19 protocols (e.g., using public, commercial transport) after waiting in vain for an ambulance. This was no surprise as Ghana has less than 400 functional ambulances for a population of 30 million. A team of contact tracers were recruited and trained to complement Ghana Health Service internal capacity to undertake enhanced contact tracing. This process of enhanced contact tracing was minimised when the partial lockdown was eased.[4]

Health infrastructure also improved. At the onset of Covid-19, only two laboratories, namely the University of Ghana Noguchi Memorial Institute for Medical Research in Accra and the Kumasi Centre for Collaborative Research of the KNUST existed. However, the facilities increased to sixteen, with four private ones. Fourteen of the facilities are in Southern

[4] Interview with GHS official.

Ghana, mainly Accra, Kumasi, Ho and Takoradi. Only two are sited at the northern Ghana, precisely Tamale and Navrongo (GHS, 2021).

Covid-19 case management Apps were invented during the period. They include the Covid-19 tracker App launched by the Ministry of Communication, Covid-19 TECHBOT developed at the Kwame Nkrumah University of Science and Technology (KNUST), and the Covid Connect App developed by the University of Ghana Medical Centre (University of Ghana, 2020). However, the uptake of these Apps remains unknown. Recruitment of more health sector workers, including retired health professionals, boosted the personnel numbers, although this was still inadequate.

The government implemented several support measures to mitigate the fallouts from the pandemic. Health workers received tax incentives in the health sector to recognise their frontline vulnerability. Economic specific measures include a stimulus package for small and medium-scale enterprises and another package for private schools, and other tax incentives. Universally applied schemes such as water and electricity subsidies were implemented short-termly. Reduction in communication tax was also applied while food distribution to vulnerable street dwellers in some cities and final year pupils in Junior High Schools was also implemented. The programmes have been critiqued for the continuum of transparency, accountability, non-targeting, inadequacy, and corruption. Thus, the following section analysed the Covid-19 mitigation measures and their accompanying socioeconomic support programmes using equity assessment tools.

EQUITY ASSESSMENT OF COVID-19 MEASURES

The measures were taken to contain the spread of Covid-19, and those designed to mitigate the negative socioeconomic consequences have differentiated effects on Ghanaian citizens, with some being especially vulnerable due to the intersectionality of their socioeconomic and political identities. We used three vulnerable social groups, namely residents of Chorkor in Accra, Kayayei, a northern migrant head porters on the streets of Accra and market traders in Bolgatabga, to demonstrate the differentiated impact of Covid-19 on vulnerable social groups. The selection is based first on geography, where two case studies were picked from the South, where the highest numbers of Covid-19 cases were recorded and the Upper East characterised by structural inequalities and higher poverty rates. Second, we focused on gender issues where female workers were deliberately included as they were especially vulnerable due to their dual work-family responsibilities, both affected by Covid-19. The third element is age, where young and older informal workers were included to reveal differentiated vulnerabilities. Table 4.2 summarises the background characteristics of the three social groups selected.

Background Characteristics

Chorkor is a densely populated fishing village falling under the constituency of the Accra Metropolitan Assembly (AMA). Most residents are from the Ga-Dangme ethnic group or migrants from other areas in Ghana or neighbouring countries. The Ga-Dangme are a minority group in Ghana and the Greater Accra Region indigenes. Chorkor is an important fish landing site and is famous for its smoked fish (the neighbourhood gave the name to the chorkor oven), but fish populations have been decreasing, resulting in residents now also engaging in other livelihood activities such as petty trading. Chorkor is especially vulnerable to Covid-19 due to high population density making social distancing difficult; informal housing which generally lacks connection to water pipelines or electricity; and the halt of economic activities during the lockdown in Accra.

Kayayei are female head porters who work in Ghana's large cities such as Kumasi and Accra and are predominantly migrants from Ghana's Northern regions. The women are often young and see head porterage as a temporary livelihood strategy to save money to get married, enter skill training, finish their education or start their businesses. Their work involves carrying goods for market women to and from their stalls or shoppers at the market. They often group at specific places in front of the market, and they share rented apartments in the city (in Accra, many live in Aglogbloshie) or sleep on the street (Yeboah et al., 2015). The *Kayayei's* lives are intertwined with movement between the city and their home villages, where they sometimes leave their children with relatives. A *Kayayei* earns approximately 30 Ghana Cedis a day or the equivalent of 5 US dollars.

The *Kayayei* were especially vulnerable during the Covid-19 pandemic due to: a decrease in economic activity during the lockdown and afterwards because of the "slowness" of the market; impossibility to travel back home due to restrictions of mobility between regions; poor housing

Table 4.2   Vulnerable groups selected for equity assessment

Backgrounds	Chorkor Residents	Kayayei	Market Women
Number of respondents	17	26	10
Gender	8 male and 9 female	All female	All female
Number with children	17	16	10
Location	Accra metropolitan Area	Work in the Central Business District of Accra and live in Agloboshie, Accra Metropolitan Area	Bolgatanga, Upper East Region
Type of work	Traders-8 Fishermen-4 Pensioners -4 Student-1	Head porters who carry goods for market women or for buyers in the market	Market women sell various goods (food, provisions, cloth, cosmetics, …) they have shops and "roam" (sell on the street) 1 market woman was also (a now unemployed) private school teacher
Prohibited from working during lockdown	Yes, exceptions to food vendors	Yes, all	No. The market was closed on two market days, but market women went to sell on non-market days to compensate (there was no lockdown in Bolgatanga)
Received support from government?	One received food Five benefitted from free water One had top-ups in their pensions 50% reduction in electricity for three months	Three received food on two to three occasions	One received a reduction of electricity bill for three months; the rest lived in rented accommodation, including utility bills

situation, which did not allow them to benefit from government water or electricity subsidies; predisposition to various types of abuse due to existing gender inequalities.

The market women in Bolgatanga were specifically vulnerable to Covid-19. They experienced a decreased income due to prolonged border closures with Togo and Burkina Faso. Furthermore, the informality of their businesses leaves them without social protection. In addition, the Covid-19 social protection measures, such as food distribution, did not reach the Northern regions. Also, since most lived in rented houses, they did not benefit from electricity or water subsidies. As women, they are affected by school closures and related halt of the school feeding programme, limited representation and political marginalisation as citizens of Northern Ghana.

Despite the importance of Ghana's markets in terms of employment creation and economic activity, market women are still in many ways discriminated against and excluded from policymaking on local and national levels (Osei-Boateng, 2019).[5] While there are considerable differences between market women in terms of socioeconomic status, ethnic backgrounds and levels of education, the informal nature of their work underpins their shared vulnerability. The structural issues make them vulnerable to shocks as social protection programmes do not cover them. Although market women most often do not fall into the category of the extreme poor, they are among a group who "*fall between the social protection gap*".[6] The Central Market in Bolgatanga is a critical economic hub for cross-border traders (Burkina Faso and Togo) as well as trade with the Southern regions of the country. It is open every three days.

EQUITY ASSESSMENTS OF COVID-19 MEASURES

Covid-19 has impacted the material and relational well-being of social groups. Its impacts manifest both in the short and long term. Similar to previous studies, the research team found that the pandemic has had a more significant economic than health impact on all three vulnerable groups included in the research (see e.g., Durizzo et al., 2020; Rahman &

---

[5] 28.1% of Ghana's informal workers work in trade or sales (GSS, 2011), with women representing 22.4% and men 5.7%, while 88% of street traders are women, and Ghana's trade sector is good for 6.3% of the country's GDP (Osei-Boateng 2019).

[6] Interview social protection officer DFID Ghana.

Matin, 2020, Sumner et al., 2020). A decrease in income was a share impact cited during Focus Group Discussion sessions held with the three groups at separate locations. The following statements reiterated the impact of Covid-19 on the groups studied,

> Even though we can now work, it is not like before. The market is not as busy as before, and the few shoppers are not engaging us. We roam from morning till evening but barely go home with GHS5-10 per day. Before Corona, we could go home with between GHS20-40 per day (*Kayayei*, Agbogbloshie, Accra)
>
> We barely make GHS40-50 a day compared to GHS200 pre- Corona. People are afraid of catching the virus and so are avoiding street food. So, I have stopped hawking (Chorkor resident, Accra)

During the three-week lockdown in Accra, *Kayayei* and most of the residents of Chorkor engaged in this research could not go to work. Even those that could sell, such as food vendors, closed for two weeks due to low patronage. Many of the respondents in Chorkor mentioned they used up all their savings, and some had to shift to buying goods on credit and repaying once they made their sales. Our findings are similar to other findings from surveys conducted by GSS (2020) and IPA (2020). GSS found that 47.4% of respondents relied on their savings as coping mechanisms, while IPA (2020) stated that almost half of the respondents had to deplete their savings to cover basic needs and up to 58.6% in the Upper East. For *Kakayei*, the situation was even bleaker as most do not have savings to fall back onto as they live from hand to mouth. In Bolgatanga, where lockdown was not imposed, some market women were relocated to allow for more social distancing, while others had to close their shops because they had no goods to sell due to border closures. They were also forced to increase their prices due to the increased cost of goods which slowed down the market. Due to fear of contagion, there were also significantly fewer buyers in markets, with many women complaining that their sales had dropped significantly. Most women also stated they fell back on their savings, and some have shifted to roaming or street vending because they could no longer afford their market stall. Not only did the border closure prevent traders from buying new goods, but some women who had already purchased goods could not retrieve them, resulting in a considerable loss of income. A trader reiterated some of the concerns,

My shop is empty, and I have used all my money to feed my family. Now I have nothing again. I used to have a small place to sit, but now I do not sit anymore but roam (Market woman, Bolgatanga, Upper East).

Covid-19 has affected not only poor people in economic terms but also their relational well-being. The contagious nature of the virus and preventive measures such as social distancing, wearing of face masks, restriction of mobility and closures of school to name a few, have also changed people's social relations at work and home or among friends. While *Kayayei* is used to gathering to work and share living spaces with up to 18 colleagues, the confinement in their tiny apartments during lockdown was extremely hard on them. The movement restrictions between regions severely affected their relations with their family and children and is highlighted in the following statement,

> On a typical day, everyone is out working and only comes back at night. However, because we could not go out during the lockdown, all of us were crowded in the room with no space to move. It was traumatizing (*Kayayei*, Agbogloshie, Accra)

Some *Kayayei* tried to return home clandestinely in cargo trucks. However, they were captured and sent back to Accra, raising public discontent, and initiating the government to provide food support to the urban poor, of which ironically, only three out of twenty-six *Kayayei* interviewed benefitted. Moreover, those that were able to return home were confronted with other difficulties as their parents and families (who usually rely on the meagre income they sent from the South) now found themselves with more mouths to feed.

The focus groups with Chorkor residents mostly raised the impacts of school closures on children, including children loitering and the issues of security, teenage pregnancy and increasing child labour, among others. However, some were happy about school closures because they could not pay school fees. In Chorkor, people generally send their children to low-cost private schools due to the lack of public schools. Respondents were generally not open to discussing their lives at home and personal relations. In the North, the stigmatisation of Covid-19 patients was also raised. A woman lamented that a market woman who had recovered from Covid-19 had been bullied out of the market. Furthermore, stones had been thrown at her children.

SUBJECTIVE WELL-BEING

The impact on the material and relational well-being of the people interviewed resonates in the way people feel about their lives. For example, the market women in Bolgatanga stated their lives improved a year before Covid-19. However, in a self-assessment of their situation, they referred to a reversal of fortunes compared with the previous year. Since most have depleted their saving, they do not know what to do again. This uncertainty was also found in that conversations with *Kayayei*, who stated they were only doing this work for survival. These findings resonate with the research by Durizzo et al. (2020, p. 5), who conducted a telephone survey of 1034 urban poor in Accra, of whom 37% stated they were feeling down, depressed, or hopeless. The additional stresses include the presence of children at home and the cost of feeding them. A market woman in Bolgatanga emphasised this by saying, *"the children are at home. We feed them from morning to evening"*.

"We were excited that the lockdown was lifted early so we could go out and feed ourselves and get away from the crowded rooms" (*Kayayei*, Agloboshie, Accra).

The pandemic, however, did not wholly dent their aspirations. Among the market women in Bolgatanga, traders and fishers in Chorkor, and Kayayei in Agloboshie, there was forward-looking energy with all groups hoping for government or philanthropic support for their economic activities.

Besides the direct short-term impact on the well-being of the poor, Covid-19 or the measures taken to manage the health crises will have long-term implications on existing inequalities in Ghana. The analysis below focuses on the longer-term impact on work and income, access to essential services and political empowerment.

ACCESS TO BASIC SERVICES

Ghana's inequalities have been most accentuated in access to basic services, and it is also here where the government has made the least consideration in terms of equity. The government's mitigation measures in education, water, and electricity were all blind-sighted in terms of the realities of the poor.

The subsidies for water were only primarily accessed by households connected to the national water pipeline, while the same counts for electricity. Water tankers were deployed in Chorkor and other communities in the South, but this did not occur in the North. Even if water tankers were provided, many residents did not want to go through the hassle of getting water due to the large crowds. For the older adults, this was certainly out of the question. Although government officials stated that people selling water would be fined, many respondents stated they paid the same or even higher prices for water. Those using public washrooms saw no reduction in charges despite accessing free water.

Similar issues occurred with the electricity subsidies. Almost all the poor people interviewed lived in rented houses, of which their electricity bill was added to their monthly rent. None of them noted a decrease in rent due to the electricity subsidies. It implied that house owners were sharing in on the subsidies at the expense of the vulnerable. It demonstrates the unequal power relations between landlords and tenants and the lack of legal protection for the poor.

The government's response to school closures also exemplified the disconnection between policy makers/implementers and poor and vulnerable populations. Whereas the government rapidly broadcasts a 24-hour learning television channel, the fact that it was only available on digital TV was regrettable considering that many poor households either had no television or satellite dishes to access the digital channels. While significant lobbying by CSOs resulted in the introduction of the radio programme, the content and continuity were disappointing, demonstrating a lack of political will. The North–South inequalities were also very apparent here as the connectivity to television, internet or even electricity was significantly lower in the Northern regions. In addition, the school feeding programme was abandoned entirely because of school closures was regrettable as many parents counted on these daily meals during "normal" times and now, faced with economic hardship, had to feed much more mouths on a smaller family budget.

Political Empowerment

Even though aspirations for the opposite, Covid-19 seems to have strengthened existing unequal power relations rather than addressed them. The northern regions of the country have been very much disadvantaged by the governance of the government's responses. Although one might argue this to be natural since the spread of Covid-19 was much higher in Accra and Kumasi, the reality is that poor people in the North, too, have suffered a lot in both material, relational, and subjective terms. Nevertheless, minimal measures were made available to them. The disappointment towards the government and politicians in Bolgatanga was rampant, and the distrust was very high. Some market women in Bolgatanga state that they demonstrated to voice their concerns but added that nobody listened. Others said they did not see the advantage of demonstrating on an empty stomach, and it was often mentioned that "others" got some support, but they did not get anything. The long-term political implications of this sense of exclusion cannot be underestimated as it feeds into the Northerners' deep story, a term Hochshild (2016) of political neglect, which in other countries has led to the rise of right-wing extremist regimes. A participant reiterated the neglect by saying, *"The Gender Ministry came here at the onset of the pandemic to write names of vulnerable people, including pensioners but never came back"(Household of two pensioners, Chorkor).*

This sense of voicelessness was also found among the *Kayayei* and Chorkor residents. There was a shared perception that nobody would listen if they were to voice their concerns. The exception was the fishers who were part of an association. They mentioned they attended a meeting at the Accra Metropolitan Assembly to discuss the pandemic issue but added that only a few of their concerns were taken seriously, and little was implemented. Similarly, the Minister of Gender, Children, and Social Protection visited Chorkor to request a list of the elderly, but later nothing more was heard from them. The association of *Kayayei* was also asked to compile a list of possible beneficiaries but never heard back from the ministry. These unfulfilled promises also resonated in Bolgatanga with market women expressing how politicians only come to promise things during election campaigns and later only think of their own "stomachs".

CONCLUSION

Like many African countries, Covid-19 impacts on Ghana have been more in economic terms than health-wise. The pandemic has seen the worsening of deprivation for the extremely poor and vulnerable groups due to the disproportionate economic impacts and failure to provide inclusive social protection. For some people, this has meant exhausting the little savings or going to bed on an empty stomach, while others have been pushed into precarious employment for survival, and this has been the case for informal sector workers such as traders in Bolgatanga, residents of Chorkor and *Kayayei* in Ghana's capital Accra.

While we argue that that the mitigation measures were appropriate, we also emphasis the fact that some of them could have been modified over time to target the most vulnerable. For instance, the prolonged closure of land borders has affected the economic activities of small-scale traders, particularly women in the northern parts of the country, and has exacerbated their already vulnerable conditions. In addition, the closure of schools significantly increased inequality. The question is whether instituting Covid-19 prevention infrastructures in schools and border-crossings would not have been more equitable.

Given the large informal sector in Ghana, the social cost of a longer lockdown would have been too high. Similarly, hardships imposed by the restrictions to curtail the spread of the virus have been high without effective social interventions to mitigate the same. The government's attempt to mitigate the impact of these measures on the poor and vulnerable has been affected by existing structural inequalities, the lack of data on the poor and Presidential and Parliamentary elections held in December 2020, among others. The results have been further alienation of the most vulnerable and political mistrust among those who needed the interventions the most, particularly among populations far removed from the centre, like market women in Bolgatanga. Perhaps, political considerations were more paramount in the decision to centralise governance of response than the fact that Accra was an epicentre, but the effect has been less involvement of District Assemblies and CSOs closest to the citizenry.

The measures were poorly targeted, and a centralised approach further affected service delivery. In 2018, about 81% of Ghanaians had access to electricity, according to the World Bank. However, even those who had access lived in rented houses with landlords as gatekeepers who decided on whether to grant the subsidy to their tenants. The study established that *Kayayei* and some residents of Chorkor and market women in Bolgatanga paid rent inclusive of electricity usage during the period the subsidy was implemented. Again, residents of Chorkor, market women in Bolgatanga and *Kayayei* reported buying water due to lack of access or inadequate supply even when the state continues to provide free access. Due to structural inequalities, the water and electricity subsidies benefitted wealthier households and not the poor.

Recommendations

With the above analysis of Ghana's Covid-19 responses, we recommend the need for:

- Strong institutional structures to collect robust data which should be used for targeting of beneficiaries of social protection programmes which consider gender, generational, geographical, and occupational differentiated vulnerabilities. By this, the Ghana National Household Registry (GNHR) should be strengthened to expand its reach and scope of data collection.
- Bottom-up approach to crisis management and support system programme implementation through decentralised structures and the involvement of community members and CSOs.
- Promote savings among low-income earners and ensure regulations that build citizens' confidence in the banking system.
- Stimulate the creation of workers and community-based associations which at least provide governments with a conversation partner and opportunity to voice concerns (e.g., in the case of the *Kayayei* Association and fishers association) even though they do not often lead to a change in policies.

References

Afram, A., & Tsekpo, K. (2017). Missing numbers in Ghana's election 2016: Low turnout or a bloated register?. Retrieved from https://www.pambazuka.org/democracy-governance/missing-numbers-ghana%E2%80%99s-election-2016-low-turnout-or-bloated-register

Afrobarometer Ghana (2016–2020). Retrieved from http://afrobarometer.rg/countries/ghana-1

Amankwaa, G., & Ampratwum, E. F. (2020). COVID-19 'free water' initiatives in the Global South: What does the Ghanaian case mean for equitable and sustainable water services? *Water International.* https://doi.org/10.108 0/025 8060.2020.1845076

Bonful, H. A., Addo-Lartey, A., Aheto, J. M. K., Ganle, J. K., Sarfo, B., & Aryeetey, R. (2020). Limiting spread of COVID-19 in Ghana Compliance audit of selected transportation stations in the Greater Accra region of Ghana. *PLoS ONE, 15*(9), e023897. https://doi.org/10.137/journal.pone.0238971

Bourguignon, F. (2015). *The Globalisation of Inequality*. Prin eton. Princeton University Press. ISBN: 9780691160528

Chaplin, D., Twig, J., & Lovell, E. (2017). *Intersectional approaches to vulnerablity reduction and resilience-building*. Resilience Intel, 12. BRA ED

Civil Society Platform on Sustainable Development Goal. (2020). Citizens' Assessment of Ghana's Covid 19 Response Report.

CNR (2020). *Police intercept Walewale-bound truck at Ejisu with kayayei 'packed like sardines'*. Retrieved from https://citinewsroom.com/2020/03/police-intercept-walewale-bound-truck-at-ejisu-with-kayayei-packed-like-sardines/

Durizzo, K., Asiedu, E., Van der Merwe, A., Van Niekerk, A., & Günther, I. (2021). Managing the COVID-19 pandemic in poor urban neighborhoods: The case of Accra and Johannesburg. *World Development, 137*, 1–14.

FAAPA. (2020). *Parliament passes Imposition of Restr ctions Bill, 2020*. Retrieved from http://www.faapa.infoen/2020/03/21/parliament-passes-imposition-of-restrictions-bill-2020/.

Ghana Statistical Services. (2018). *Ghana Living Standard Survey Round 7 Report*. Retrieved from http://www2.statsghan.gov.gh/nada/index.php/cat alog/97/study-description

Ghana Statistical Services (2019). *Ghana Poverty Report*. Retrieved from http://www2.statsghaa.gov.gh/docfiles/publications/GLSS7/Poverty%20Profile%20Report_2005%20-%202017.pdf

Ghana Health Service (2020). COVID-19 Updates. Retrieved from https://ghanahealthservice.org/covid19/ (accessed in May 2020)

Ghana Statistical Services (2020a). *Brief on COVID-19 Households and Jobs Tracker Wave 1*. Retrieved from https://statsghana.go.gh/covidtracker/HH_tracker_wave_1_weighted_update_v6.pdf

Ghana Statistical Services (2020b). *How COVID-19 is affecting firms in Gh na Results fromthe Business Tracker Survey*. Retrieved from https://statsghana.ov.gh/covidtracker/Business%20Tracker%20Brief%20Report_GSS_web.pdf

Ghana Health Service. (2021). COVID-19 Updates. Retrieved from https://ghanahealthservice.org/covid19/ (Accessed in Feb 2021)

Ghana Health Service (2021). Accredited laboratories. Retrieved from https://www.ghanaheathservice.org/covid19/accredited_labs.php

Harding, R. (2015). Attribution and accountability: Voting for roads in Ghana. *World Politics, 67*(4), 656–689.

IPA. (2020). *Research for Effective COVID-19 Respo ses (RECOVR) Survey Analysis Rwanda*. Retrieved from https://www.poverty-acion.org/recovr

Lamptey, S. D, Baffour A. A., Senkyire, E., & Ameyaw, J. (2020). Knowledge, risk perception and prepa edness towards coronavirus disease-2019 (COVID-19) outbreak among Ghanaians: A quick online cross-sectional survey. *Pan African Medical Journal, 35*. 10.1604/pamj.supp.2020.35.2.22630.

Lindberg, S. I., & Morrison, M. K. C. (2008). *Are African Voters Really Ethnic or Clientelistic? Survey Evidence from Ghana. Political Science Quarterly Volume 12 Number 1 2008.* Available at http://www.brandonkendh amer.com/pols441_fall_2011/wp-content/uploads/2011/08/Lindberg-Morrison-2008-Are-African-Voters-Really-Ethnic-or-Clientelistic-Survey-Evi dence-from-Ghana.pdf (Accessed in September 2020).

Mcgregor, J. A., & Pouw, N. (2017). Towards an economics of well-being. *Cambridge Journal of Economics, 41*, 123–1142. https://doi.org/10.1093/cje/bew044

MoH. (2020). P ess Release Update on Preparedness n 2019 Novel Corona Virus Outbreak. Retrieved from https://www.ghanahealthservice.org/cov id19/downloads/covid_19_press_release_31_Jan.pdf

Nana Akufo Addo. (2020a). Update https://www.facebook.com/watch/?v=281 0558329044598

Nana Akufo Addo. (2020a). Update 19. Retrieved from https://web.facebook.com/nakufoaddo/photos/pb.7893934835.-2207520000../101587874210 59836/?type=3&theater&_rdc=1&_rdr

Nana Akufo Addo. (2020b). Update 23. Retrieved from https://web.fac ebook.com/nakufoaddo/photos/pcb.10158998318969836/101589983182 24836?_rdc=1&_rdr

Nana Akufo Addo (2020c). *President Akufo-Addo National Address ahead of commencement of Voter Registration Exercise.* Retrieved from https://www.facebook.com/nakufoaddo/videos/196105675111205

Natanson, J. (2016). *Contra la igualdad de oportunidades.* Le Monde Diplomatique, 199, retrieved from https://www.eldiplo.org/199-america-latina-gira-a-laderecha/contra-la-igualdad-de-oportunidades

Oduro, A. D., Arhin, A. A., Domfe, G., Alidu, S., Agyeman, F. S. K., Asimadu, D. E., Walker, J., Gibson, L., Mariotti, C., & Hall, S. (2018). *Building a more equal Ghana.* Oxfam International.

OECD. (2014). *Focus on Inequality and Growt—December 2014.* OECD. Retrieved from www.oecd.org/social/inequality-and-poverty.htm

Ofori-Atta, K. (2020). The presentation of the Mid-Year Revi w of the Budget Statement and Economic Policy of the Government of Ghana and Supplementary Estimates for the 2020 Financial Year. Available at https://thebftonl ine.com24/07/2020/govts-2020-gdp-growth-revised-to-0–9-from-6–8/

Osei-Boateng, C. (2019). *Informal Workers and Social Dialogue n Ghana, the case of UNIWA and the Accra Metropolitan Assembly.* Mondiaal FNV.

Our World in Data (2020). *Ghana: Coronavirus Pandemic Country Profile.* Retrieved from https://ourworldindat.org/coronavirus/country/ghana?cou ntry=~GHA

Piketty, T. (2014). *Capital in the Twenty-First Century.* Arvard. Belknap Press.

The Presidency, Republic of Ghana. (2020). Briefing Room: Speeches. Retrieved from http://presidency.gv.gh/index.php/briefing-room/speeches

Saba, . & Nzeh, J., Addy, F., & Akosua, B. (2020). *COVID-19: Knowledge, perceptions and attitudes of residents in the Northern Region of Ghana, West Africa.* Preprints 2020, 2020080060. 10.2 944/preprints202008.0060.v1

Sen, A. (1984). Well-being, agency and freedom: The Dewey lectures. *The Journal of Philosophy, 82*(4), 169–221.

Sumner, A., Hoy, C. & Ortiz-Juarez, E. (2020). *Estimates of the impact of COVID-19 onglobal poverty.* UNU-WIDER Working Paper 2020/43. Hels nki, Finland: United Nations Un versity.

University of Ghana (2020). Launch of COVID-CONNECT – UGMC. Retri ved from https://www.ug.edu.g/announcements/launch-covid-con nect-ugmc

World Bank. (2018). Ghana Priorities for Ending P verty a d Boosting Shared Prosperity. In *Ghana Priorities for Ending Poverty and Boosting Shared Prosperity.* https://doi.org/10.1596/30974

Yeboah, T., Owusu, L., Arhin, A. A., & Kumi, E. (2015). Fighting poverty from the street: Perspectives of some female informal sector workers on gendered poverty and livelihood portfolios in southern Ghana. *Journal of Economic and Social Studie, 5*(1), 239–267.

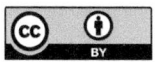

CHAPTER 5

Mali

Ousmane Z. Traoré and Djénéba Diarra

INTRODUCTION

In Mali, Covid-19 had caused the deaths of 357 of the 8470 infected persons as of March 4, 2021 (INSP, March 2021). According to OCHA (September 2020), the pandemic had spread to nine administrative regions and 36 of Mali's 75 health districts by August 30, 2020. Most cases of Covid-19 contamination were seen in Bamako (49.6%), followed by the regions of Timbuktu (18.5%), Mopti and Koulikoro (8.3%) (UNICEF, September 2020). Well before the declaration of the health emergency in Mali and the emergence of the first positive case on March 25, 2020, the Malian government, following the example of other countries in Africa and elsewhere in the world, introduced a range of preventive measures effective March 17, 2020, to prevent and slow the spread of coronavirus and mitigating the impact on public health.

O. Z. Traoré (✉)
Department of Agricultural Economics and Consumer Science, Groupe de Recherche en Économie Appliquée Et Théorique (GREAT), Laval University, Québec, Canada
e-mail: ousmane-z.traore.1@ulaval.ca

D. Diarra
Groupe de Recherche en Économie Appliquée Et Théorique (GREAT), Bamako, Mali

A. Altaf et al. (eds.), *EQUITY IN COVID-19*, EADI Global Development Series, https://doi.org/10.1007/978-3-031-58588-3_5

The Malian population were already under immense stress before the pandemic. In 2017, half the Malian population were already deprived of about four basic social facilities or services in health, water, electricity, or financial services/goods (Afrobarometer, 2017). That deprivation affected three times as many rural inhabitants as their urban counterparts and certainly had more effect on the poorest and most vulnerable individuals (e.g., women, young people) in both areas. According to EMOP[1] Data collected by INSTAT (November 2019), food insecurity affected three of ten households (30.6%) in Mali in 2019. Food insecurity was most prevalent in the Kayes (55.2%), followed by the Mopti (44.6%) and Gao (44.5%) regions. Rural households paid a higher price for food insecurity than urban households (33.3% versus 23.8%). Furthermore, INSTAT (November 2019) reveals to us that the phenomena of unemployment in Mali were particularly more prevalent among young people aged 15–49 and women. The unemployment rate for young people aged 15 to 49 was 20.2% with more young women (6.1%) affected than men (4.9%). The rate was more pronounced in the Gao region (30.5%), followed by Koulikoro (13.1%) and Kidal (10.7%). The lowest unemployment rates were recorded in Mopti (4.1%), Kayes (2.4%), Sikasso and Ségou (2.1%) and Timbuktu (1.2%). Another inequality present in Mali before the pandemic is income distribution. Indeed, the average quarterly expenditures/income per capita was twice as much higher in the urban area (FCFA 126 509) than in the rural zone (FCFA 60 872).

According to projections from FAO (June 2020), coronavirus disease and the restrictive measures adopted by the Malian government will increase the number of people affected by food insecurity to 280,000. In addition, it should be noted that, because of the military conflicts and their impact on communities, the FAO had already predicted that more than one million people in Mali would be affected by severe food insecurity. Since January 2012, the country has been experiencing unprecedented security and political crisis that has gradually affected its Northern regions (Gao, Timbuktu, and Kidal) and those of the Center (Mopti and Segou). This unstable situation has been exacerbated by the advent of Covid-19 and a recent military coup on August 18, 2020.

---

[1] EMOP, a modular and permanent household survey, is a survey carried out since April 2011 annually in four rounds and each round lasts three months of collection. It contains demographics, housing, education, health, employment, food security, consumer spending, etc.

Several recent studies have demonstrated that the preventive measures have been effective in controlling the pandemic, particularly the closing of the borders (Burns et al., 2020), quarantine (Nussbaumer-Streit et al., 2020), social distancing (Ebrahim et al., 2020) and the wearing of masks and visors (Chu et al., 2020; de Bruin et al., 2020, etc.). In Africa, Djooue et al. (2020) used a simulation model to show that isolating exposed people, a general lockdown, monitoring people living in high-risk areas, wearing masks, and respecting hygiene rules have slowed the outbreak of the pandemic.

However, although these measures would seem to be effective in terms of managing the spread of the virus, one of the more important questions remains as to how and to what extent the socioeconomic circumstances of vulnerable households and affected sectors have been considered in the formulation and implementation of these responses. In particular, the lockdown of Malian's economy due to the pandemic has direct or indirect social and economic consequences for households. There are many studies (FAO, June 2020; INSTAT, June, July, and August 2020; Han et al., 2020; Laborde et al., 2020; Martin et al., 2020; Mukumbang et al., 2020; Patel et al., 2020) that support that these consequences could be more significant for vulnerable households or individuals since they amplify socioeconomic inequality and food insecurity. For instance, measures for the prevention of Covid-19 could negatively affect the livelihoods of poor households and vulnerable individuals (e.g., women and young people), especially regarding limited access to essential commodities and basic social services, jobs, and income losses. As a result, they could exacerbate the socioeconomic vulnerability of marginalised households or individuals.

In the context of this case study, we are particularly interested in the socioeconomic vulnerability of households and individuals, which refers to the loss of economic resources (income, employment, etc.) and essential social services such as food, health care, water, education and electricity among others (de Oliveira Mendes, 2009; Fallah Aliabadi, Sarsangi, & Modiri, 2015; Fatemi et al., 2017; Martins et al., 2012).

In our analysis, we will focus on how the pandemic and the subsequent preventive measures have exacerbated inequalities between poor and non-poor households, rural and urban households, and between female and male-headed households. This introduction is followed by methodology. Section 5.3 presents the government's preventive and social protection measures. Finally, Sect. 5.4 examines the impact of the measures on vulnerable households.

METHODOLOGY

For this study, the methodological approach initially involved conducting a systemic review of Covid-19 literature to identify the preventive and economic support measures adopted by the Malian government and other stakeholders in response to the pandemic in Mali. To this end, a comprehensive literature survey was conducted on Covid-19 in Mali to collect policy documents and reports, analysis reports from national and international institutions, scientific articles, media journals, databases, and other relevant documents relating to the pandemic in Mali. Completing this literature survey resulted in the identification of the preventive measures and support measures for households and workers in the health, security, and economic sectors. In addition, the literature survey also allowed for identifying the sectors most affected by Covid-19 in Mali. The sectors identified in this way guided the selection of key informants for the semi-structured interviews.

To understand better how the Malian government and other stakeholders are addressing inequalities in their policy responses to Covid-19, semi-structured interviews were conducted with community leaders and other key informants from several public and private institutions in all the sectors affected by Covid-19 in Mali from 3 to September 16, 2020. The opinions of 33 key informants in total were collected on various themes. The primary focus was on their role in the process of developing and implementing prevention and social support measures, the impact of Covid-19 and preventive measures on workers in the health sector and the economy, the resiliency measures adopted, the level of stakeholder participation and how stakeholders perceived the government response to the pandemic.

The methodological approach combined qualitative and quantitative methods to assess the impact on vulnerable households of the adopted measures. It initially consisted of using a content analysis to investigate statements made by the key informants and the textual content of different documents obtained during the literature survey. This context analysis related to the roles played by the stakeholders, the socioeconomic impact of Covid-19 and preventive measures, and the resiliency measures adopted by stakeholders and the stakeholders' perceptions of the effectiveness of policy responses to the pandemic. The next step was to complement the results of these analyses with the results obtained from the statistical analyses of the data available on Covid-19 in Mali from

INSTAT and the World Bank. Those data were collected as part of an extensive triple-phase study of the effects of the Covid-19 pandemic on the living conditions of households in Mali. The first phase of this survey was conducted with computer-assisted phone calls from May 11 to June 3, 2020. A sample of 2270 households was surveyed and selected from the database of the Harmonised Survey of Household Living Conditions (EHCVM). The second data collection phase was from June 17 to July 3, 2020. This survey also covers the district of Bamako, the capital, and other urban cities, and rural areas of Mali. They are representative of the national and regional levels, place of residence, and poverty status. Data from the first two phases available at the time of the study were used in the analyses.

Preventive Measures and Social Protection Measures

As part of the fight against coronavirus disease (Covid-19), the government of Mali, working through a range of ministries, introduced preventive measures and social protection policies. These measures aimed to counter the spread of the disease and mitigate the impact of the pandemic on living conditions, particularly of the most vulnerable groups.

Long before the health emergency was declared in Mali by the Ministry of Health and Social Affairs on March 25, 2020, and in response to the outbreak of the first cases of Covid-19 in neighbouring countries, the government took several preventive measures. The measures were adopted after an extraordinary session of the Supreme Council of National Defence on March 17, 2020, and took effect on Thursday, March 19, 2020. First, bans and restrictions have been imposed on large gatherings and movement. This resulted in limited activity or total closure of such places. The government also imposed a 5 am–9 pm curfew and suspended gold mining. In addition, the government also introduced cordons on the land borders. There were periodical definition and adjustment of the prevention and response strategy. The state raised awareness and orchestrated stakeholders at all levels to prepare the response to the pandemic and empowered crisis and epidemic control committees and rapid response teams at all levels of the health pyramid. Simulation exercises to test the effectiveness of the arrangements and strengthening epidemiological surveillance were also organised. Table 5.1 summarises the measures and their timelines.

Table 5.1 Measures to prevent the spread of Covid-19

No.	Measures	Sources	Effective date	Date of suspension
1	Suspension of all public gatherings, including workshops, conferences, seminars, and large meetings	Government of the Republic of Mali, Extraordinary Session of the Higher Council of National Defence of March 17, 2020	March 19, 2020	
2	Suspension of commercial flights from affected countries, except for freight transport	Government of the Republic of Mali, Extraordinary Session of the Higher Council of National Defence of March 17, 2020	March 19, 2020	July 25, 2020
3	Closure of public, private, and denominational schools (nursery, primary, secondary, and higher education), including the madrasas	Government of the Republic of Mali, Extraordinary Session of the Higher Council of National Defence of March 17, 2020	March 19, 2020	June 2, 2020, for examination classes (DEF, Bac, Cap, BT, IFM) and September 14 for all classes
4	Closure of nightclubs and dance halls	Government of the Republic of Mali, Extraordinary Session of the Higher Council of National Defence of March 17, 2020	March 19, 2020	
5	Prohibition of any sporting, social, cultural, or political gathering with more than 50 people, such as weddings, baptisms, or funerals, subject to compliance with preventive measures	Government of the Republic of Mali, Extraordinary Session of the Higher Council of National Defence of March 17, 2020	March 19, 2020	

(continued)

Table 5.1 (continued)

No.	Measures	Sources	Effective date	Date of suspension
6	Introduction of curfew	Government of the Republic of Mali, Decree N°2020–0170/P-RM of March 25, 2020	March 26, 2020	
7	Closure of international stations	Government of the Republic of Mali for the attention of transport professionals and travellers	March 26, 2020	July 31, 2020
8	Suspension of gold mining	Interministerial Order N°2020–1197/ MMP-MATD-MSPC-MEADD-SG of March 27, 2020	March 27, 2020	September 30, 2020
9	Restricted working hours (from 7.30 am to 2 pm) in all public services except the national defence, security, and health services	Government of the Republic of Mali	April 1, 2020	August 1, 2020
10	Opening and closing times for markets	Government of the Republic of Mali Decision N°2020 50 MIC-SG of April 7, 2020	April 7, 2020	June 30, 2020
11	Establishment of the technical committee for the management of the crisis	Government of the Republic of Mali Decree N°2020–0200/ PM-RM of April 10, 2020	April 10, 2020	

Source Authors based on the literature survey, 2020

According to INSTAT (June 2020)[2] overall, most Malian people said that they complied[3] with the preventive measures taken by the Malian government in response to the pandemic. Indeed, nearly nine over ten households (88.6%) washed their hands more often than usual, while 61.7% of households reduced their use of places of worship. INSTAT (June 2020) also reported that 12.9% of households respect all social distancing behaviours.

[2] Round 1 of *the COVID-19 Panel Phone Survey of Households* of Mali was carried out by INSTAT in June 2020 and founding by World Bank.

[3] This is not an effective behaviour but what people say they do.

ECONOMIC SUPPORT MEASURES

Preventive strategies taken to counter the spread of coronavirus disease have had an impact, especially on vulnerable households. As a result, the government instituted measures to mitigate the socioeconomic fallouts of the pandemic and its response measures. Table 5.2 summarises the measures and their relevant details. The social protection policies come in two categories. The first relates to physical individuals/population groups. These are the first six measures. The second focuses more on formal entities/companies, comprising the last five measures.

About the measures targeting physical individuals, it is essential to note that the payment of water and electricity bills for April and May 2020 throughout the area covered by the SOMAGEP and EDM essentially targeted the most deprived households. In practical terms, in the case of water bills, these are customers whose monthly consumption is between 0 and 10 cubic metres (m^3) and those with standpipes. This implies that the standpipe operators will provide water free of charge to this vulnerable group during the period covered by the measure. In practice, all poor or non-poor households have benefited from the measure, with customers consuming more than 10 m^3 having to pay for the surplus. Domestic connections in the SOMAGEP network were included in this range. This measure benefited just over 200,000 customers or about 4 million people.

Electricity subsidy covered customers using between 1 and 100 kwh a month, whether with a conventional or Isago metre. Isago metre customers received free credits of up to 100 kwh a month during the period covered by the measure (two months). The bills of subscribers with conventional metres were paid directly by the State. The latter category consisted of 370,000 clients or approximately 3,700,000 affected people.

The special fund set up in Mali's 703 communes consists of making cash transfers to each household in the form of monthly allowances in a single category. The social safety net programme determines the monthly cash transfer amount, which is XOF 15,000 per household. As a result, each selected household in a single category should receive six months of monthly allowances, or 90,000, in a single instalment to cover its basic needs. The beneficiaries of this social protection measure were households registered in the Mali Unified Social Register (RSU).

In addition, several other partners such as UNICEF, the World Bank, and the Food and Agriculture Organization of the United Nations (FAO)

Table 5.2 Economic measures for social protection in response to Covid-19

No.	Measures	Cost (XOF)	Beneficiaries	Qualification arrangements	Document title	Sources	Effective date	Date of suspension
1	Free distribution of 56,000 tonnes of cereals and 16,000 tonnes of cattle feed	15 billion[4]	Vulnerable populations	All Households affected by Covid-19	Government announcement	Government announcement in the speech by the President on April 10, 2020	April 17, 2020	
2	Reduction of customs duties for necessities, in particular, rice and milk	7 billion	All consumers	None	Government announcement	Government announcement in the speech by the President on April 10, 2020	April 2020	June 2020

(continued)

[4] The United Nations synthesis report confirmed the costs of the first five (5) measures, *Summary analysis of the socioeconomic impacts of COVID-19 in Mali was* conducted by UNDP and UNICEF in May 2020.

Table 5.2 (continued)

No.	Measures	Cost (XOF)	Beneficiaries	Qualification arrangements	Document title	Sources	Effective date	Date of suspension
3	Payment of electricity and water bills for April and May 2020	7 billion	Poorest households	Households consuming from 0 to 10 m3/month (water) for home connections; Standpipes (serving 200,056 subscribers, or approximately 4 million people); Households that use between 1 and 100 kWh/month whether with conventional or Isago metres (electricity) (370,000 customers, or approximately 3,700,000 people)	Ministerial announcement	SOMAGEP-SA and EDM-SA briefing memoranda of April 17, 2020; Government announcement in the speech by the President on April 10, 2020	April 2020	May 2020

No.	Measures	Cost (XOF)	Beneficiaries	Qualification arrangements	Document title	Sources	Effective date	Date of suspension
4	VAT exemption on electricity and water bills for April, May and June 2020	9 billion	All consumers/clients (private, business, and industry)	None	Letter on implementation modalities	Government of the Republic of Mali, Letter No. 01671/MEF-SG of April 2,8 2020	April 2020	June 2020
5	Establishment of a special fund for Mali's 703 communes administered in a collegial and transparent way with the public authorities, village and neighbourhood chiefs, civil society, and the moral authorities designated by the beneficiaries themselves	100 billion	Most vulnerable families	Households on the Unified Social Register (RSU)[5]	Government announcement	Social Safety Net Programme in Mali; Government announcement in the speech by the President on April 10, 2020	April 2020	

(continued)

5 The RSU is an information system with a national database of social security beneficiaries: https://rsu.gouv.ml/portail/

Table 5.2 (continued)

No.	Measures	Cost (XOF)	Beneficiaries	Qualification arrangements	Document title	Sources	Effective date	Date of suspension
6	Payment of a unique premium to health personnel and components of the security and defence forces for monitoring the curfew and possible crowd locations		Health workers and security and defence forces	Deployed health staff, security and defence forces deployed to monitor the curfew and possible crowd locations	Government announcement	Government announcement in the speech by the President on April 10, 2020	April 2020	
7	The establishment of a guarantee fund for the private sector to underpin the financing needs of companies affected by the pandemic	20 billion	SMEs, decentralised financial systems, industry, and some large companies	Companies affected by the pandemic	Government announcement	Government announcement in the speech by the President on April 10, 2020	April 2020	

No.	Measures	Cost (XOF)	Beneficiaries	Qualification arrangements	Document title	Sources	Effective date	Date of suspension
8	Waiving of domestic debt due on December 31, 2019	110 billion	Companies		The announcement by the Prime Minister	Government announcement in the speech by the Prime Minister on May 9, 2020	May 1 2020	December 31 2020
9	Payment of money orders for the financial year 2020	100 billion	Companies		Government announcement	Government announcement in the speech by the President on April 10, 2020	January 2020	December 2020
10	Restructuring of credit for companies affected by Covid-19		Companies	Companies affected by coronavirus disease	Government announcement	Government announcement in the speech by the President on April 10, 2020		
11	Tax rebates, on a case-by-case and sector-by-sector basis, for private companies affected by the Covid-19 prevention measures		Tourism (hotels, travel, and catering), cultural and transport industries	Private companies affected by the Covid-19 prevention measures	Letter on implementation modalities	Government of the Republic of Mali, Letter No. 01671/ MEF-SG of April 28, 2020	April 2020	December 2020

Source Authors based on the literature survey, 2020

have also provided the State of Mali with assistance for its response to the Covid-19 pandemic. These different target segments of the population. For example, UNICEF targeted support for children while the FAO's grant of USD 10 million was used to support the food security needs of vulnerable households. The World Bank's USD 25.8 million assistance was used to provide resources for the health sector.

According to INSTAT (June 2020), about one over five (19.2%) households were dissatisfied with the government's response to the Covid-19 pandemic, especially those related to social protection measures. In all, 40.3% of households cited a lack of financial assistance from the government as the reason for their dissatisfaction. The rest of the reasons include the government's late response (21.0%) and the shortage of medical supplies (4.7%).

Loss of Income Related to Covid-19 Prevention Measures

This section describes the number of respondents who lost their jobs because of Covid-19. Looking at households, Table 5.3 shows that agricultural workers, traders, and wage workers have been most affected by Covid-19. In the agricultural sector, more than half of the income losses (52.8% in the first phase and 55.9% in the second phase) can be attributed to Covid-19. Similarly, 56.9% of people in the lost income in the first phase and 57.7% in the second phase. Covid-19-induced income losses also included a reduction in remittances, unemployment benefits, income from real estate investment, pension income, and government and non-government aid. Table 5.3 also summarises the extent of income loss according to household poverty status. It emerged clearly that the loss of agricultural and business income resulting from Covid-19 is much greater in poor households than in non-poor households and for female-headed households than in male-headed households. Given that agriculture and small informal businesses are the primary sources of income for poor people and women, it, therefore, emerged that the effects of Covid-19 and isolation measures had disproportionately impacted these two sectors.

Table 5.3 Loss of income linked to Covid-19 prevention measures (in %)

	All households		Poor		Non-poor		Rural		Urban		Men		Women	
	P1	P2	P1	P2	P1	P2	P1	P2	P1	P2	P1	P2	P1	P2
Agricultural income	52.8	55.9	75.7	77.1	45	48.1	85.6	81.9	38.1	35.9	55.7	35.6	58.4	50.2
Business income	56.9	57.7	63.8	64.5	54.6	55.2	62.5	60.7	54.4	50.9	57.1	54.3	58.1	56.7
Salary	32	30.3	16.1	14.3	37.5	36.2	17	15	38.8	35	32.4	24.2	31.1	31.8
Unemployment benefit	2.3	3.4	1.1	1.9	2.7	3.9	0.5	1.5	3.1	3.8	1.6	2.7	3.4	3.0
Money transfers	12.1	11.5	8.9	8.9	13.1	12.5	13.5	12.8	11.4	10 ara>	10.5	20.5	10.4	13.5
Family	12.5	12.2	12.7	12.8	12.4	12.1	14.1	13	11.8	11	10.0	16.9	11.7	14.7
Other support	4.8	4.1	3.4	2.9	5.2	4.6	2.9	2.9	5.6	4.8	4.8	5.9	3.9	4.7
Real-estate investment	2.5	2.1	0.7	0.6	3.1	2.6	1.3	0.9	3	2.6	2.2	3.2	1.9	2.8
Pensions	6	5.5	2.5	1.6	7.2	7	1.5	1.3	8	7.3	6.3	11.4	4.8	5.7
Government aid	0.7	0.6	0.9	0.6	0.6	0.6	0.5	0.5	0.7	0.7	0.8	0.0	0.7	0.5
NGO	0.8	1	2	1.7	0.5	0.7	1.7	1.7	0.5	0.6	0,7	0,5	1,1	1,0
Other aid	7.6	8.2	6	8.1	8.1	8.2	4	4.8	9.2	9.1	7,5	5,9	8,5	7,6

Source Authors, Survey Covid-19 Panel Phone Survey of Households 2020 of Mali
Note P1 = First phase, P2 = Second phase

FINANCIAL ASSISTANCE FOR HOUSEHOLDS IN RESPONSE TO COVID-19

To help vulnerable households to cope with the health crisis, the State and its partners provided some social support such as free food provision and direct cash transfers. Looking at the value of the total financial support received by the population, our results show that the financial aid received by poor households is between XOF 1000 and 200,000, while non-poor households received between XOF 250 and 380,000. On average, poor households received aid amounting to XOFF 30,710, while the average for non-poor households was XOF 31,821, a difference of more than XOF 1000. This means that wealthier households received even more financial support than poorer households. Similarly, rural households received much less aid than urban households. The amount was XOF

26,902 per rural household compared with XOF 33,792 per urban household. In a similar financial aid disparity pattern, female-headed households received much less aid than male-headed households. The figures were XOF 22,108 for the former and XOF 38,847 for the latter. In conclusion, the data show a significant imbalance in the distribution of financial support compared with the effects of the crisis on income loss. The poor, rural, and female-headed households appeared to be the most affected by income loss, whereas they received relatively lower financial support.

Regarding the source of financial aid received by households, the government (32.61%) and religious organisations (30.43%) emerged as the principal sources of aid received by non-poor households. The two primary sources of aid the poor receive were from non-governmental organisations (27.27%) and other organisations (31.28%). A specific analysis shows that 78.95% of government aid was distributed to non-poor households and only 21.05% to poor households. The same applies to aid from community organisations, which finance 83.33% of non-poor households compared with only 26.67% of poor households. The funding from non-governmental organisations is distributed equitably, and only support from other organisations was channelled in favour of poor households which constituted 53.85% for poor households and 46.15% for non-poor households. The government (40%) is the principal source of financial support received by male-head households, while the primary sources of aid received by the women head households were religious organisations (34.21%). Similarly, 63.16% of government aid was distributed to male-headed households, and only 36.84% went to female-headed households. This pronounced inequality in the distribution of government and non-government aid shows that the responses exacerbated structural inequalities (Tables 5.4 and 5.5).

DIFFICULTIES WITH OBTAINING BASIC NECESSITIES ASSOCIATED WITH COVID-19

This section describes the households that reported being unable to acquire basic food and health care during the Covid-19 period in the two phases. Overall, 14.1% of households reported that they could not purchase medicines and masks as recommended by the government due to the closure of sales outlets (Table 5.6). However, this percentage dropped to 5.1% in the second phase, suggesting that government action

Table 5.4 Distribution of financial support disaggregated by source and household poverty status of households (in %)

Poverty status		The primary source of financial aid in response to Covid-19					
		1	2	3	4	5	Total
Distribution of poor and non-poor according to the principal source	Non-poor	32.61	10.87	13.04	30.43	13.04	100.00
	Poor	18.18	4.55	27.27	18.18	31.82	100.00
Distribution of funding from each source between poor and non-poor	Non-poor	78.95	83.33	50.00	77.78	46.15	67.65
	Poor	21.05	16.67	50.00	22.22	53.85	32.35
Total		27.94	8.82	17.65	26.47	19.12	100.00

Source Authors, *Covid-19 Panel Phone Survey of Households 2020* of Mali

Table 5.5 Distribution of financial aid disaggregated by sources and Sex (in %)

Sex		The primary source of financial aid in response to Covid-19					
		1	2	3	4	5	Total
Distribution of men and women according to the principal source	Men	40.00	6.67	13.33	16.67	23.33	100.00
	Women	18.42	10.53	21.05	34.21	15.79	100.00
Distribution of funding from each source between men and women	Men	63.16	33.33	33.33	27.78	53.85	44.12
	Women	36.84	66.67	66.67	72.22	46.15	55.88
Total		27.94	8.82	17.65	26.47	19.12	100.00

Source Authors, *Covid-19 Panel Phone Survey of Households 2020* of Mali
Note Sources of financial assistance: 1 = government, 2 = community organisation, 3 = non-governmental organisation, 4 = religious organisations, 5 = other organisations

improved access to these products. The same applies to the lack of availability of certain food products, particularly rice, millet, and maize, which was seen in 10.2%–16.1% in the first phase and 3.2%–6.3% in the second phase.

Looking at the products unavailable to households during the crisis, 74.74% of non-poor households and 68.18% of poor households did not say they could not obtain a product because of Covid-19 during the

Table 5.6 Difficulties obtaining basic necessities associated with Covid-19

Difficulties obtaining necessities associated with Covid-19	All households (%)	
	P1	P2
Rice	10.2	3.2
Millet	10.9	5.3
Maize	16.1	6.3
Sugar	3.4	0.8
Meat	7.3	4.6
Oil	2.9	0.8
Medicines, masks	14.1	5.1

Source Authors, *Covid-19 Panel Phone Survey of Households 2020* of Mali

first phase. In other words, 31.82% of poor households and 24.26% of non-poor households said they could not access at least one of the necessities in the first phase. Overall, the number of unavailable products was higher for poor households. The access issue is also real for the place of residence. More rural households and female-headed households suffered from shortages due to Covid-19 than urban households.

Food insecurity would seem to be quite similar for both poor and non-poor households. However, it is essential to note a fall in perceived food insecurity in the second phase of the survey. This suggests that the support measures implemented by the government, NGOs, and international partners had some positive effects. The same applies to the place of residence (Table 5.7). A relatively high levels of food insecurity were seen in both rural and urban areas. It also appears from Table 5.8 that food shortage has been more pronounced in the female-headed household than in male-headed households.

Impact of Covid-19 and the Government Response

The health system is undoubtedly under the most strain. The survey of key informants in this sector provided a picture of the effects of the disease on workers and hospitals involved in the fight against the pandemic. In terms of health and human resources, health workers were infected because of a lack of adequate protective equipment. The significant increase in workload and stress also led to psychological difficulties

Table 5.7 Perceived food insecurity due to Covid-19 disaggregated by location (in %)

Food insecurity due to Covid-19	Rural		Urban	
	P1	P2	P1	P2
Enough to eat	30.5	24.9	34.2	27.4
Foods that are nutritious and healthy	22.3	18.6	25.9	20.2
Always the same thing	17.7	13.2	21.9	14.4
Skipped meal	6.2	6.8	9.3	5.8
I do not eat as much as I should have done	9.9	11.3	14.7	9.9
There was no food left in the house	5.7	3.5	6.8	4.0
You were hungry but did not eat	6.2	4.6	6.4	3.3
You have not eaten anything all-day	2.4	1.3	2.4	0.8

Source Authors, *Covid-19 Panel Phone Survey of Households 2020* of Mali

Table 5.8 Perceived food insecurity due to Covid-19 disaggregated by sex (in %)

Food insecurity due to Covid-19	Male		Female	
	P1	P2	P1	P2
Enough to eat	13.9	3.8	14.2	5.3
Foods that are nutritious and healthy	10,7	1,6	9,7	3,4
Always the same thing	11.4	3.4	10.4	5.6
Skipped meal	16.8	6.8	15.5	6.3
I do not eat as much as I should have done	2.6	1.6	4.1	0.7
There was no food left in the house	7.4	3.7	7.1	4.7
You were hungry but did not eat	2.5	0.5	3.3	0.9
You have not eaten anything all-day	13.9	3.8	14.2	5.3

Source Authors, *Covid-19 Panel Phone Survey of Households 2020* of Mali

among medical staff and carers. In the absence of adequate health insurance and their financial inability to take care of themselves, these medical staff and carers affected by illness and stress found themselves in difficult situations that were accentuated by the spread of the virus. In some medical facilities with declining revenues, there was reduced remuneration for health workers. The financial consequence of the pandemic triggered a 70% fall in health service access particularly for health care, consultations, surgery, testing, and radiography. The decline was due to the fear of infection. As a result, the turnover of hospitals declined thereby reducing their capacity to finance themselves and, above all, safeguard certain essential services for some patients including antiretroviral drugs for HIV-positive and essential drugs for pregnant women.

At the organisational level, there have been significant changes in hospital operating procedures to cope with the disease, including the transfer of hospital activities and resources to treatment centres, a change in budgeting strategies and the suspension of specific activities in certain hospitals due to the transfer of equipment to the treatment centres. The health resource reallocation has led to health resources being transferred from some hospitals in rural areas to urban areas where infections were higher. Despite the low incidence of Covid-19 in rural areas, rural dwellers remain vulnerable to other endemic diseases such as malaria, which wreaks havoc, particularly on poor households.

The closure of the borders has also severely affected the freight transport sector. Given that Mali predominantly relies on imports for necessities, the lockdown of the economy and the cessation of international freight transport have led to shortages of necessities and an increased risk of food insecurity among poor households. Employment in the transport sector also fell significantly due to the decline in customer base. The curfew imposed resulted in a reduction in working hours and therefore less income for workers in the transport sector, making the families of these workers, who are already in a difficult situation, more vulnerable. The public transport system (buses, taxis, etc.) has also suffered a significant downturn because of the social distancing measures recommended by the health authorities.

Traders have been severely affected by the pandemic and the closure of the markets. In addition to a fall in the number of customers seen in outlets, and the difficulties affecting supplies of various products, several businesses went into bankruptcy during the lockdown of the economy. Official figures indicate that 4,500 workers have lost their jobs because of the pandemic. Unrecorded job losses in the informal sector are much higher, and they primarily affect low-income families whose livelihoods depend on small businesses in local markets. In addition, providers of some services (parties, weddings, etc.) have suffered huge losses due to the cancellation of ceremonies. In the hospitality sector, the decline in the customer base forced some hotels and similar establishments to dismiss a significant number of their employees. Several permanent staff members, particularly permanent staff, were laid off. In addition, introducing a curfew and social distancing measures have hurt companies in the catering sector, which have suffered a drastic reduction in their turnover. Informal sector restaurant workers who depend on daily food sales have been most affected by the loss of their livelihood. As a result, food insecurity has increased among these vulnerable households. Furthermore, the flow of goods was affected by border closures, and local demand for goods declined, resulting in revenue losses.

The mining sector is an essential part of the Malian economy. It relies heavily on foreign partners from North America and African countries. The closure of the borders resulted in a temporary shutdown of activities. Some projects funded by partners to benefit local populations also suffered delays in implementation. The lockdown and the curfew resulted in shorter working hours in gold mining and, therefore, lower earnings for workers who find themselves in a vulnerable situation because of their inability to support their families, with the associated increase in vulnerability and food security at home. Some mines introduced wage bonuses for their employees to incentivise them to stay and work. In addition, employees who took the risk of staying on received a 50% risk premium for continuing to work in the mines during the pandemic. The banking sector was also affected.

The pandemic-related measures led to a reduction in the volume of transactions, a fall in net banking income, and an increase in the cost of risk. At the international level, banks were affected by a fall in international transfers and lower interest rates on loans.

SECTORAL SUPPORT MEASURES

Generally, common support measures across sectors were mainly in hygiene and sanitation item provision. Specific measures applied to some sectors, however. For example, the health sector received multiple support measures. These include shift and risk allowances and food supply (e.g., rice, sugar, meat). Health facilities providing care for Covid-19 patients received equipment and training to manage the pandemic better. In addition, mobile phone operators such as Orange Mali organised phone credit offers for medical staff (XOF 100,000/doctor, or 100 million for all hospitals valid for one month). Some hospitals provided psycho-social support for the medical staff affected by Covid-19. To reduce operational costs, the electricity company of Mali also reduced electricity charges for hospitals for three months. Regarding the criteria for beneficiaries, all staff qualified in proportion to their level of involvement, including administrative and financial staff, hospital crisis committee members, on-call nurses and doctors, and the on-call team. The distribution of aid prioritised staff in direct contact with patients. As for food, distribution was often based on staff income prioritising low-income staff.

The transportation sector, although essential, suffered disruptions due to travel restrictions. The government, working through the CMTR (the road hauliers council of Mali), provided hauliers with equipment allowing them to comply with hygiene and other measures (hand washing kits and masks). These resiliency measures were introduced for urban and inter-urban transport. A Covid-19 fund to help businesses hard hit by the curfew and the closing of the borders was also instituted. The beneficiaries of the fund were all members of the transport companies' union (SET) and particularly vulnerable workers who had lost their jobs or had seen a decline in their operations. These resiliency measures were temporary as they were implemented during the lockdown from April to June 2020.

Tax relief measures were the most common in the sector. Sector players argued that there was little support for import and export sectors and that few measures were universally applied. In the hospitality sector, the focus was on providing hygiene items and PPE. Several hotels were selected to house people from other countries. This situation allowed some hotels to recall some of their staff who had been laid off. These resiliency measures related to hotel owners who had agreed to accommodate quarantined persons who were repatriated to Mali. They lasted between 28 and 45 days. However, it has been reported that the State has not honoured its commitments to pay the corresponding bills immediately, stretching the cash position of the hotels concerned. Rotational working arrangements were implemented in the industrial sector. In addition, the State introduced a reduction in taxes paid by industrial companies until the end of the year and the suspension of VAT for industrial companies for two months (May and June 2020). These measures related primarily to SMEs, which received more flexible access to credit and a suspension of VAT payments to the State. Since this is untargeted, it made access weak for informal sector actors. In the banking sector, the reduction by half of the transfer charges for customers over a period of three months was implemented.

Regarding consultation, the Malian state had more consultative engagements with some formal private sector actors, such as mining, banking, and insurance than the informal sector. The actors in the hospitality industry complained that the measures that concerned them were parachuted and imposed on them.

CONCLUSION AND RECOMMENDATIONS

The overall aim of this study was to systematically reconstruct, document, and analyse the response of the Malian government and other stakeholders, considering the inclusiveness of the responses to Covid-19. The Malian government had appropriately reacted and has early (since March 17, 2020, before the first case on March 25, 2020) introduced a range of measures to prevent and slow the spread of Covid-19 and mitigate its impact. The main preventive measures taken were the closure of air and land borders except for the transport of goods; the closure of schools, bars, and restaurants; measures relating to conduct such as social distancing; a curfew from 5am to 9 pm and a ban on any gathering of more than fifty people.

The Malian State implemented several economic mitigation measures such as tax rebates, guarantee funds, and waiving of domestic debt, among others. However, it is to be stressed that the support measures in the financial sector specifically targeted the formal sector to the detriment of informal businesses.

The social protection measures of the Malian government and non-governmental organisations did not benefit the affected people proportionally. Consequently, they contributed to exacerbating the already significant levels of inequality (deprivation of essential social services, food insecurity, and unemployment) in Mali. For instance, before Covid-19, women (6.1%) were more affected by unemployment than men (4.9%). Furthermore, the average expenditures/income per capita was twice as less in rural areas (FCFA 60 872) than in urban areas (FCFA 126 509). However, the support measures were not properly targeted.

In terms of the effects of the pandemic on social groups, the income poor, female-headed households, and rural households were the most affected by the pandemic and its subsequent preventive measures in terms of job and income losses, difficulties with obtaining essential social services (drinking water and education), and food insecurity.

A critical examination of both the responses and support measures showed that they were poorly targeted and decisions non-inclusive. Also, the eligibility criteria for support measures were, in most cases, too general, inaccessible, or unknown to the intended beneficiaries. Three action areas are needed to guide future pandemic management. Firstly, there is a need for a robust mechanism of identifying eligible people with clear and accessible criteria to help target the most vulnerable social groups. Secondly, a collaboration between the State and non-state actors in the professional circles must be strengthened to enhance the implementation of policies. Finally, the State must enhance the coordination of financial aid and the provision of, and access to, essential social services for more vulnerable households with humanitarian organisations and NGOs, especially for those affected by food insecurity and job and income losses.

References

de Bruin, Y. B., Lequarre, A. S., McCourt, J., Clevestig, P., Pigazzani, F., Jeddi, M. Z., Colosio, C., & Goulart, M. (2020). Initial impacts of global risk mitigation measures taken during the combatting of the COVID-19 pandemic. *Safety Science*, 104773.

Chu, D. K., Akl, E. A., Duda, S., Solo, K., Yaacoub, S., Schünemann, H. J., El-Harakeh, A., Bognanni, A., Lotfi, T., Loeb, M., & Hajizadeh, A. (2020). Physical distancing, face masks, and eye protection to prevent person-to-person transmission of SARS-CoV-2 and COVID-19: A systematic review and meta-analysis. The Lancet.

de Oliveira Mendes, J. M. (2009). Social vulnerability indexes as planning tools: Beyond the preparedness paradigm. *Journal of Risk Research, 12*(1), 43–58. https://doi.org/10.1080/13669870802447962

Ebrahim, S. H., Ahmed, Q. A., Gozzer, E., Schlagenhauf, P., & Memish, Z. A. (2020). Covid-19 and community mitigation strategies in a pandemic. BMJ: *British Medical Journal* (Online), 368.

Fallah Aliabadi, S., Sarsangi, A., & Modiri, E. (2015). The social and physical vulnerability assessment of old texture against earthquake (case study: Fahadan district in Yazd City), *8*(12), 10775–10787. https://doi.org/10.1007/s12 517-015-1939-8.

Fatemi, F., Ardalan, A., Aguirre, B., Mansouri, N., & Mohammadfam, I. (2017). Social vulnerability indicators in disasters: Findings from a systematic review. *International Journal of Disaster Risk Reduction, 22*, 219–227. https://doi. org/10.1016/j.ijdrr.2016.09.006

Han, J., Meyer, B. D., & Sullivan, J. X. (2020). Income and poverty in the COVID-19 pandemic (No. w27729). National Bureau of Economic Research.

Laborde, D., Martin, W., & Vos, R. (2020). Poverty and food insecurity could grow dramatically as COVID-19 spreads. International Food Policy Research Institute (IFPRI).

Martin, A., Markhvida, M., Hallegatte, S., & Walsh, B. (2020). Socioeconomic impacts of COVID-19 on household consumption and poverty. *Economics of Disasters and Climate Change, 4*(3), 453–479.

Martins, V. N., Silva, D. S., & Cabral, P. (2012). Social vulnerability assessment to seismic risk using multicriteria analysis: The case study of Vila Franca do Campo (São Miguel Island, Azores, Portugal). *Natural Hazards, 62*(2), 385–404. https://doi.org/10.1007/s11069-012-0084-x

Mukumbang, F. C., Ambe, A. N., & Adebiyi, B. O. (2020). Unspoken inequality: How COVID-19 has exacerbated existing vulnerabilities of asylum-seekers, refugees, and undocumented migrants in South Africa. *International Journal for Equity in Health, 19*(1), 1–7.

Nussbaumer-Streit, B., Mayr, V., Dobrescu, A. I., Chapman, A., Persad, E., Klerings, I., Wagner, G., Siebert, U., Ledinger, D., Zachariah, C., & Gartlehner, G. (2020). Quarantine alone or combined with other public health measures to control COVID-19: A rapid review. *Cochrane Database of Systematic Reviews, 9*.

Patel, J. A., Nielsen, F. B. H., Badiani, A. A., Assi, S., Unadkat, V. A., Patel, B., Ravindrane, R., &Wardle, H. (2020). Poverty, inequality, and COVID-19: The forgotten vulnerable, *183*(110).

Reports from Institutions

Afrobarometer. (2017). Enquête Afrobarometer Round 7 au Mali. https://afrobarometer.org/fr/publications [consulté le 7 novembre 2020]

Food and Agriculture Organization of the United Nations (FAO). (June 2020). Mali: Response Overview, two pages. http://www.fao.org/resilience/resources/ressources-detail/fr/c/1296624/. [consulté le 13 août 2020].

Institut national de santé publique (INSP). (4 mars 2021). Communiqué Numéro 367 du 4 mars 2021 sur le suivi des actions de prévention et de riposte à la maladie à coronavirus, p.1. http://www.sante.gov.ml/index.php/actualites/communiques/item/6016-communique-n-367-du-ministere-de-la-sante-et-du-developpement-social-sur-le-suivi-des-actions-de-prevention-et-de-riposte-face-a-la-maladie-a-coronavirus. [consulté le 4 mars 2021].

Institut Nationale de la Statistique (INSTAT). (août 2020). Rapport mensuel de l'enquête sur l'impact de coronavirus sur les conditions de vie des ménages du mali, p. 33. http://www.instat-mali.org/ [consulté le 4 août 2020].

Institut Nationale de la Statistique (INSTAT). (Juillet 2020). Rapport mensuel de l'enquête sur l'impact de coronavirus sur les conditions de vie des ménages du mali, p. 33. http://www.instat-mali.org/ [consulté le 4 août 2020].

Institut Nationale de la Statistique (INSTAT). (Juin 2020). Rapport mensuel de l'enquête sur l'impact de coronavirus sur les conditions de vie des ménages du mali, p. 39. http://www.instat-mali.org/ [consulté le 4 août 2020].

Institut Nationale de la Statistique (INSTAT). (novembre 2019). Rapport d'analyse d'enquête modulaire et permanente auprès des ménages, p. 74. https://instat-mali.org/fr/publications/enquete-modulaire-et-perman ente-aupres-des-menages-emop [Consulté le 18 février 2021].

UNICEF (septembre 2020). Mali: COVID-19 Situation Report - #07, Reporting period 1st-30 September 2020. Numéro 07, p. 7. www.unicef.org [consulté le 3 août 2020].

UNICEF. (août 2020). Mali Humanitarian Situation Report, #08, Reporting period 1st-30 August 2020, p. 7. https://reliefweb.int/report/mali/uni cef-mali-humanitarian-situation-report-no-8-01-31-august-2020 [consulté le 7 novembre 2020].

UNOCHA. (septembre 2020). Mali: COVID-19 Rapport de situation #11 7 pages. www.unocha.org [consulté le 7 novembre 2020].

World Bank. (2020). The Covid-19 Emergency Response project in Mali. https://www.worldbank.org/en/news/press-release/2020/04/10/mali-to-receive-25-8-million-for-Covid-19-response [consulté le 7 novembre 2020].

LAWS, DECREES AND ORDERS

Mali Ref, Decree N°2020–0263/PM-RM of June 10, 2020, on the monitoring committee's creation, organisation and modality of operation: Government of the Republic of Mali, 2020.

Mali Ref, Ministerial Decree N°2020–0170/P-RM of March 25 2020, establishing a curfew: Government of the Republic of Mali, 2020.

Mali Ref, Decision N°2020 50 MIC-SG of April 7 2020, setting opening and closing times for markets: Government of the Republic of Mali, 2020.

Mali Ref, Decree N°2020–0200/PM-RM of April 10 2020, creating the technical committee for crisis management: Government of the Republic of Mali, 2020.

Mali Ref, Interministerial order No. 2020–1197//MMP-MATD-MSPC-MEADD-SG of March 27 2020, suspending gold mining: Government of the Republic of Mali, 2020.

Mali, Government announcement of March 17 2020. An extraordinary session of the Superior Council of National Defence instituting the first preventive measures against coronavirus disease, COVID-19, in Mali: Government of the Republic of Mali, 2020.

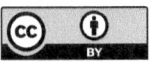

CHAPTER 6

Niger

Rahmane Idrissa

INTRODUCTION

Prior to Covid-19, the socioeconomic indicators of Niger were very depressed. Niger's economy, security, and governance systems were severely threatened due to the Islamic insurgency with security implications for the country. Niger is a landlocked country with the largest landmass in West Africa (1.267 million km^2), much of which is desert or arid land. The bulk of its twenty million population lives in the southern strip of arable land. Most of them reside and work in rural areas, as Niger has the lowest urbanization rate (19%) in the region, a detail that is important for this study because urban areas were the hardest hit, and government restrictions were imposed on urban, not rural areas.

Niger's economy is small, undiversified, and marked by a largely traditional and informal sector that employs more than 90% of the workforce. Although GDP growth has been consistently high during the past decade (between 5 and 6%), it has little impact on the structures of the economy and does not cope well with a very high population growth rate (4%). Niger has ranked at the bottom of the UNDP's Human Development Index, despite a moderate decrease in the poverty rate (from 48% in 2011

R. Idrissa (✉)
EPGA, Niamey, Niger
e-mail: a.idrissa.abdoulaye@asc.leidenuniv.nl

© The Author(s) 2024
A. Altaf et al. (eds.), *EQUITY IN COVID-19*, EADI Global
Development Series, https://doi.org/10.1007/978-3-031-58588-3_6

to 41% in 2019) in recent years. At the time of study, Niger was formally a democracy that tended to slide back into authoritarianism. The leadership in power since 2011 had been mired in a string of financial scandals which had considerably reduced the level of trust in Government in the country, a fact explored in this study concerning government management of the pandemic crisis.

Some border areas of Niger (west-north corner and south-east) are war zones in which various militant forces operate, including Boko Haram and the Islamic State in the Greater Sahara. Most Nigeriens are active in the traditional (over 80%) and informal (over 15%) sectors of the economy. The traditional sector is prevalent in the rural areas and the informal in the urban centres. 'Traditional' and 'informal' may be lumped together into a category which India's political economists call 'the unorganized sector,[1]' a term that works well in the conditions of Niger. The unorganized sector may be defined, by and large, as consisting of the sectors of economic activity that are marginalized because rules and policies that comprehensively organize credit, investment, and social protection under the aegis of the state either do not apply to them or apply only occasionally and minimally.

Prior to the pandemic, Niger's healthcare system did not meet the objectives that the state had set for itself. Niger did not spend 15% of public revenue on the health sector, which translates into much fewer health personnel, weaker institutional capacities, poorer infrastructures, and starker inequality between urban centres and rural areas. Today, Niger has 2467 rural infirmaries (in small towns and villages), 1285 integrated health centres (in secondary towns and the neighbourhoods of larger towns), 56 private hospitals and clinics, 70 public hospitals, 346 pharmacies and laboratories, and 484 small private health centres. Before the pandemic, there were all 9828 hospital beds in the system, and only 52% of the population had ready access (less than 5 km distance) to a healthcare facility of any type. Indeed, data from the Direction of Human Resources of the Health Ministry show that, in 2015, 76% of all health personnel worked in the urban centres, which have only 20% of the country's total population. The city of Niamey, which has 7% of Niger's population, concentrates 34% of the health personnel. These service inequalities and imbalances are reinforced by the fact that health

---

[1] See https://vikaspedia.in/social-welfare/unorganised-sector-1/unorganized-sector-informal-sector.

insurance and social protection are mainly tied to jobs in the organized sector.

Acute awareness of this gross inadequacy of the country's equipment regarding Covid-19 infections explains the fearful reaction of the Government, and why measures were taken even before there was a single confirmed case in Niger. As we shall see, Niger, assisted by an array of aid agencies and organizations, ramped up pandemic preparedness in the health sector, although the task of reaching standards required to cope with the pandemic at levels observed in the industrialized countries was hopeless. Moreover, this effort affected the healthcare system regarding inclusion and exclusion.

The study uses a political economy framework to analyse Niger's pandemic response, impacts, and reactions from the population. These are situated in the country's context of a distressed economy and existing sectoral and locational inequalities in access to services. A brief description of the methodology follows this introduction. It is followed by an analysis of government responses, impacts on different sectors, and the responses from different social groups; the last sections conclude and make policy recommendations.

METHODOLOGY

The methodological approach in this study is qualitative. We have used three methods: documentary research, interviews (structured and open-ended), and media analysis. The choice of a qualitative approach is determined by the focus and context of the study. The context is critical since our methodology shifted during fieldwork. For instance, initially, we had planned to apply a survey questionnaire (quantitative method) to the study of the informal sector.

Nevertheless, during the pre-test, we realized that it was fragmented into subsectors that were differentially impacted by the Government's restrictions. The initial sample was thus broken into smaller sub-samples, making it more useful (and manageable) to apply to it the structured-interviews method, instead of questionnaires. Given that the pandemic crisis is a phenomenon with no precedent, qualitative data collection, with its knack for uncovering unexpected information, ultimately appeared to us more pertinent than quantitative. Nevertheless, it relies on small samples, making it critically important to provide contextual information through which the results may be analysed and related to general conditions. Some results have been presented in a 'quantitative' (i.e., numerical) format. Nevertheless, this is to convey information in a short and rapid medium, and there is no claim of any statistical significance attached to the tables: they illustrate empirical qualitative findings.

COVID-19 RESPONSE MEASURES

On 12 March, following the WHO declaration of Covid-19 as a pandemic (11 March), a series of prevention measures were taken. On 17 March 2020, when there were still no confirmed Covid-19 cases in Niger, President Mahamadou Issoufou made a televised speech to explain and justify the measures of prevention adopted five days before, as well as the additional measures, taken that day. 'On our continent, Africa,' he said, '27 countries, meaning 50%, are affected by a pandemic that is making even the most powerful powerless and defenceless. Their healthcare systems, in particular their reanimation systems, are overwhelmed. Currently, there is neither treatment nor vaccine against this virus. The only weapon that exists today is prevention.' At the end of the speech, he said, 'I repeat it: there is neither treatment nor vaccine. Our only weapon is prevention.[2]

Swift measures were taken from then on. Between the 13 and 17 of March, Niger's international airports were closed and land borders shut, and it was recommended to avoid large gatherings. On 19 March, Prime Minister Brigi Rafini was in the middle of a consultation meeting with religious leaders (Muslims and Christians) when the health minister whispered to his ear that there was a first confirmed Covid-19 case in Niger. The next day, many of the measures that had only been recommended became compulsory (including the one about 'gatherings'), and a slew of rules and policies were adopted under a state of a health emergency. As a result, the measures graduated from the beginning and relaxed as the cases dropped. However, in all, restrictions on movement, a 7 pm to 6 am curfew in the capital Niamey, a ban on large gatherings and safety protocols were announced and enforced strictly and or anecdotally. Perhaps partly because of these measures, the pandemic has had little effect in Niger. At the time of research (September–October), official

---

[2] See France 24, 'Exclusif: Mahamadou Issoufou sur France 24: « Oui, le virus peut tuer des millions de personnes en Afrique.»' https://www.france24.com/fr/video/202 00403-exclusif-mahamadou-issoufou-sur-france-24-oui-le-virus-peut-tuer-des-millions-de-personnes-en-afrique.

tallies indicated that total case numbers were 2258 confirmed cases, with 80 dead and 1292 recovered. This is a statistically insignificant impact in a country where the primary killer disease remains malaria.[3] However, the socioeconomic impact of the disease is more significant, even though the Government trod much more carefully in the economy than in other sectors (religion, education). The measures were in full force in March–May 2020. Afterwards, they were considerably relaxed, either officially or in terms of their implementation. By August–September, they had become anecdotal, although they have left behind a trail of economic misery.

In terms of managing the pandemic, the Government created a so-called *dispositif de riposte* ('response system') with a pyramidal chain of command and responsibilities and several technical commissions. At the top sat the decision-making *comité d'orientation* (orientation committee), chaired by the head of state, and an Inter-ministerial Committee for the Management and Response to the Covid-19 pandemic, which served to coordinate response among the different ministries and the sectors in which they were in charge. This body's role in the decision-making process was to centralize information required to design the response measures and propose them to the council of ministers. Besides a consultative committee, which advised on non-technical matters, the committee spoke with the One Health technical committee, eight regional technical committees (one for each region), and seven commissions (logistics, communication, monitoring, laboratories, etc.) that constituted the administrative side of the response system.

While the decision-making process was national, in some sectors (financial especially), it was coordinated with countries of the West African Economic and Monetary Union (WAEMU) grouping. Other influence came from the WHO and consultation with countries of the Economic Community of West African States (ECOWAS). In each country in the region—and such was the case of Niger too—international NGOs and aid agencies also played a significant role in the funding and organization of emergency social support measures thanks to their installed capacities in supplying humanitarian aid.

---

[3] According to the WHO, Niger had 3,358,058 confirmed malaria cases in 2018 (WHO World Malaria Report for 2019).

COMPENSATORY MEASURES

According to a study from the Chamber of Commerce and Industry of Niger, the Government took two types of compensatory measures. The first type was economical and fiscal support, which included tax exemptions, waivers and reductions, suspension of statutory payments and suspension of prosecution of tax defaulters, among others. Aside from the national measures, Niger was a party to measures taken at the level of the regional grouping WAEMU. These measures essentially aimed at boosting the financial resilience of member states. They included an increase of 340 bn. Cfa Francs (533.5 million euros) in the volume of liquidities the central bank BCEAO would inject weekly on the money market for the community banking sector, rising it to 4750 bn. Cfa Francs; a broadening of refinancing facilities to include 1700 different businesses across the community; financial interventions of the central bank and the WAEMU Commission aimed at raising concessional resources for member states; the granting of a concessional loan of 15 bn. Cfa Francs to each member state of WAEMU by the West African Development Bank (WADB). In the case of Niger specifically, the WADB decided a moratorium on the country's debts of 13.2 bn. Cfa Francs.

The economic and fiscal measures concerned the formal sector exclusively. Aside from the tax exemptions and other measures of fiscal relief, resources mobilized through the WAEMU-BCEAO-WADB system led to support plans for the formal private sector via the national banking sector. A financing mechanism in the amount of 150 bn. Cfa Franc was thus set up to supply credit to businesses affected by the Covid-19 crisis. This was divided into a 50 bn—envelope for SMEs and a 100 bn. one for larger enterprises. The monies secured via these loans were to be earmarked for payroll and quarterly fixed expenses only. After the crisis has ended, stimulus credit would be supplied based on files and paperwork prepared by applicants. Access to this aid (both relief and stimulus) was and would be contingent on the production of paper evidence (trade registration, contracts of employees, evidence of loss attributable to the pandemic based on a comparison between turnover documentation in the previous year and since April 2020, etc.). In addition, verification of use and management of the loaned funds required further bureaucracy.

As these details indicate, businesses outside the formal sector or with limited formal management capacities were de facto excluded from the facility. Yet, these were most businesses in Niger, and the most fragile and the ones that employed the greater number of people. On 17 June, a group of business associations and organizations put together a consortium of economic and social actors and addressed a memorandum to the finance minister, asking for a mechanism tailored to the needs of businesses in the informal sector. At the time of research, their advocacy did not lead to significant decisions.

The second type of compensatory support concerned social support, which estimated a need for a total financing sum of 597 bn—Cfa Francs (over 910 million euros). The programmes included waiver of household water and electricity bills for April and May, free food, and reduced food price to strengthen the yearly plan of social support for vulnerable people, adoption of a price ceiling for certain products such as grains and household necessities and early release of 1540 prisoners (older, juvenile, women, ill). The waiving of utility bills was a relief chiefly for middle-class households; and the 'strengthening' or broadening of the yearly support plan, which included one-off cash payments in some cases, was an 'empirical' extension of established social measures, not measures explicitly designed for conditions arising from the pandemic—in part because such conditions were not well-known. The measure of price ceiling was the object of discussion with import–export traders and was not always applied. For example, in the region of Maradi, where I conducted fieldwork in October, traders convinced the authorities that, in the depressed conditions that then existed and especially given restrictions on transborder trade from both Nigeria and Niger, competition between traders actually would tend to produce lower prices than the price fixed by government order. As a result, the measure was discontinued in the region, and perhaps elsewhere.

THE PANDEMIC HAVOC

Since the Government's compensatory measures relied essentially on credit and institutional social protection, the consequences for the unorganized sector—especially for the (urban) informal sector—are not hard to fathom. The urban informal sector was hard hit by the measures but could not receive relief to the same extent—or even to any extent—as the organized sector. The urban informal sector includes marketplace, street, and network retail trade; eateries and catering (many makeshift); handicraft and makers of household goods; mechanics; city public transportation (most of it); inter-city public transportation (some of it);

personal services (barbershops, etc.); domestics; carting and distribution (of water, e.g.); and casual workers. This sector employs the vast majority of urbanites. It is partly integrated with the traditional sector since some of the goods and products sold on the markets and some of the raw materials used in some of the activities (food, e.g.) come from the rural areas. Moreover, workers in the city send remittances to the rural areas and invest there in local trade (e.g.: animals, grains).

The unorganized sector is heterogeneous as it is also a place of capital accumulation that leads some to great wealth, not just survival. Indeed, the wealthiest social layer of Nigeriens, the merchant capitalists, begin their journey 'from rags to riches' in the unorganized sector and remain active there. The sector is arguably more divided along gender lines than the organized sector. For example, none of those wealthy traders is a woman, whereas women are remarkably successful in the top reaches of the organized sector.[4] Owing to conservative Islamic values, Nigerien women are more active in petty network trade than in the more rewarding marketplace trade (in contrast, for example, with women in the Gulf of Guinea). The customary rules that apply in the unorganized sector— given the vanishing act played by official rules and policies—also favour men and, especially in some rural areas, high 'caste' men and women. Recognizing the importance of the urban informal sector in the livelihood of most Nigeriens, the Government did not apply any real lockdown measure to it.

RESTAURANTS

Restaurants in the formal sector suffered from the measures significantly less than eateries in the informal sector. Restaurants have hours of operation that were less affected by the curfew. Even if they lost dinner customs, their lunch hours stayed busy. They could more easily implement social distancing and hygiene measures and organize catering and food delivery. They could also set up furlough plans for their staff with the support of government services, including in applications for relief credit. After the end of the curfew period, their activity snapped back into its former self with no lasting damage. The picture for eateries in the

---

[4] See Clarisse Juompan-Yakam, 'Au Niger, le business est (aussi) une affaire de femme,' in Jeune Afrique (22 October 2016): https://www.jeuneafrique.com/mag/270940/eco nomie/au-niger-le-business-est-aussi-une-affaire-de-femmes/

informal sector was and is very different. Due to the dominant lifestyle in Niamey, the busiest time for their activity is from 2 pm (or later) to 1 am. Daytime eateries are usually snack suppliers, especially grilled meat and skewers. The big business happens after dusk. People unwind as the night sets in, which is when turnover is made in eateries, especially around the city's many 'night markets.'

We interviewed ten owners of eateries, including five women and five men. Their businesses range from those that are more restaurant-like (with premises, furniture, and a staff) to those that are makeshift installations. Figures of daily turnover losses starkly indicate that the more profitable businesses tend to be those owned by men, which reflects well the general context in Niamey (Table 6.1). Indeed, although the data are about a small group of people, trends and structures in the unorganized sector are more favourable to men than to women.

The stories behind these figures show the ramifications of these losses. People with the higher daily turnovers also employed a comparatively large staff, which they had to lay off almost entirely in all cases. Although they have rehired afterwards, their staff is smaller today ('things still have not gone back to normal,' 'this is true poverty, sister.[5]'). In one case, we learn that the curfew has upended a classic plan of immigrant social integration. Many of the owners of these businesses are immigrants from

Table 6.1 Daily turnover of eateries and restaurants in Niamey

Gender	Estimated daily turnover loss under curfew, in Euros
M	305
M	300
M	106
M	92
M	61
F	61
F	53
F	30
F	15
F	15

Source Author's filed work, 2020

[5] The EPGA researcher for this sector was female.

the rural areas. One of them, the man who lost 92 € daily turnovers, is a 25-years old who had just got married and came to town in search of opportunities to help him support the family he was starting. Now, he said, he was unable to send remittances to his newlywed, whom he had left back at the village, and whom he had planned to bring to town once his business had flourished enough. Others said they had stopped sending food (rice) 'back home,' i.e., to the rural areas. None reported any kind of support from the authorities. They do not understand the measures ('So is it that the virus moves about only at nighttime?', a woman asked). In most cases, they survived by dipping into their savings or receiving help from friends and relatives. In all cases, they had to cut on some life necessities, including food.

Unlike the eateries sector, the arts and crafts sector in Niamey is self-organized. Artisans and workers in this sector can be divided into two groups: those who have a spot in artisan centres, i.e., the *Village Artisanal de Wadata* and the *Musée National Boubou Hama*; and those who have shops in the city. They are generally registered with the Niger Chamber of Arts and Crafts (CMANI in the French acronym), which gives them a toehold in the formal sector. Those in the *Village Artisanal* and the *Musée National* are also members of those centres' cooperatives.

The arts and crafts industry has typically larger turnovers than other industries in the urban informal sector, although this varies enormously. The more successful artisans can make hundreds of thousands of Cfa Francs per month, in contrast to a few tens of thousands for those at the bottom. Success is highly dependent on tourism. Artisans already suffered in the past when the first terror attacks in the Sahel curtailed tourism in Niger in the early 2010s. At that point, many travelled outside Niger and the Sahel to make their wares available to tourists. Those who did not travel entrusted their productions to those who did, and hence, business travels became a central part of the business for many artisans in Niamey. These trips led them to festivals, shows, and fairs across West Africa, and a few even found their way to Europe. The measure that hit the hardest is therefore, the closure of borders: not only are tourists no longer travelling in, but artisans cannot travel out. They also complained of the curfew, which, by limiting times of operation, also automatically limited the sales opportunities that remained.

We interviewed ten artisans, all men (the industry appears to be entirely populated by men). Estimated turnover losses confirm the fact that artisans belong to very different leagues (Table 6.2).

Table 6.2 Turnover of Artisans

High earners estimated turnover losses due to restrictions from late March to October (€)
18,000 +
15,000 +
10,000 +
10,000 +
9000 +
Low earners estimated turnover losses due to restrictions since late March to October (€)
1200 +
1000 +
530 +
460 +
380 +

Source Author's fieldwork

Despite the differences in earnings, reported hardships are very similar. If low earners have cut dramatically in their spending ('I went from about 2000 francs [3€] a day to 500 [0.7 €],' reported one), the income stoppage also has dramatic consequences for high earners due to their higher spending and fixed costs (rent, utilities). High earners employed paid apprentices, whom they had to lay off. The man who reported the highest losses and regularly attended lucrative events in France found a way to export artsy masks there and has kept one paid apprentice out of eight: 'I had to let the others go because there were things I was no longer being able to take care of in my household.' Others in both categories have tried their hand at different activities, but with little luck: 'I tried,' said one, 'but unfortunately, I realized that the Covid-19 has made things harder in all activities.' 'I opened a small shop at my door and tried selling rice, but that really was not my area, I was a bit confused about it.' They also tried cutting their prices and directly contacting customers. The results, they said, were lacklustre.

Unlike workers in the eateries sector, everyone reported having received food aid, either through the cooperatives or through CMANI. These organizations give artisans a voice in meetings with the authorities and donors, even though they are not set up in such a way that they could organize group solidarity.

PUBLIC TRANSPORTATION I: TAXIS AND 'FABA'

Niamey has a unique—relative to other towns in Niger—city public transportation system that combines buses (a formal-sector company), taxis and minibuses known as *'faba'* ('succour,' in the local Zarma language). These two are the main city public transportation, given that the bus network has limited reach. Taxis and *faba* are registered at city hall, paying the imposts tied to trade vehicles. This gives them a certain formality that has enabled their drivers to unionize, and at times, to organize strikes—mainly against petrol price increases. The measures that affected taxis and *faba* are the curfew and the social distancing prescriptions. These measures limited the number of passengers, but the fare rate remained the same. Profit margins for taximen, especially those who work for an owner, are thin and volatile, requiring them to make constant calculations of fare, distance, and petrol consumption to save the day. The social distancing measure threw a wrench in those calculations. Owners have little patience when taximen do not make the daily payments, and this was the case even under the special conditions of the pandemic. Owners must spend money on maintaining the car and paying its taxes. Many owners have small incomes. Six out of the ten taximen we interviewed said they lost their contract during the pandemic (one, only for three months). Even though the sample is tiny, it is still significant considering that the proportion is actually even higher (i.e., 6/8) because two of the ten interviewees were the owners of their taxis. The social repercussions of such loss of income are significant, given that many taximen support relatives in the rural areas. In one case, a taximan-owner told us: 'I host several high school students from our village because it doesn't have a high school. However, this year, I told them not to come to my house, save for just one, because I have no means to support all of them.' Another one had to divorce at the age of 56 (box 1).

There is no programme to help taximen. Their union was able to secure food aid during the duration of the restrictions (April–May), but it was offered only to hired taximen. Not only did taximen-owners receive nothing, but city authorities declined to give them relief on taxes and fees beyond a stated time. The man who could no longer host school students from his village told us he had to park his car and work as a substitute driver because his straitened circumstances did not allow him to sort the bureaucratic payments.

Box 1: Pandemic Experiences of Taximen

Taximen under stress.

The car has gone. Well, the crisis has meant that the car has gone, the owner took it back. That's because of the curfew. I worked for that person on the afternoon and evening shift, which means from 1 to 6 pm, and after an hour break, I worked again from 7 pm until late at night. Nevertheless, with the curfew, I couldn't make the payments, and also had a colleague who worked in the morning, but he was no longer able to do it. So the owner could rely only on my payments, which I couldn't make. See, the thing is, before, I always managed to make 5000 francs [7.6 €] a day after I made the payment, but during the curfew, that was impossible. The owner was losing money, so of course, he took the car back. So I became a porter; I am able to give to my wife 1000 francs each day, that's half what I gave her before. I have back rent of 140,000 francs. The taxi drivers' union got us some food aid, I was told about it and went to get my share. But when I got there, they told me my name wasn't on the list. Frankly, the Government has destroyed me.

It's getting better. I couldn't work as much as I used to, so it kind of broke me financially. You know, with the social distancing, and the curfew, this was a great deal less to have in one's pocket. The owner was understanding to some extent. He reduced my daily payment from 7000 francs to 5000 francs. Moreover, I cut on spending at home. It wasn't too bad, I just spent less. I did get some food aid, the union drew up lists and gave us tickets, and officers of the Water and Forestry Authority distributed the food. But I thank God, it's getting better now.

It's all pain. I worked the night shift, so with the curfew, the owner just fired me. At the time, if I subtract the payment to the owner and petrol costs, I made 3000 francs a day. And all of a sudden, I was making nothing. I could no longer help the family back home, in the village, which I used to do. But with the loss of income, my wife became very angry at me, and eventually, she left me. I feel completely helpless. When I find something, I do it, and when there's nothing I am patient. The union gave me tickets for food aid, and the Water and Forestry Authority handed it out. This was 50 kg of millet, 50 kg of maize, and 20 kg of black-eyed peas per month. We got it twice until they lifted the curfew. But in the meantime, I have become a man with no job and no wife. It's all pain.

You just cannot not work. With the pandemic, customers became very wary. And then there were the measures from the Government. These created hardship but in the end, I think they were efficient. Because they prevented the fast spread of the virus, didn't they? Anyway, I used to make 10,000 francs and even more before, I mean, after I made the payment and paid the petrol. This went down to just 2000 francs, pretty steep. And then at some point, it became impossible to make any payment to the owner. The owner got fed up and sold the car. That was tough. You know, I was in the habit of bringing fruits to the kids each day at the end of my shift. But then I became so embarrassed that I could no longer do that that I started to be back home after their sleeping time. I also got into debt. A taximan just cannot not work. I worked really hard to keep that car, but it didn't happen. I got some food aid through the union, and I am mostly doing substitute driving. Things are a bit better now that the measures have been lifted. Of course, I no longer have a car, but it is better than when the measures were in force.

PUBLIC TRANSPORTATION II: 'BUSH TAXIS'

Bush taxis are intercity public vehicles, usually with 17 passengers' seats (although the practice is to take in 18 people by adding a spot in the front cabin). In the case of Niamey, these minibuses connect the city to other towns in Niger and foreign towns, especially in northern Mali, Burkina Faso, and Benin. In recent years, the development of bus transportation (formal sector companies) has tended to crowd them out of the more popular international destinations in the ECOWAS region. They are much cheaper than the buses and popular with people in the rural areas and the more impoverished social categories. Their organization is very similar to urban taxis, where their owners drive some, others by hired drivers who must make payments after each trip. They are registered in the transportation system and must pay taxes and car insurance. However, they are not unionized.

During the sanitary isolation of Niamey (from late March to mid-May), the activity was virtually dead due to land border closures and a decline in passenger flow. Unlike the taximen, bush taxi drivers did not receive any food aid during the period, which can be ascribed to the fact that they are not unionized. The union offers a level of formality which could help the authorities identify legitimate aid recipients, and it could also talk with the Government. Without such an organization, the bush taxi drivers were only part of the mass of the needy, most of whom would only receive, by luck, some occasional humanitarian aid. Given the limited reach of such aid, it had no impact on the situation of bush taxi drivers.

For some, though, this proved to be a boon *after* the sanitary isolation of Niamey was lifted. At that point, the only restriction left—aside from the shut borders—was the social distancing measure which cut the number of persons admitted in a minibus from 20 to 10 (driver and 'apprentice' included). Due to this measure, steep increases in fares (generally more than three times higher) were allowed. However, since the police had ended the patrols, which only aimed at enforcing the isolation of Niamey, some drivers resumed the practice of rendezvousing with passengers in the open country. As a result, these drivers could fill their car at a much higher fare than before. One interviewee who was particularly successful at this business was straightforward about the result: 'the fact is, the crisis has given a big boost to my profit.' Nevertheless, given government regulation, this was still a risk, and those who tended to take it were drivers who were also owners (which was the case of that interviewee).

The period was a time of misery for many more. It was a time of dishonour:

> The only option left to me was debt, but since I cannot repay it, I live in dishonour.' My wife cannot accept that I cannot provide, she's angry, yells at me, and I cannot respond because I am not providing. Therefore, the Government has dishonoured me in the eye of my wife.

A time of helplessness,

I just go to the station, sit, and wait, and nothing happens, so I come back home, friends and kind-hearted people support us.' 'Now I am picking wood and selling it on a cart, and it is that or nothing.

This is the fate of hired drivers, who were laid off since the vehicles were no longer profitable. Nevertheless, many driver-owners also suffered a similar situation. After having spent their savings and gotten into debt, the bureaucratic costs of running the business became unbearable: 'I could not pay the papers, so I parked my car, and now I am doing substitute driving when I get the chance.' The crisis disrupted the industry's organization and habits, with one result being that travellers deserted the minibus stations. Some drivers therefore started to park at unconventional spots, where the custom was more easily found. However, they were harassed by the police. One of them was fined a hefty sum (73 €) when the EPGA researcher interviewed him at one such location. This kind of lack of understanding from the authorities deepens the sense that *'le gouvernement s'en fout de nous'* ('the government does not care a fig about us').

Moreover, they must contend with the competition of the big bus companies, which travel to secondary towns. Before, such minor destinations were left to the bush taxis. As long as the borders were shut, this competition continued.

The social and economic consequences of the crisis extended beyond the misery of transportation workers. Usually, these workers are breadwinners for their families and relatives in the rural areas. One very successful driver-owner possessed six minibuses. Although childless, he calculated that he had over 40 persons directly under his care in Niamey and his village, all of whom suffered from income stoppage. The minibuses are also a critical factor in petty trade, especially between the rural areas, secondary towns, and Niamey. Many of these precarious ventures were broken because the bush taxis could no longer move goods around. The freezing of minibus stations wrecked the street trading of small retailers, coaxers, and snack vendors that flourished around them.

In May, the Government ended some of the restrictions and calculated that 85 bn. Cfa francs were needed to restore the passenger transportation system to its former self[6]: Nevertheless, this estimate was based on the needs of the formal sector. The latter is a dynamic and booming sector of Niger's service economy, with 18 bus companies connecting all the country's main towns and destinations across West Africa, specializing in postal service and intercity and international instant cash transfer. Some of these enterprises belong to Niger's wealthiest businessmen—including notorious tax evader Mohamed Rhissa Ali of 'Panama Papers' fame[7]—and the diversification of their activities means that, while they indeed reeled from the restrictions,[8] they did not lack the sinews to rebound when international borders reopened. On the contrary, they, not the bush taxis, were set to reap the benefits of the stimulus policy that the Government planned for after the pandemic.

Petty Trade: MKK and Buckets

Petty trade is an everyday activity in the unorganized sector, either to add to income on the side or as principal activity. It ranges from established small-size shops to street hawkers and peddlers. We studied them to understand how people in the sector were affected or profited from the pandemic. For this, we conducted fieldwork in Maradi, which borders Nigeria enjoys a vibrant transborder trade or piggyback on trade with the large Nigerian cities of Katsina and Kano; and Niamey, the capital. The Nigerian transborder trade is organised in a scheme, 'the special transit,' whereby merchants in the three cities of Maradi, Katsina and Kano import consumer goods and equipment via Niger's docks in Cotonou and ferry them through southern Niger and into northern Nigeria, paying only

---

[6] See Morgane Le Cam, '« La route est vitale pour nous»: au Niger, le secteur des transports au bord du gouffre,' in Le Monde (11 November 2020): https://www.lem onde.fr/afrique/article/2020/11/11/la-route-est-vitale-pour-nous-au-niger-le-secteur-des-transports-au-bord-du-gouffre_6059376_3212.html.

[7] See https://panamapapers.investigativecenters.org/niger-2/

[8] We interviewed the director of one of those companies, Société des Transports Moderne (STM), which has 650 employees. He reports a loss in turnover of 40% caused by the restrictions and salary payments of 50% in May. However, the company's capital allowed them to maintain their infrastructure (including station buildings rented across Niger and some West African countries), and if costs were cut on running bills, employees are now paid in full, partly on shareholders' dime. In the universe of Niger's bus companies, STM is middle-ranked. The lower-ranked ones suffer more from the pandemic havoc, including non-payment of salaries.

transit taxes. Under cover of the Nigerian imports, merchants in Maradi could also import goods at the same reduced tax rates.

Moreover, Maradi is part of the trade corridor known as MKK (Maradi-Katsina-Kano), a trade route with its own office at Maradi's chamber of commerce. In this commercial system, Maradi exports agricultural and pastoral products and buys consumer goods and equipment, a fraction of which is manufactured in Nigeria. If the rate of profits depends a good deal on the exchange rate between the Naira and the Cfa Franc,[9] goods bought in Nigeria are, at any rate, cheap by Nigerien standards since conditions in the enormous Nigerian market tend to generate low prices compared with those in Niger.

This trade—the most intensive at any border region in Niger and, in fact, in any part of the country—has many effects, including the fact that many among Maradi working and pauper classes earn a living through petty trade. This activity was damaged by the Covid-19-related border closure. Nigeria and Niger froze passenger-car traffic, and the border was effectively sealed. The 'Corona closure,' as it was known, stopped the flow of trade and turned Maradi into a ghost town.

The stories we collected from petty traders and shopkeepers describe effects reminiscent of those attending a natural disaster. The border closure brought hardship to the smaller traders, who, given their dependence on short spurts of cash flow, had to make several trips to Nigeria a week (for some, a day) to sustain their activity. When these trips became impossible, they were utterly deprived of income. Nevertheless, on the other hand, those who could make stocks (shopkeepers and suppliers of certain types of goods, for example, plastic bags to make water pouches.[10]) benefited from the higher prices created by penury. However, according to testimonies, this was counterbalanced by the fact that these traders frequently had to sell on credit or—in the case of commodities such as water bags—at a loss when it came to habitual customers.

Petty trade differs from other occupations by its adaptability, as was shown by the case of hygiene kit sellers in Niamey. Most of those we

---

[9] They are, at present, favorable to Niger due to the depression in the global petroleum market. However, many in Maradi deplore the loss in value of the Naira because it depresses commercial activities in Nigeria and, by repercussion, in Maradi.

[10] In the indigent economy, water pouches initially played the role of bottled water in more affluent economies. However, they have become a standard on the market for retailing drinking water in most African countries.

interviewed were small retailers (shopkeepers) who found themselves in difficulty when their customers dwindled in number and re-stocking became a challenge. A case in point is that of a shopkeeper successful enough to run two shops, one of which he entrusted to a brother brought from the village. Given the fall in business that came with the curfew, travel restrictions, and border closure, he closed his shop, sent his brother back to the village, took over that other shop, and turned it into a selling point for buckets. That article had become popular due to the Government's hygiene campaign. Soon afterwards, he learned how to turn buckets into hygiene kits (a bucket set in a high-legged metal basket and sporting a faucet and a soap dish on the sides). 'I went from being a seller of wrappers and women's articles to being a seller of hygiene kits and all that goes with that,' he said. Another trader said that such conversion came from the simple fact that they saw sales of buckets going from two to three units per day to several dozen almost overnight. 'The crisis,' he said, 'has created some temporary jobs, such as making and selling masks. However, I think these hygiene kits are here to stay, and we know how to make them.' The hygiene kits were adopted by many eateries and may become an essential article in those businesses or in households.

RURAL AREAS

At the time of writing, the pandemic did not spread significantly in rural areas, but they felt its economic impact. According to a study by Save the Children, the Food Economy Group, and the USAID, two million people (70%) in rural areas would face livelihood and survival deficits due to Covid-19. The studies estimated that the many Covid-19 restrictions could affect 40% of the sale of animals and animal products, 40% of the supply of agricultural workforce, cut seasonal cash transfer from urban areas, reduce the sale of garden products, reduce trade incomes, and increase the cost of agricultural input. They also considered that the 'rural areas' are complex regions with different 'livelihood zones.' Thus, its findings remind us that the rural areas are not isolated from the country's general welfare.

Public Responses to Covid-19 Measures

The public responded in variable ways, according to social milieu, economic activity, and type of measure. For this study, we conducted a social media analysis that gave us access to opinions in the Francophone social milieu, Islamic religious circles, the informal sector, especially public transportation, petty trade arenas, and among the pauper classes in Niamey.[11]. The situation in Niger moved from public fear of a health crisis of unprecedented proportions in March–April–May; to a period of cautious hopes, in June–July, that this might not come to pass; to a growing conviction that the Covid-19 disease was not a severe threat. This evolution is particularly well-reflected in attitudes in the Francophone social milieu, which, in turn, showed a greater responsivity to government discourse—distinctly because this milieu is also the one from which government staff and decision-makers overwhelmingly come.

In the first phase (March–May), the curfew and the closing of mosques to significant prayer events triggered resistance across the country, including riots and acts of rebellion. Such resistance came principally from people in the country's large lower classes. In some cases, police stations were attacked, and in Mirriah, a town in the region of Zinder (centre-east) at the border with Nigeria, a school was torched after the arrest of a cleric who was calling for disobedience. In many cases, incidents were avoided because the police forces sent to guard mosques successfully resorted to negotiation. In practice, the mosque control measures were relaxed or unenforced by the end of April due to the onset of the fasting month of Ramadan (23 April–23 May). Indeed, they were formally ended on 13 May. Nevertheless, among the more compliant Francophones and the more restive lower classes, mistrust of the Government ran high, though it was expressed in very different ways and led to quite different attitudes.

The educated class, referred to as 'Francophones,' refers to the socio-cultural group of people who have gone through the different levels of schooling—in French—and would generally work in the formal or modern sector of the economy. The better off in this group is the country's middle class, and the others would, at any rate, aspire to that social condition. Perhaps ten per cent of Nigeriens belong to this social category. Although this social class were more responsive to the government's responses with the belief of the peril of the crisis, a section faulted the

---

[11] Data for the pauper classes are missing at the time of writing.

Government's heavy-handedness, civil right abuses connected to crisis management, lack of transparency, accountability, corruption, and issues about priorities on the management of the pandemic.

Reactions by the majority of Muslims are essential to note. Over 98% of Nigeriens are Muslims, but Islam is not a monolithic reality in the country. It is shaped by history, sociology, and external influences. Most Nigeriens are Sunni Muslims and most also belong to the lower classes (urban low-income and paupers, rural poor). Closing mosques and other places of worship was a decision that most, if not all, West African states took in the early months of the pandemic. What distinguished Niger was that, unlike many of its neighbours, it did not close the markets as well; and, unlike the countries of the Francophone Sahel (Burkina Faso, Mali, Senegal), with which it has so much in common, it is under the influence of opinion trends in northern Nigeria. These two facts combined made the measures that tried to restrict religious gatherings more controversial in Niger than in neighbouring countries. While citizens, even religious leaders, praised the Government (if grudgingly) for keeping the markets open, they also were struck by the inconsistency of having these day-long, crowded areas going while mosques were told to shut.

Moreover, the general mistrust of a government that was not known to care very much for the living conditions of the working and pauper classes was heightened, in Niger, by the widespread belief, sourced from northern Nigeria, that the Government was a stooge of the West, seen as the enemy of Islam. This is an ideological belief which is not moved by contradictions: thus, an interviewee who mentioned the (perceived) government inaction during a cholera epidemic as proof of its lack of care, stressed that the population was saved in the instance by an emergency health centre built by Médecins Sans Frontières, a Western organization: yet, he kept assuming that the West was hostile to the Muslim people of Niger. Because these clerics are more influential among the working and pauper classes, these ideological beliefs are more prevalent there too.

This context says a lot about the level of mistrust the Islamic leadership feels toward the Government.[12] The top-down approach the Government adopted in relation to the faithful, as opposed to working with all layers of the Islamic religious leadership, ultimately proved ineffective in controlling the faithful.

---

[12] In Niger, traditional chiefs are state agents under the ministry of the Interior. The higher-ranked (sultans, chiefs of province and canton) have salaries and perquisites.

CONCLUSION AND RECOMMENDATIONS

This study reviews how the Government and the public responded to the Covid-19 pandemic in Niger, focusing on issues of trust and inclusion/exclusion. It tells the story of how, following a warning from the World Health Organization and taking into consideration the minimal resources of the national healthcare system, the Niger's Government was on alert at a very early stage and took Covid-19 prevention measures before there was a single confirmed case in the country. This responsivity was inspired by fears stemming from the conviction that Niger faced a humanitarian disaster of untold proportions. The study shows that the strategy that was followed relied on the concept of 'prevention,' meaning slowing down as much as feasible the introduction and then the propagation of the virus in the country. The main steps in this view included the closure of national borders, the 'sanitary isolation' of the capital (seen as the main point of entry of the pandemic), the banning of crowd congregations across the country, and the freezing of passenger travels. Controversially, banning crowd congregations allowed congregations in the marketplace but not in places of worship. This led to many incidents, including riots. The study also reviews Niger's healthcare system and how the Government attempted overhauling it in the hope of coping somewhat with the expected waves of Covid-19 patients. Alongside these emergency measures, the Government took compensatory measures, which are also studied.

The study relies on the results of fieldwork conducted in Niamey and Maradi, in August-October 2020. Reports, studies, and other documents were also collected and used. Thus, the study goes into the details of the government policy, and the grain of public response and experience, in the religious sphere and the urban informal sector. The latter is analysed from the abovementioned perspectives: trust and inclusion/exclusion.

The study argues that trust in the Government, which had been low before the epidemic, remained so, but in different ways depending on socio-cultural categories. The middle-class 'Francophones' were critical of government corruption, and incompetence and consistently believed in the conspiracy theory that the official epidemic figures—at many points in time the lowest in West Africa—were inflated by the Government, which, it was thought, hoped to secure aid funds, and embezzle it. People from the lower classes, outraged by the closure of mosques in a country where the Islamic faith is often tinged with ideological convictions imported from northern Nigeria, accused the Government of being a stooge of the West, which would have created the 'Corona' scare to undermine the practice of Islam. However, mistrust did not hurt compliance. This outcome is mainly due to the counterbalancing effects of an intensive campaign of persuasion that enlisted even figures traditionally opposed to the Government.

Concerning inclusion/exclusion, the study found that the epidemic and its response revealed a form of bias that is based not so much on discrimination as on structure. Professional groups and social categories whose needs are amenable to bureaucratic governance are more easily and consistently included in relief schemes than those in the 'unorganized sector,' i.e., the informal and traditional sectors. This is the case even though the latter are more vulnerable to and suffer more from the restrictions imposed by the Government. Humanitarian aid, which has fewer bureaucratic demands than processive policy, reaches them better but has fewer long-lasting effects.

There are lessons that the Government in Niger and other Sub-Saharan African countries may draw from this.

Regarding the issue of trust, governments—aside from the ideal point of developing better financial ethics—must become more adept at using tools of persuasion rather than coercion. If, despite the high level of mistrust, Nigeriens were by and large compliant, this is due mainly to the efforts put into sensitization campaigns, including resources allocated to the training of media workers and frequent interventions of usually more distant state officials.

Regarding the issue of structural inclusion/exclusion, changing the structures to eliminate the problem would be ideal but appears like an unrealistic tall order. It seems better to adapt to them by establishing levels of correspondence between the 'unorganized' and state/formal bureaucratic order. Pragmatic solutions, including through reliance on technology, may be fleshed out. Moreover, the mobilization of actors to boost the healthcare system in response to the emergency of the pandemic showed that it could be far more inclusive than it usually is. Lessons should be drawn to study how one could integrate the observed efficiencies into the regular operation of the healthcare system.

CHAPTER 7

Nigeria

Thelma Obiakor, Chimere Iheonu, and Ezra Ihezi

INTRODUCTION

On February 27, 2020, Nigeria reported its first case of the coronavirus (COVID-19) disease (Ehanire, 2020), and by the third week of March, the total number of cases had risen to 22 across Nigeria. Healthcare expenditure in Nigeria was low pre-COVID-19. In 2018, the per capita government expenditure on health care was 3.89% of GDP, below the regional average of 5.1% (World Bank, 2018). As of 2019, there were 0.381 physicians per 1000 people (World Bank, 2018), meaning that traditional medicine still plays a significant role in meeting people's health needs, especially in rural areas (Antail, 2010).

Before the pandemic, the Nigerian economy had been grappling with a weak recovery from the earlier 2014 oil price shock. In 2019, GDP growth hovered around 2.3%. In February 2020, the IMF revised its initial forecasted 2020 GDP growth rate from 2.5% to 2% (Fouda, 2020) to reflect the impact of lower international oil prices and limited fiscal

T. Obiakor (✉) · C. Iheonu · E. Ihezi
Centre for the Study of the Economies of Africa (CSEA), Abuja, Nigeria
e-mail: tobiakor@cseaafrica.org

E. Ihezi
e-mail: eihezie@cseaafrica.org

© The Author(s) 2024   147
A. Altaf et al. (eds.), *EQUITY IN COVID-19*, EADI Global
Development Series, https://doi.org/10.1007/978-3-031-58588-3_7

space. A high debt profile further impeded the economic growth trajectory. As of the end of 2019, the total public debt portfolio stood at USD 84 billion (NGN 27.40 trillion). Nigeria's overdependence on crude oil also resulted in a gloomy revenue outlook for the year. To reflect the oil output cut by the Organisation of the Petroleum Exporting Countries (OPEC), in Q1 2020, the Nigerian crude oil production volume was revised from the 2.18 million barrels per day (mbdp) used to create the 2020 budget to 1.9 mbdp (Federal Ministry of Finance Budget & National Planning, 2020). This revision resulted in an estimated budget shortfall of about USD17 billion. Given these constraining factors, coupled with deteriorating terms of trade, the outlook for Nigeria's economy pre-COVID-19 was fragile (Federal Ministry of Finance Budget & National Planning, 2020).

In addition to its oil dependency, another essential feature of the Nigerian economy is its huge informal sector, which contributes 65% to GDP and, COVID-19, 80% of employment (ILO, 2020). PricewaterhouseCoopers (PwC) estimates that about 96% of all enterprises in the country are categorised as MSMEs, contributing 84% of national employment (PwC, 2020). The informal sector absorbs a disproportionate number of women, young workers, and migrants—all of whom face socio-cultural barriers that often place them in precarious economic conditions.

Inequality of educational opportunities and learning outcomes are also stark, and educational attainment is correlated with poverty incidence. Households headed by individuals with little or no education experience the highest depths of poverty in Nigeria (Ojowu et al., 2007). Despite an increase in school enrolment figures, with 9 out of 10 children enrolled in school (NPC, 2010), there are still 10.5 million children out of school, and more boys than girls are enrolled in school.

While Nigeria is the largest economy in Africa, poverty and inequality are pervasive. According to data from the National Bureau of Statistics, NBS (2019), 40% of the total population lives below the country's poverty line of USD381.75 (137 430 Naira) per year. Stark disparities exist between the rural and urban areas in Nigeria. In 2019, urban poverty was 18% compared to rural poverty of 52%. Income inequality is also high at a Gini coefficient of 35.1 with a ratio of 32. Eight in rural compared to 31.9 for urban areas.

Lack of access to basic infrastructure and services is a crucial driver of poverty in Nigeria. Access to electricity remains low at 45% (36% rural and 55% urban) and a paltry generating capacity of about 4000 MW

(USAID, 2020; World Bank, 2020a, 2020b, 2020c) with a current access rate of 45%. Even when there is access to electricity, electricity in Nigeria is erratic, and vulnerable households find it difficult to pay electric bills. Additionally, due to the exchange rate crises in Nigeria, it has become expensive to afford generators. For those households who own generators, fuel prices have increased significantly over the years, leading to reduced usage.

METHODOLOGY

This research draws on both primary and secondary research carried out between August and November 2020. The literature review provides the backdrop of the evolving socio-economic context in the following chapters. We culled data from the National Longitudinal Phone Survey (NLPS) 2020 (World Bank, 2020a, 2020b, 2020c) conducted jointly by the NBS and the World Bank to monitor, in real-time, the socio-economic effects of the COVID-19 crisis on households and individuals in Nigeria. A nationally representative sample of 1950 households was drawn from the selected households interviewed in the 2018/2019 General Household Survey-Panel (GHS-Panel). This survey provided detailed background information that we leveraged to assess the differential impacts of the pandemic in the country. The survey has been conducted monthly, beginning in April, with the survey questions revised monthly to accommodate the crises' evolving nature. For this report, we utilised data from the survey collected over three rounds—April/May, June, and July.

Primary data was collected to provide some depth to understanding the full socio-economic implications of the COVID-19 pandemic. The primary data collection aimed to understand better the impact of COVID-19 and the containment measures and restrictions implemented by the government and to assess the accessibility and impact of the mitigation measures on micro and small enterprises, the informally employed, and students, particularly the most vulnerable groups. We collected primary data through two methods: surveys/questionnaires and Focus Group Discussions (FGD).

The survey data were from the four states with federally imposed lockdowns—Abuja, Kano, Lagos, and Ogun. The field surveys were administered in rural and urban communities. Participants were interviewed using a structured questionnaire, including both open and closed-ended questions. The questionnaire's objective was to assess the gender context, social protection coverage, the potential for learning loss, and distance learning coverage deeply. Two separate questionnaires were administered, one channelled toward garnering information on the impact on the informal economy and the other on the basic education sector (primary and secondary schools). Therefore, we discuss the findings in individual sections in the following chapters. For both questionnaires, a purposive sampling technique was employed to select informants, including business owners and workers in the Micro, Small, and Medium Enterprises (MSME) sector, and parents, students, and teachers.

A cross-sectional technique was employed, and the interviews were conducted in person, using a Computer Assisted Interview (CAPI) method. For the NLPS survey, majority of the respondents worked in the agriculture sector (51.3% on average in the months of interest), followed distantly by workers involved in buying and selling (18% average) and personal services (15% average). To make up for this agricultural sector bias, the field survey covered a small percentage of agricultural sector workers (7%), focusing more on wholesale retail and trade (buying and selling, 56%). We also purposefully selected respondents who worked in sectors with substantial informal sector representation.

Cumulatively, we conducted four FDGs at two selected sites in Abuja—Mpape and Gishiri, two remote and rural areas in Abuja. The participants were all-women groups drawn from the communities, a cross-section of mothers, informal and micro-enterprises business owners or workers, and schoolteachers or owners.

Policy Responses to COVID-19 Health Crisis: Costs and Impacts

The first recorded case of COVID-19 in sub-Saharan Africa (SSA) occurred in Lagos State on February 27, 2020, (NCDC, 2020) when the health system was under stress. In June 2020, Nigeria's capacity for COVID-19 testing was about 2,500 samples daily (Dixit et al., 2020). However, only 50% of this capacity was utilised due to constraints in the availability of testing kits, laboratories, and human resources. As of June 30, 2020, only 0.07% of the Nigerian population had been tested for the virus—138,462 individuals in a population of 200 million. Before the outbreak, Nigeria had only 350 ventilators and 350 Intensive Care Unit (ICU) beds. However, in April 2020, 100 additional ventilators were acquired. An additional 200 ventilators were donated by the government of the United States of America (Federal Ministry of Health, 2020). Also, ICUs have been provided across various states in the six geopolitical zones of Nigeria (devex, n.d.).

To ensure a coordinated emergency response to the virus, in February 2020, a Level 3 Emergency Operations Centre (EOC) was activated by the Nigeria Centre for Disease Control (NCDC). Before the outbreak, the NCDC had established EOCs in 23 Nigerian states. These centres have continued to serve as the state level's coordination point since the confirmation of the first case. Furthermore, state governments established isolation centres to provide the necessary care and social distance for COVID-19 patients. The NCDC has also deployed rapid response teams across the states in Nigeria and has continued to work with and receive support from the African Centre for Disease Control, the World Health Organisation (WHO), and the West Africa Health Organisation (NCDC, 2020).

Furthermore, the Nigerian government provided grants to all the states in Nigeria and the FCT via the COVID-19 Preparedness and Response Project (CoPREP) to support the fight against the virus through containment and mitigation strategies. CoPREP aimed to improve the capacity for detecting the virus by providing technical expertise, diagnosis, and case management in the 36 states in Nigeria. It also aimed at strengthening response capacity through frontline healthcare workers' training, among other aims.

The swiftness of the responses perhaps limited the spread of infections in the country. Rapid Response Teams (RRT) were also deployed across the country, with individual states charged with lead contract tracing and other health response activities within their states. On the 9th of March, the Federal Government commissioned a Presidential Task Force (PTF) on COVID-19, which was supposed to work collaboratively with NCDC to provide crucial and uniform guidelines for dealing with the pandemic at the national level. Immediately, the PTF began issuing policy guidelines to control the virus's spread within the country. The measures include a federally Sanctioned lockdown implemented in the three states most affected states such as Lagos, Ogun, and the Federal Capital Territory, by the end of March, school closures, travel bans, closure of airports, and restrictions on interstate movement and border closures. The government made some exceptions to accommodate essential services to facilitate food movement within states and across the country.

FALLOUTS OF COVID-19 IN NIGERIA

Several fallouts of the COVID-19 measures are essential to note. The implementation and enforcement of the lockdown policy ultimately proved controversial and fatal in Nigeria. Security operatives, military and paramilitary personnel were drafted to execute the lockdown order in the Federal Capital Territory and several states with state-imposed lockdowns. Despite the increase in inter-agency cooperation between the police and other institutions, the enforcement of Phase 1 of the lockdown amplified existing challenges around human rights abuses and corruption within these institutions and the nation. Between March 30 and April 15, the first two weeks of the lockdown, eight reports of extrajudicial killings were directly related to the enforcement of the lockdown regulations, leading to eighteen deaths (Africanews, 2020a, 2020b, 2020c). Stark, when juxtaposed with the fact that the COVID-19 virus had led to only eleven deaths in the country (NHRC, 2020). Various human rights violations were reported during the monitoring period, induced by corruption, misuse/abuse of power, excessive use of force, and non-adherence to national and human rights laws. They include thirty-three instances of torture, degrading, and inhumane treatments, twenty-seven cases of breach of the right to the freedom of movement, unlawful detentions, and arrest, nineteen cases of unauthorised seizures/confiscation of properties, thirteen cases of bribery and extortion (profiteering from the lockdown), and sexual abuse (Odigbo et al., 2020; Obaji, 2020). The security agencies were also accused of profiteering from the lockdown by extorting money from motorists in exchange for passage at established checkpoints (The Guardian, 2020a).

In addition, there was an initial spike in crime and unrest in the affected lockdown states due to lockdown hardships and inmates' release from correctional facilities across all states (Odita, 2020). Within the first two weeks, 200 people were reportedly arrested on counts of robbing and raping young girls. The increase in local crime rates, especially in residential areas, resulted in impromptu vigilante groups springing up in residential areas as residents tried to secure themselves (Benson, 2020). There was also an increase in other forms of crime during the first month of the lockdown (Asimi, 2020). Intelligence from Interpol headquarters revealed that fraudsters had set up fraudulent websites, e-commerce platforms, and social media accounts claiming they retail COVID-19 medical products.

The incidence of domestic and gender-based violence also escalated. For example, in June 2020, Lagos state government-run Domestic and Gender Violence Response Team said it had been inundated with increased sexual and domestic violence reports since the lockdown began at the end of March (DSVRT, 2020). On average, the team received 13 new calls daily, and by the end of March, had 390 reports. Cumulatively, domestic violence, sexual violence, and physical child abuse cases increased by 60, 30, and 10%, respectively, compared to the months before the lockdown was implemented. Although the lockdown restrictions were relaxed in May, this upsurge persisted through the other phases of the lockdown, as many offices and schools stayed closed until September 2020. Additionally, people's financial difficulties during and beyond the complete lockdown contributed to the upsurge (Global Biosecurity, 2020).

COVID-19 and Job Losses

The lockdown measures led to the fall in economic activities across all industries and segments of the economy, causing a spike in unemployment rates. As of July 2020, the first three rounds of the NLPS 2020 survey revealed that since mid-March, 11% of the respondents had not engaged in any work, and 39%, 36% and 14% were able to return to work in April/May, June, and July respectively. Similarly, 27.5% of field survey respondents reported that they had experienced unemployment due to COVID-19, with 17% of the total respondents reporting that they were yet to find suitable employment at the time the surveys were conducted. In terms of sectors, 28.8% were in food services 11.6% were in wholesale and retail sectors. The NLPS 2020 survey shows that by June, 45% of Nigerians surveyed had stopped working.

At the household level, labour income losses were ubiquitous. Eighty percent of NLPS respondents reported some level of income loss. The decrease in household income was prominent for households engaged in non-farm activities. For the field survey, 93% of respondents reported an income decrease of at least 50% in current incomes. For informal sector respondents, this reflected 95% compared to 86% of formal sector respondents. All respondents operating in the agricultural, fishing, poultry, food service, construction, and domestic work sectors reported a decline in income. In all other sectors under review, above 90% of respondents reported a loss in individual and household incomes.

The findings from NLPS 2020 and the field survey reveal two things: First the compliance of Nigerians with the government's policies to curb the spread of the virus and second, for the people who were most affected by the pandemic, recovery has been slow. Although the partial reopening of the economy began in May 2020, the dampening effects of Phase 1 of the lockdown on the livelihoods persisted. According to the NLPS 2020, 56% of people with formal urban jobs had stopped working as of June 2020, compared to 40% of rural workers. Thirty percent of the field survey respondents who identified as employees in the informal sector revealed that they had experienced unemployment due to the lockdown, compared to 20% in the formal sector.

Furthermore, this is particularly dire for family-run businesses whose shutdown affects the members. Recovery was slow as 80% of respondents cited disruptions in supply chains as a significant constraint. Other essential factors to note are an increase in raw material and input costs, as was reported by 45% of survey respondents.

Youth were more vulnerable to job losses, and the most impoverished people were most susceptible to high-income losses. The age bracket of respondents with the highest unemployment due to the COVID-19 was youth between 18 and 25 years old. An overwhelming majority of respondents (90%) reported that their incomes had been severely affected since the lockdown. While all income groups reported a loss, those who fell in the first wealth quintile, less than the minimum wage of USD 78.70 (NGN 30,000), reported the most significant losses, at almost 80%.

Food insecurity issues were exacerbated during lockdown periods, and the effects have persisted. Though the significant lockdowns affected urban areas more than agricultural producing rural areas, restrictions on interstate movement, panic buying, and border closures caused bottlenecks in the food supply, driving up prices. According to NLPS 2020, more than 80% of the surveyed households could not purchase staple food during Phase 1 of the lockdown because of the lack of income. Fifty-one percent of field data respondents reported that their food consumption had substantially compared to the pre-COVID-19 period. Eight percent attributed this to lack of income, while 19% blamed it on food unavailability. The problem was exacerbated by food inflation which rose steadily between March and September. According to the Central Bank of Nigeria (CBN), food prices increased by 0.52 percentage points between July 2020 and August 2020 (CBN, n.d.). According to NLPS 2020, 85% of households experienced increased prices of staple foods, while 55% dealt with income shocks by consuming less food. All survey respondents had to adjust food consumption as a result.

During the lockdown phases, women were just as likely to lose their jobs and have their incomes affected as men. Most (97.5%) of female field survey respondents compared to males (93%) reported that the lockdown negatively affected their incomes. Similarly, 15% of females, compared with 12%, reported losing their jobs during the lockdown. However, the most significant impact of COVID-19 on women was the increased time spent providing unpaid care work. Even though the economy began to reopen in May 2020, schools remained closed until September 2020, which meant an increase in demand for childcare within homes. Women were disproportionately affected by the increased time spent doing unpaid care work. Many female participants during the FGD reported reducing their work hours or quitting their jobs or businesses to focus on childcare because schools were closed until mid-September. Many (75%) of all field survey respondents acknowledged an increase in the amount of time spent performing non-paid childcare, and the burden for providing care was on a female household member. Similarly, 74% of respondents reported that there was also an increase in the amount of time spent caring for an ill member of the household, and female household members provided 70% of the care. As a result, the recovery for women has been far slower than for men.

EDUCATION: IMPACTS ON ACCESS TO LEARNING FOR VULNERABLE STUDENTS

According to the United Nations Education, Scientific and Cultural Organisation (UNESCO), the shutdown of schools affected about 35.9 million (91%) primary and secondary school students in Nigeria. Out of these, over 91% are primary and secondary school learners (Adelakun, 2020), of which 84% were public school students (Obiakor & Adeniran, 2020). Aside from the missed learning opportunities, the school shutdowns have resulted in a more significant crisis for this group of vulnerable young students. For the most vulnerable young students, formal education provided more than basic educational needs; it provided these groups with daily meals, social protection, and other vital school-provided services.

The NLPS 2020 showed that the COVID-19 pandemic reduced children's learning opportunities. Over the three months in review, it was revealed that 38% of pre-pandemic in-school children did not engage in any educational activity for the last seven days preceding the survey. Moreover, educational activities were lower for poorer households (35%) than their wealthier counterparts (65%). Similarly, urban-based children reported more activities (70%) than their rural counterparts (48%).

The most significant barrier to learning was the lack of access to appropriate tools and infrastructure, which was the case for 84% of all students surveyed. Unavailability of resources and digital infrastructure (60%) and support/help (25%) constituted the main constraints to learning. Additionally, over 20% of the parents reported that their children either did not study during the school closures or did not study for up to an hour per day because the children had to be engaged in other income-generating activities to support their families. Lack of access to adequate nutrition also affected learning.

Mitigation Measures

One of the most immediate and predominant impacts of the COVID-19 policies in Nigeria was its impact on economic outcomes and society. However, the impacts continue to persist beyond the lockdown. Unfortunately, the first to bear the effect were vulnerable individuals, including students, women, micro and small enterprises, and daily wage earners operating in the formal and informal sectors. For these groups, the combined effects of the severity of the pandemic and the uncertainty of everyday normalcy deepened inequality and further entrenched poverty. To mitigate some of the socio-economic impacts, the Federal Government introduced a range of short-term interventions to absorb some of the shocks experienced by different social groups. Several ministries coordinated these efforts at the national level, in partnerships with state governments nationwide.

The income and livelihood support programmes include conditional cash transfer, social protection, in-kind support, a CBN USD 129.95 million (NGN50billion) credit facility and tax support for MSMEs. In terms of income support, on April 1st, the government announced a conditional cash transfer (CCT) programme of 51.58 USD (NGN 20,000) monthly for four months beginning in April and targeted the poorest and most vulnerable households (Obiakor, 2020). The CCT was an extension of an existing CCT program, introduced in 2016 as part of the President's Social Investment Program (SIP). The initial itera-tion of the CCT programme involved payments of 12.90 USD (NGN 5,000) paid bi-monthly to the poorest and most vulnerable people in Nigeria (primarily residing in rural areas), as identified in the National Social Register (NSR) (Sanni, 2020). The CCT is funded through three combined sources, namely recovered loot from Switzerland belonging to former president Sani Abacha (USD322million), credit from the Work Bank USD500million, and National SIP USD 1.289billion captured in the Federal government budget (Sanni, 2020).

A three-stage targeting process based on geographical targeting, community-based validation, and proxy-means-testing (PMT) was used to identify the poorest and most vulnerable households in the NSR (Okoye & Adeniran, 2020). Before COVID-19, the NSR contained 2.6 million households (Obiakor, 2020), covering a mere 2% of the over 80 million Nigerians living in extreme poverty. However, the government announced plans to expand the coverage by 1 million households during the first month of the lockdown; given the rural bias of the initial NSR, the following criteria were set for selecting the individuals/families to be included (Chafe, 2020):

- Urban low-income individuals/households with an account balance of USD 12.90 (NGN 5,000) or less.
- Individuals across Nigeria who regularly top up their mobile phones with between USD 0.26–0.52 (NGN 100–200).
- Daily wage earners and people who live with a disability.

Disbursement started in earnest on April 1, 2020. The Humani-tarian Affairs Ministry started the disbursement of 51.58 USD (NGN 20,000) to families registered in the NSR (Human Rights Watch, 2020). Despite this timeliness, the CCT programme underperformed regarding its comprehensiveness, targeting, and coverage.

The size, scope, and reach of the CCT were insignificant, given the scope of the problem. The total amount allocated per household was also inadequate to cover the basic needs for a family of five, the average number in a Nigerian home (World Bank, 2018). Additionally, the NSR, through which the fund recipients are determined, excludes most people living in extreme poverty in Nigeria. The NSR consists of about 11 million people from about 2.6 million households. Unfortunately, this does not begin to scrape the bottom of the barrel, especially as, pre-COVID-19 and the lockdown, it was estimated that around 87 million Nigerians lived in poverty (Kharas, Hamel & Hofer, 2018). The pandemic and ensuing movement restrictions likely increased the number of people in extreme poverty.

Heeding the public outcry that the NSR did not truly capture the most vulnerable people affected by the lockdown, on April 13, the government announced plans to expand the NSR by including an additional one million households based on the criteria mentioned above. However, the process was shrouded in mystery as the government failed to disclose any necessary details of the programme or the process of profiling new households. Confirmation of the expansion did not come till August 2020 (The Guardian, 2020c), when the ministry announced that the NSR had been expanded to 3.7 million households (15.5 million individuals) as of June 2020 (three months after the most profound impacts of the lockdown had been felt). However, in terms of reach and coverage, this expansion paled insignificance, as it only covered 19% of people living in poverty in Nigeria.

Secondly, there is the issue of poor targeting. The use of the NSR as the method for identifying the recipients of the CCT was uninformed. Their approach used the NSR to identify the poorest 30% of households in states with the highest poverty levels, the majority of which were not significantly impacted by the initial lockdown (Okoye & Adeniran, 2020). Since the lockdown affected the three most urbanised cities, this identification approach excluded the urban poor and informal sector workers who suffered the shocks in livelihoods due to the restrictions on movement (Okoye & Adeniran, 2020). Unfortunately, this population was largely excluded from the potential pool of beneficiaries.

Some other systematic issues also limited the program's effectiveness. Nigeria lacks a robust information management system, or comprehensive database on informal workers, making digital payments difficult. As a result, people had to receive the funds at physical locations; given the movement restrictions, many people in the NSR who were due to receive payments could not do so. On a governance level, the government did not make any announcements on crucial details of the intervention, limiting the scope for accountability. Additionally, no information is known about who is getting the money, and no data is collected on the national level on the impact of the transfers during the lockdown.

Fuel and electricity subsidies were other crucial social protection programmes implemented to mitigate the pandemic effect on the population. Fuel price was reduced from USD 0.37 to 0.32 (NGN 145–125) in March (Olisa, 2020) and USD 0.28 (NGN 108) in May. In April, the Nigerian Electricity Regulatory Commission (NERC) suspended the payment of the new electricity tariff scheduled to commence on April 2nd till 2021, citing the impact of COVID-19 as one of the reasons for the suspension (Nigerian Electricity Regulatory Commission, 2020). However, given that the electricity supply in Nigeria is low and erratic, the reductions were less likely to impact the poorest and most vulnerable households directly. About 97 million Nigerians are yet to connect to the electricity grid, of whom an overwhelming majority reside in rural areas or urban slums (Energy Central, 2020). Given the relationship between access to electricity and vulnerability, it is evident that the poor and vulnerable people were not the beneficiaries of these reductions. As with electricity, the poor and vulnerable consume relatively less fuel directly. Therefore, reducing fuel prices could only benefit them indirectly through other channels, such as reduced transportation costs or increased food security. However, given the unique challenges of COVID-19 and the ensuing lockdown, those channels were also affected by other market forces.

As of June 2020, the government removed the long-held price cap on the fuel prices (fuel subsidy), causing fuel prices to rise to a high of USD 0.43 (NGN 162) as of December 2020 (BBC, 2020). In September, the implementation of the new electricity tariffs, which were suspended in April, was reinstated. With the removal of the electricity subsidy, the electricity tariff increased from USD 0.079 (NGN 30.23) to USD 0.16 (NGN 62.23) for all consumers with an electricity supply above 12 hours per day. Fuel and electricity subsidies were removed due to the decline in government revenues over the year.

Temporary food supply to vulnerable groups was also implemented. On April 8, 2020, the Federal Government announced the distribution of 77,000 metric tons of food to vulnerable households in the three affected lockdown states (Obiakor, 2020). However, the distribution modalities were not precise at the time, and the process was impaired by low transparency and accountability (African Arguments, 2020). The lockdown led to a mass hunger crisis in Nigeria induced by reduced incomes, food shortages, and the hike in food prices. A survey conducted during the first week of the lockdown revealed that 72% of Nigerians were mainly concerned about the lockdown because of hunger (NOIPolls, 2020), 40% were worried that there would be a lack of food for the poor, 21% worried that people would die of hunger, and 5% worried that the cost of food would rise. Given the sheer scale of the crisis, 77,000 metric tons of food could not likely tend to the needs of a significant proportion of people that lacked adequate food. It was alleged at specific points that the food palliatives were hijacked by state politicians (Eranga, 2020). In October 2020, it was revealed that many state governments had been hoarding COVID-19 food palliatives. The loot was discovered when citizens overran several government-owned warehouses and found food meant to be distributed to households across many states in Nigeria during the lockdowns.

Finally, in response to housing and electricity challenges faced by vulnerable households during the pandemic, the government announced a USD 818.3 billion (NGN 317.29 billion) Mass Housing Program (MHP) (Olarewaju, 2020). The strategy was revealed to have two tracks. Track one involved building 300,000 homes across the country within a year, and track 2, was to leverage existing institutions to develop an additional 25,515 houses across the country within the same period (KPMG, 2020a). In addition, the programme also proposed installing Solar Home Systems (SHS) for 5 million households across Nigeria (Olarewaju, 2020). Funding for the MHP will be derived from the USD 5.93 billion (NGN2.3trillion) National Economic Sustainability Plan (a bouncing back plan for Nigeria) approved by the Federal Executive Council on June 24th. While well-conceived, these programmes had no immediate impact on people during the different phases of the lockdown, as they were not being delivered immediately.

There were stimulus packages for MSMEs such as loans, tax waivers, and loan term restructuring, among others. On March 23, the Central Bank of Nigeria (CBN) announced a targeted credit facility of USD 128.95 million (50 billion NGN) available for households and SMEs that were impacted by the pandemic (CBN, 2020). The credit facility was financed through the Micro, Small and Medium Enterprises Development Fund (MSMEDF). Through the fund, eligible households can access up to USD 7,737.06 (NGN 3million), while businesses can access up to USD 64,475.48 (NGN 24 million) (CBN, 2020). The CBN also announced regulatory forbearance for the restructuring loans, allowing a one-year moratorium for CBN intervention facilities, and granting leave to Other Financial Institutions (OFIs) to consider restructuring loan terms and tenor for businesses/households affected by the pandemic. A key strength of this credit was that the funds are available to businesses and households impacted by the COVID-19 induced restrictions and are gender-neutral. The credit facility avails up to USD 7737.06 (NGN3 million) each for low-income families and USD 64,475.48 (NGN25million) each for impacted businesses (CBN, 2020). However, the critical challenge was that this credit facility was targeted at the formal urban sector, having no impact on the informal sector.

The application procedures are, at best, limiting and, at worst, exclusionary. The lower literacy levels and access to banking services for poor households and businesses in the informal sector limit their access to formal credit facilities. The applications are made available through an online portal that requires all intending applicants to access a phone/computer and internet facilities and the know-how to navigate the portal. For the poorest and most vulnerable households and businesses, this limits their access to this opportunity. Additionally, the application is required to contain Bank Verification Numbers (BVN), business registration documents (for businesses), and a business plan with clear evidence of the adverse effects of the pandemic and the opportunity that the funding will provide—all considerable barriers for informal sector workers to access the package. The constraints raise several issues, mainly because obtaining a BVN requires access to a bank account, which only about 40% of Nigerians have. Getting a BVN also requires a valid form of national identification, which 21% (Salazar, 2018) of Nigerians (consisting of the most excluded and vulnerable) currently lack access to. The requirement of a business registration document immediately precludes informal sector businesses. The business plan aspect blurs channels of accountability, allowing individuals to be refused the loan based on someone's appraisal of their plan.

Finally, access to the loans also requires proof of collateral, such as property documents or moveable assets registered in the National Collateral Registry, and it is not interest-free. Communications around the availability of and access the loans are also insufficient, excluding many low-income households, businesses, and the informal sector.

The Federal Inland Revenue Services (FIRS) released a tax relief plan, which included delaying tax filing deadlines (KPMG, 2020b), waiving late returns penalty for personal or corporate income taxpayers who pay their tax liability early, suspension of field audits, 50% tax rebate to all Nigerian companies who retain their workers from 1 March to 31 December

2020, and leniency for taxpayers facing challenges in sourcing FOREX to settle their tax liability (KPMG, 2020c). However, for the tax waivers and rebates made available by FIRS, the benefits are available to businesses registered under the Companies and Allied Matters Act, accruing only to businesses in the formal sector, exhibiting another urban formal sector bias. While necessary and beneficial to formal sector business, this bill provides no support for informal sector businesses (who contribute 65% of Nigeria's total GDP and employ 80% of the labour force).

In March, the CBN announced the extension of USD 257.9million (NGN100 billion) credit facilities to equip businesses in the health sector to deal with the pandemic's challenges. Those eligible for this credit programme include health product manufacturers, health service providers, pharmaceutical and medical product distributors, and logistics services. The programme covers all products and services they provide, and the credit assistant is designed to run from April till December 31, 2030, (KPMG, 2020a). This scheme was funded by the CBN's Real Sector Support Facility-Differentiated Cash Reserves Requirement (RSSF-DCRR) (George Etomi & Partners, 2020). Pharmaceutical companies also received six-month import duty waivers on medical (KPMG, 2020d).

The health sector intervention highlights the urban formal sector bias of the interventions. Given that the health sector is an overly regulated and standardised field, and the informal sector is characterised by the absence of health insurance plans, credit assistance for the health industry, and import duty waivers for pharmaceutical firms did not accrue to the informal sector directly. Essentially, given the nature of informality in the country and the poor understanding of the make-up of the informal sector, the government did not/were unable to provide any support that was created directly to fit the landscape of informality and address the issues being faced.

The socio-economic impact of COVID-19 on the Nigerian education system limited over 35 million children from accessing learning. Before the pandemic, students attending public schools in Nigeria were granted daily access to meals provided by the federally-funded school-feeding programmes (Obiakor & Adeniran, 2020) introduced in 2016 as part of the government SIP to support feeding 24 million school children. According to the World Food Programme's estimate, in 2019, over 9 million students in over 40,000 public schools were provided with daily meals. In addition to feeding, this initiative also provides students access to essential health services such as immunisation. To mitigate this, the government continued the school-feeding programme during the school closures; the programme spent over NGN523.3 million (Federal Ministry of Education, 2020). However, there were no clear policies on its implementation and targeted beneficiaries.

Powered by UNESCO and the Universal Basic Education Commission (UBEC), the Federal Ministry of Education (FME) developed a Learn at Home Programme (LHP) geared toward reducing the effects of school closures on learning for Nigerian students. Through the LHP—in collaboration with educational technology companies—the FME developed virtual learning platforms, distributed links to e-learning resources, strengthened states' radio and television education programmes, and provided printed take-home materials for student activity books, worksheets, and assessment cards. The learning mitigation responses did not provide clear-cut actions on responding to learning disruptions for children or addressing the digital literacy and infrastructure divide.

IMPACTS, GAPS, AND CHALLENGES OF MITIGATION RESPONSE

While these mitigation measures show pro-poor concerns by national policymakers, an analysis of the modalities around the relief measures/mechanisms presents several gaps that hindered the equitability of the government's response. These obstacles revolve around the deficiencies and knowledge gaps inherent in the formation and implementation of the mitigation measures, resulting in poor access and impact for the people most affected by the COVID-19 shock. The poverty-targeted CCT was poorly targeted because its provision was skewed toward the rural households, who were less likely to be negatively affected by the lockdown's immediate impact than the urban poor, who were the first to feel the brunt of the lockdown. Despite increasing coverage by including more urban poor households in the NSR, the CCT only reached a minority of families (Okoye & Adeniran, 2020). No survey beneficiary accessed CCT.

Challenges with targeting also stem from limited information and data on the large informal sector in Nigeria. This deficiency complicates targeting support schemes to the most vulnerable during this crisis. It limits the government's ability to provide relief for individuals engaged in the undocumented informal economy. Therefore, most of the government's assistance schemes targeted the formal economy, providing limited coverage for informal economy workers. As a result of poor targeting, inherent weaknesses inadvertently create barriers that exclude the most vulnerable sections of the population. The majority (98%) of the field survey respondents who had reported knowing about government support mentioned that they could not access the support because the terms and conditions of the support were exclusionary. Those who met the eligibility criteria reported that the application process was demanding. The many bureaucratic access processes also meant that many poor women could not access them.

Another problem worth noting is the weaknesses in the delivery channel of programmes. This was especially pertinent in the education sector. The government's available distance learning modalities, including low-tech options (TV, radio), and high-tech options (online), posed challenges for ensuring inclusive and quality learning, given Nigeria's literacy levels and infrastructure challenges. The delivery system for the poverty-targeted support schemes was also inadequate due to inadequate information on intended beneficiaries, a lack of adequate database, and inadequate digital payment systems. For example, the CCT and food rations were disbursed in person at specified locations, beginning during the first week of the lockdown. On the one hand, given the strictness with which security officials enforced the lockdown, it would have been difficult to access the collection point at best, difficult and dangerous. On the other hand, this delivery method was prone to amplify the risk of disease transmission during collection.

Many of the support schemes implemented in response to COVID-19 were insufficient for meeting essential needs, supporting struggling households and businesses, or mitigating the learning loss induced by the school closures. For example, despite expanding the CCT, the benefits only accrued to only approximately 13% of the poorest individuals.

The lack of adequate consultation with stakeholders was another challenge to the programme delivery. While half of the respondents of the education questionnaire for the field survey acknowledged that they were aware of the government's various distance learning programmes, only 10% approved of their effectiveness. Also, 80% reported a lack of access to resources to support. Almost all respondents who acknowledged the government's provisions reported that the guidelines to co-opt available options were not helpful. Eighty per cent of respondents mentioned that the government did not provide access to any tools to support the distance learning measures they made available.

Majority of the teachers (90%), parents (93%) and students (90%) surveyed reported that their government did not involve them or engage in the decisions to close schools or during the process of developing a COVID-19 education contingency plan. The lack of consultation of critical stakeholders underpins power and accountability relations between decision-makers and the poorest and vulnerable people in society. Another reason for the inadequacy is the government's preparedness to deal with a crisis of this magnitude. One of the essential criticisms was that the government's response effort was the evidence of poor planning and the failure to consult and engage necessary stakeholders in developing their response strategy.

The pandemic and its policies also highlight the social contract and trust issues between citizens and the government. Most of the field survey respondents and FGD participants acknowledged that they trusted the government's initial response to close schools and ban movement was necessary to curb the virus's spread. However, as the months passed, there was evidence that some government actions have only served to erode the initial trust they might have built during the early phase of government policy response. Some key actions and events stand out. First, it is essential to note that Nigerians had low trust levels in their government before the pandemic. During the FGDs conducted in Abuja, one resounding comment was that the people had no government expectations as they had been disappointed multiple times. Instead, when asked for recommendations on what can be improved to ensure better access to social protection, all participants called on the private sector, civil society organisations, non-governmental organisations, and well-meaning Nigerians to devise ways to support them. Overall, citizens' trust in government declined even further.

CONCLUSION AND POLICY IMPLICATIONS

Globally, the COVID-19 pandemic has created one of the worst economic crises since the great depression, and the evidence points to the fact that the economic fallout will long outpace the health crisis. Economies worldwide face the adverse economic impact of the lockdown and a global economic slowdown. However, for Nigeria, the effect was intensified by a third factor, the decline in commodity prices that preceded the lockdown measures. Given the pre-COVID-19 conditions, with falling per capita income, high inflation, and an overdependence on oil, the pandemic has placed the nation at a critical juncture. The impacts of the pandemic are not short-term only but will endure. Overall, the crisis has unevenly impacted different segments of the population. The worst has been the poor in urban and rural areas, which are not the most covered with many programmes.

The pandemic has become a crisis of uneven and ephemeral responses. While the government quickly implemented several support schemes, the response has been chiefly inadequate and unevenly distributed. Social safety nets have primarily benefited the rural poor, while support schemes targeted toward businesses have wholly excluded the most vulnerable sector—MSMEs operating in the informal economy. There was no direct effort to target workers in this sector. This population's lack of social protection makes them especially vulnerable to shocks as they cannot count on protection provided by poverty-targeted support schemes or social insurance.

Additionally, the schemes have been transient, mostly stop-gap emergency responses that were not accompanied by adequate policy and institutional structures that provide long-term social protection for informal economy workers. There is no evidence that the government is picking the suitable lessons from the crisis, focusing on recovering the economy instead of revamping it to be more inclusive. In the absence of data, stakeholder dialogue is critical to garnering information. Unfortunately, they did not consult or get the necessary input from critical stakeholders or scheme users in forming and implementing the socio-economic support schemes. The government's poor use of evidence and inclusive social dialogue hindered its policy and mitigation responses.

The neutrality of mitigation strategies implemented to address the pandemic's socio-economic impacts could deepen poverty and inequality in Nigeria. The consequences are already evident and will continue to linger unless conscious action is taken. As the threat of a second wave looms, social protection must be built around any health responses. The COVID-19 crisis has revealed gaps in Nigeria's social protection systems and stressed the importance of developing robust national social protection systems, establishing social protection floors, and covering working in all forms of employment. The awareness of these gaps has created the impetus for policymakers to reflect on the space social protection should occupy in their socio-economic models. Longer-term strategies for extending social protection and support should be part of broader, integrated strategies to promote inclusive development. When developed and implemented correctly, social protection can contribute to more comprehensive recovery plans and policies that simultaneously address structural socio-economic weaknesses. While mobilising the resources will be difficult, the cost of inaction would be detrimental to the country. In this light, we recommend designing context-specific solutions to pandemic crises considering existing inequalities to provide inclusive solutions. For this to be effective, there is the need for a robust database of vulnerable citizens, particularly in its high informal sector. In addition, permanent physical, technological, and policy structures must be built to support the informal sector. Finally, for the listed recommendations to be approved by citizens, social dialogue between the state and citizens must be improved.

REFERENCES

AA. (2020). Nigeria: Madagascar's herbal cannot cure COVID-19. Retrieved from https://www.aa.com.tr/en/africa/nigeria-madagascars-herbal-drink-can not-cure-covid-19/1915948

Adelakun, I. S. (2020). Coronavirus (COVID-19) and Nigerian education system: Impacts, management, responses, and way forward. *Education Journal, 3*(4), 88–102. Retrieved from https://www.researchgate.net/pub lication/344115847_Coronavirus_COVID-19_and_Nigerian_Education_Sys tem_Impacts_Management_Responses_and_Way_Forward

Africanews. (2020c). Nigeria receives Madagascar's COVID-Organics, efficacy tests ordered. Retrieved from https://www.africanews.com/2020/05/17/ ecowas-rejects-covid-organics-madagascar//

Africanews. (2020b). Coronavirus is a product of evil: Boko Haram leader jabs Trump mocks social distancing. Retrieved from: https://www.africanews. com/2020/04/15/coronavirus-is-product-of-evil-boko-haram-leader-jabs-trump-mocks-social//

Africanews. (2020). *18 dead in the enforcement of Nigeria's COVID-19 lockdown.* https://www.africanews.com/2020/04/17/18-dead-in-enforcement-of-nigeria-covid-19-lockdown-report/

Allafrica (2020). *Nigeria: NBS - Only 18 Million Nigerians Have Access to Water, Sanitation.* Retrieved from https://allafrica.com/stories/202011120 208.html

Antai, D. (2010). *Social context, social position and child survival: Social determinants of child health inequalities in Nigeria'.* Department of Epidemiology, University of Stokholm.

Asimi, S. (2020). *In Nigeria, COVID-19 brings home the need for effective criminal justice complaint channels.* Retrieved from https://www.transpare ncy.org/en/blog/in-nigeria-covid-19-brings-home-the-need-for-effective-cri minal-justice-complaint-channels

BBC. (2020). 'Fuel price in Nigeria: Goment reduce money to N162.44 per litre'. Retrieved from:https://www.bbc.com/pidgin/tori-55227380

Benson, E.A. (2020). *Lagosians groan as criminals terrorise neighbourhoods during Covid-19 lockdown*. Retrieved from https://nairametrics.com/2020/04/13/lagosians-groan-as-criminals-terrorise-neighbourhoods-during-covid-19-lockdown/

Energy Central. (2020). Electricity: 97 Million Nigerians Yet To Connect To Grid. Retrieved from: https://energycentral.com/news/electricity-97-million-nigerians-yet-connect-grid

Central Bank of Nigeria. (2020). *Guidelines for the Implementation of the N50 Billion Targeted Credit Facility*. Retrieved from https://www.cbn.gov.ng/Out/2020/FPRD/N50%20Billion%20Combined.pdf

Central Bank of Nigeria (n.d.). Inflation Rates (Percent). Retrieved from https://www.cbn.gov.ng/rates/inflrates.asp

Chafe, I. (2020). 3 classes of Nigerians to benefit from Buhari's cash transfer: Minister. Retrieved from https://www.pmnewsnigeria.com/2020/04/15/3-classes-of-nigerians-to-benefit-from-buharis-cash-transfer-minister/

devex(n.d.). *Coalition against COVID-19 (CACOVID)*. Retrieved from https://www.devex.com/organizations/coalition-against-covid-19-cacovid-150517

Dixit, S., Ogundeji, Y. K. & Onwujekwe, O. (2020). How well has Nigeria responded to COVID-19?. The center for policy impact in global health. Retrieved from https://centerforpolicyimpact.org/2020/07/28/how-well-has-nigeria-responded-to-covid-19/

Domestic and Gender Violence Response Team(2020). https://dsvrtlagos.org

Ehanire, D. (2020). *Nigeria Centre for Disease Control*. Retrieved from https://ncdc.gov.ng/news/227/first-case-of-corona-virus-disease-confirmed-in-nigeria

Eranga, I. O. (2020). COVID-19 Pandemic in Nigeria: Palliative measures and the politics of vulnerability. *International Journal of Maternal and Child Health and AIDS*, 9(2), 220–222. Retrieved from https://www.researchgate.net/publication/342813156_COVID-19_Pandemic_in_Nigeria_Palliative_Measures_and_the_Politics_of_Vulnerability

Federal Ministry of Health. (2020). COVID-19: US donates 200 life saving ventilators to Nigeria. Retrieved from https://www.health.gov.ng/index.php?option=com_k2&view=item&id=739:covid-19-us-donates-200-life-saving-ventilators-to-nigeria

Federal Ministry of Education. (2020). *Education Coordinated COVID-19 Response Strategy*. Retrieved from https://education.gov.ng/education-coordinated-covid-19-response-strategy/

Federal Ministry of Finance Budget and National Planning, Nigeria. (2020). *2021–2023 Medium Term Expenditure Framework and Fiscal Strategy*

Paper. Retrieved from https://www.budgetoffice.gov.ng/index.php/2021-2023-mtef-fsp?task=document.viewdoc&id=814

Forbes. (2020). Terrorist organizations use COVID-19 lockdown to expand territory. Retrieved from: https://www.forbes.com/sites/ewelinaochab/2020/05/18/terrorist-organizations-use-covid-19-lockdown-to-expand-territory/?sh=31a3381454bb

Fouda, L. (2020). *IMF Staff Concludes Article IV Consultation to Nigeria*. Retrieved from https://www.imf.org/en/News/Articles/2020/02/17/pr2053-IMF-Staff-Concludes-Article-IV-Consultation-to-Nigeria

George Etomi and Partners. (2020). *CBN N100 Billion Credit Support Scheme for the Healthcare Sector*. Lexology. Retrieved from https://www.lexology.com/library/detail.aspx?g=5422d349-6aef-4e2a-8332-6800c3db8805

Global biosecurity. (2020). Domestic violence amid the COVID-19 lockdown: a threat to individual safety. Retrieved from: https://jglobalbiosecurity.com/articles/https://doi.org/10.31646/gbio.94/

Human Rights Watch. (2020). Nigeria: Protect Most Vulnerable in COVID-19 Response. Retrieved from: https://www.hrw.org/news/2020/04/14/nigeria-protect-most-vulnerable-covid-19-response

International Labour Office, Geneva. (2020). *Women and men in the informal economy: A statistical picture*. Retrieved from https://www.wiego.org/sites/default/files/publications/files/Women%20and%20Men%20in%20the%20Informal%20Economy%203rd%20Edition%202018.pdf

International Monetary Fund. (n.d.). Nigeria. Retrieved from https://www.imf.org/en/Countries/NGA

Kharas, H., Hamel, K., & Hofer, M. (2018). *The start of a new poverty narrative*. Brookings. Retrieved from https://www.brookings.edu/blog/future-development/2018/06/19/the-start-of-a-new-poverty-narrative/

KPMG. (2020b). Nigeria: *Extended deadline for filing Lagos State tax returns (COVID-19)*. Retrieved from https://home.kpmg/us/en/home/insights/2020/05/tnf-nigeria-extended-deadline-for-filing-lagos-state-tax-returns-covid019.html

KPMG. (2020c). *Nigeria: Tax relief, responding to coronavirus (COVID-19)*. Retrieved from https://home.kpmg/us/en/home/insights/2020/03/tnf-nigeria-tax-relief-responding-to-coronavirus.html

KPMG. (2020a). *Government and institution measures in response to COVID-19*. Retrieved from https://home.kpmg/xx/en/home/insights/2020/04/nigeria-government-and-institution-measures-in-response-to-covid.html

KPMG. (2020d). Nigeria: Medical supplies exempted from VAT and import duty (COVID-19). Retrieved from https://home.kpmg/us/en/home/insights/2020/05/tnf-nigeria-medical-supplies-exempted-from-vat-and-import-duty-covid-19.html

National Bureau of Statistics. (2019). *Poverty and Inequality in Nigeria*. Retrieved from https://nigerianstat.gov.ng/download/1092

Nigeria Centre for Disease Control. (2020). *First Case Of Coronavirus Disease Confirmed In Nigeria*. Retrieved from https://ncdc.gov.ng/news/227/first-case-of-corona-virus-disease-confirmed-in-nigeria

Nigeria Centre for Disease Control. (2020). 100 Days of Nigeria COVID-19 Response. Retrieved from https://ncdc.gov.ng/news/253/100-days-of-nigeria-covid-19-response

Nigerian Electricity Regulatory Commission. (2020). *NERC Order on the Transition to Cost Reflective Tariffs in the Nigerian Electricity Supply Industry*. Retrieved from https://nerc.gov.ng/index.php/component/remository/NERC-Orders/NERC-Order-On-The-Transition-To-Cost-Reflective-Tariffs-In-The-Nigerian-Electricity-Supply-Industry/?Itemid=591

NOIPolls. (2020). COVID-19 Poll Result Release. Retrieved from https://noipolls.com/covid-19-poll-result-release-2/

Obaji, P. (2020). *Women 'abused' by police enforcing COVID-19 rules in Nigeria*. Retrieved from https://www.aljazeera.com/features/2020/9/9/women-abused-by-police-enforcing-covid-19-rules-in-nigeria

Obiakor, T., & Adeniran, A. (2020). *COVID-19: Impending situation threatens to deepen Nigeria's education crisis*. Centre for the Study of the Economies of Africa. Retrieved from https://media.africaportal.org/documents/COVID19-Impending-Situation-Threatens-to-Deepen-Nigerias-Education-.pdf

Obiakor, T. (2020). *COVID-19 and the Informal Sector in Nigeria: The Socio-Economic Cost Implications*. Centre for the Study of the Economies of Africa. Retrieved from http://cseaafrica.org/covid-19-and-the-informal-sector-in-nigeria-the-socio-economic-cost-implications/

Odigbo, B., Eze, F., & Odigbo, R. (2020). COVID-19 Lockdown controls and Human Rights abuses: The Social Marketing implications. *Emerald Open Research*. https://doi.org/10.35241/emeraldopenres.13810.1

Odita, S. (2020). *Why crime rate may rise after COVID-19*. https://guardian.ng/news/why-crime-rate-may-rise-after-covid-19/

Debt Management Office, Nigeria. (2020). *Nigeria's Total Public Debt Portfolio as of December 31, 2019*. Retrieved from https://www.dmo.gov.ng/debt-profile/total-public-debts/3123-nigeria-s-total-public-debt-stock-as-at-december-31-2019/file

Ojowu, O., Bulus, H., & Omonona, B. (2007). Nigeria Poverty Assessment'. www.pak-nigeria.org/pdfs/24_Nigeria_Poverty_Assessment_2007_Table_of_Contents_Executi.pdf

Okoye, D., & Adeniran, A. (2020). *Effective Targeting of COVID-19 Aid in Nigeria*. Centre for the Study of the Economies of Africa. Retrieved from http://cseaafrica.org/effective-targeting-covid-19-aid-in-nigeria/

Olarewaju, T. (2020). *Nigeria's post-COVID-19 recovery plan has some merit. But it misses the mark*. The Conversation. Retrieved from https://theconversation.com/nigerias-post-covid-19-recovery-plan-has-some-merit-but-it-misses-the-mark-140974

Olisa, C. (2020). Update: FG approves reduction in pump price of petrol to N125. Retrieved from https://nairametrics.com/2020/03/18/fg-approves-reduction-in-pump-price-of-petrol/

NM Partners. (2020). *Logistics in Nigeria: keeping soul of e-Commerce operational during COVID-19 pandemic.* Retrieved from https://nairametrics.com/2020/04/14/logistics-in-nigeria-keeping-the-soul-of-e-commerce-operational-during-covid-19-pandemic/

Presidency, Federal Republic of Nigeria. (2020). *The Quarantine Act (CAP Q2 LFN 2004).* https://covid19.ncdc.gov.ng/media/archives/COVID-19_REGULATIONS_2020_20200330214102_KOhShnx.pdf

Presidential Task on Covid-19 (n.d.). *Implementing Guidance for Lockdown Policy.* Retrieved from https://covid19.ncdc.gov.ng/media/archives/PTF-COVID-19-Guidance-on-implementation-of-lockdown-policy-FINAL.docx-2.pdf

Salazar, D. (2018). *Why is Financial Inclusion in Nigeria Lagging Compared to Its African Peers?.* Center for Financial Inclusion. Retrieved from https://www.centerforfinancialinclusion.org/why-is-financial-inclusion-in-nigeria-lagging-compared-to-its-african-peers

Sanni, K. (2020). Nigerian govt pays N20,000 to 5000 Abuja households—Minister. Retrieved from https://www.premiumtimesng.com/news/top-news/385440-nigerian-govt-pays-n20000-to-5000-abuja-households-minister.html

The Guardian. (2020c). FG enrolls 15.5m persons in National Social Register. Retrieved from: https://guardian.ng/news/fg-enrolls-15-5m-persons-in-national-social-register/

The Guardian. (2020a). 'How police, military extort at COVID-19 checkpoints'. Retrieved from: https://guardian.ng/news/how-police-military-extort-at-covid-19-checkpoints/

The Guardian. (2020b). 'IGP alerts Nigerians to emerging crimes over COVID-19'. Retrieved from:https://guardian.ng/news/nigeria/national/igp-alerts-nigerians-to-emerging-crimes-over-covid-19/

United Nations. (2020). *The COVID-19 Pandemic In Nigeria: Impact On Crime, Security And The Rule Of Law.* Retrieved from https://nigeria.un.org/en/49557-covid-19-pandemic-nigeria-impact-crime-security-and-rule-law-brief-10-june-15-2020

USAID. (2020). *Nigeria Energy Sector Overview.* Retrieved from https://www.usaid.gov/powerafrica/nigeria#:~:text=Nigeria%20is%20endowed%20with%20large,4%2C000%20MW%2C%20which%20is%20insufficient

World Food Programme. (2019). *The impact of school feeding programmes.* Retrieved from https://docs.wfp.org/api/documents/WFP-0000102338/download/

World Poverty Clock. (2020). *Nigeria*. Retrieved from https://worldpoverty.io/map

World Bank. (2020). COVID-19 national longitudinal phone survey 2020. *National Bureau of Statistics*. Retrieved from https://microdata.worldbank.org/index.php/catalog/3712/related-materials

World Bank. (2020a). *Access to Electricity, Rural and Urban (% of Urban Population)*. Retrieved from https://data.worldbank.org/indicator/EG.ELC.ACCS.UR.ZS?locations=NG, https://data.worldbank.org/indicator/EG.ELC.ACCS.RU.ZS?locations=NG

World Bank. (2020b). *Individuals using the Internet (% of Population)*. Retrieved from https://data.worldbank.org/indicator/IT.NET.USER.ZS

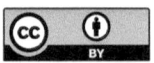

PART II

East and Southern Africa

CHAPTER 8

Ethiopia

Kassa Teshager and Tesfaye C. Cholo

INTRODUCTION

Ethiopia, Africa's second most populated country, announced its first confirmed COVID-19 on March 13, 2020. The pandemic hit the country at the time it was experiencing mixed socioeconomic fortunes. The country had an estimated population of 115 million people in 2019 (United Nations, 2019). Regarding geographical spread, the population is mainly rural, with only 21% urban dwellers. The sex composition of the population was even (Statista, 2020a).

Ethiopia's two-digit growth figures in the last decade are unevenly distributed, making equity in economic gains a key concern. According to the World Bank database, the mean economic growth was 10.5% between 2012 and 2018, driven by agricultural growth, according to the National Bank of Ethiopia (NBE). However, the agriculture sector's contribution to GDP growth has dwindled, with services taking the lead with

K. Teshager (✉) · T. C. Cholo
Department of Development Economics, Ethiopian Civil Service University,
Addis Ababa, Ethiopia
e-mail: ktshger@yahoo.com; kteshager@yahoo.com

T. C. Cholo
e-mail: tesfaye.chofana@ecsu.edu.et

A. Altaf et al. (eds.), *EQUITY IN COVID-19*, EADI Global Development Series, https://doi.org/10.1007/978-3-031-58588-3_8

a 40% share of GDP. The agricultural sector's share was 33% in 2019 (NBE, 2019). This notwithstanding, the agriculture sector employed 67% of the population in 2019.[1] Despite the substantial share of agriculture to income and employment, the sector is vulnerable to climate change impacts with long spells of droughts (Deressa, 2007). Yet, the pandemic impact on the agricultural sector was minimal compared to industry and service sectors (Degye et al., 2020).

Ethiopia's labour force participation rate was 79.6% in 2020. More men (85.8%) than women(73.56%) participated in the labour market in 2020 (ILO, 2020). With a 3% and 3.5% unemployment rate, women and youth were more likely to be unemployed (ILO, 2020). The pandemic measures that restricted mobility worsened the existing unemployment condition in the country with increased job losses in the early stages of the pandemic (Degye et al., 2020). However, the effect was unequally distributed across economic activities, geographic location, and social groups.

In 2015, 23.5% of Ethiopia population lived below the national poverty line. However, the global poverty headcount ratio is still significantly high. The population living on less than $5.5, $3.2, and $1.9 daily at international prices, respectively, were 90.7, 26.8, and 9.4% (World Bank, 2019). Although over 79% of the population working in the agricultural sector lives in rural areas, total undernourishment was 20.6% from 2016 to 2018 in Ethiopia, and the prevalence of wasting in children under age five was 10% and was the highest in Africa in 2018 (FAO et al., 2019). Child and maternal malnutrition is also high in Ethiopia; for example, 38% of children under five were stunted, 24% were underweight, and 22% of women aged 15–49 were thin with a BMI under 18.5 (WHO, 2016). It is important to note that since the agricultural sector is not insured, the coronavirus crisis is an additional bottleneck to agricultural-dependent countries like Ethiopia.

Ethiopia's health indicators show it was not ready for a pandemic, and this realisation determined its swift COVID-19 responses. The country falls below the continental average healthcare system with 0.8 midwives and nurses, 0.08 physicians, and 0.3 hospital beds in 2015—only 11.2% of its population access potable water. In terms of sanitation, 4.2% of rural people used at least one essential sanitation services in 2017. The study

---

[1] https://data.worldbank.org/indicator/sl.agr.empl.zs?locations=et

situates COVID-19 policies in Ethiopia's political and socioeconomic performance to examine their equity and inclusiveness dimensions.

METHODOLOGY

The study employed a mixed method design that combined quantitative and qualitative data to examine the equity in Ethiopia's COVID-19 mitigation and policy responses. This case study was mainly desk research based on secondary sources from national institutions, including the Ethiopian Public Health Institute, Ministry of Health, Ministry of Education, Ministry of Water and Energy, Ministry of Labor and Social Affairs, Ministry of Technology and Innovation and Ministry of Women, Children and Youth, Ethiopia Central Statistical Agency, eight Regional Health Bureaus and two city administrations (or Addis Ababa and Dire Dawa cities). Due to security problems the Tigray region was not considered in the study. The study also relied on statistics from the WHO, John Hopkins University, and the Africa Centre for Disease Control. Primary data were collected through key informant interviews in institutions. The interviews were conducted via Zoom, telephone, and in-person. National and local policies, rules, and regulations were also analysed. The analysis also culled data from the World Bank's three rounds of a telephone survey. The first-round survey was conducted between April 22 and May 13, 2020, and covered 3249 people. The second-round survey was conducted between May 14 and June 3, 2020, with 3 107 respondents. The third survey round was conducted between 4 and 26 June 2020 and had 3058 respondents.

POLICY RESPONSES TO COVID-19 IN ETHIOPIA

Despite severe economic constraints, Ethiopia took swift and bold measures in response to COVID-19 which relied on three foundations namely, solidarity and collaboration among stakeholders, coordination of resource mobilisation and the continuity of socioeconomic service delivery to the population Lia (2020). The Ethiopian government's response evolved over the period depending on the threat at stake. However, its responses can be categorised into three broad areas: public health, social, and economic interventions.

The first public health measures hinged on restrictions on movement, which covered the closure of schools, borders, and public places. The government declared a five-month state of emergency (SoE) (Proc. 3/ 2020) on April 8, 2020, and an executive task force was established. An implementation guideline was developed to implement the protocols. It provided the federal government sweeping powers to limit individual rights in favour of public health and security. The SoE transferred the ultimate government decision-making power to the Cabinet. The regulation (Regulation 466/2020) prohibited religious, government, social, or political meetings in places of worship, public institutions, hotels, meeting halls, or any other place. The regulation also prohibited regional or federal officials from giving statements to members of the press about COVID-19 without first obtaining permission from the federal committee or sub-committees at the regional level. However, exceptions were made for professional commentary on COVID-19 laws, professional medical explanations, or daily press briefings by the Ministry of Health. The regulation also prohibited disseminating information about COVID-19 and related issues that would cause "terror and undue distress among the public". The regulation requires public communication professionals and media outlets to ensure that information, analysis, or programmes on COVID-19 were "without exaggeration, appropriate and not prone to cause panic and terror among the public".

The key informants said that declaring a state of emergency improved compliance with COVID-19 protocols such as wearing nose masks, social distancing, and other hygiene protocols. Unlike some countries in the region, Ethiopia did not undergo a full lockdown. Movement across regional states was permitted and humanitarian organisations, and cargos were permitted to operate without restrictions. The measures were scaled up gradually through an assessment of their impacts.

The government postponed the national election to May 2021, which was scheduled for August 2020. The House of Federation agreed on the rescheduling following extensive research and expert consultation. However, the Tigray region held a regional election by rejecting the parliament's decision.

Public Health and Social Measures

Public health and social measures were instituted to break the chain of transmission of the virus. The key strategies included awareness raising on the pandemic and preventive measures. As the health sector strategy of the country focused on prevention via primary healthcare provision, public awareness regarding the nature of COVID-19, its symptoms, transmission, and treatment was crucial. Goshu et al. (2020), who assessed the level of public awareness of COVID-19 mitigation measures, confirmed that knowledge of the pandemic was high in the country's rural and urban areas. For example, over 83% of rural people and 95% of urban households were knowledgeable about the basic COVID-19 hygiene protocols. Moreover, over 61% of rural and 77% of urban people knew masks or gloves could prevent infections.

The Ethiopian government received support from the WHO, Africa CDC, and Jac Ma Foundation to intensify contact tracing. Under the State of Emergency (Proclamation No 3/320), the government enforced social distancing, encouraging people to stay two metres from each other in all their essential activities. However, there were barriers to social distancing measures. For example, the limited number of sleeping rooms per household illustrates the difficulty of self-isolation. Also, limited access to electricity restricted access to COVID-19 prevention messages disseminated on various channels.

EDUCATION MEASURES

Following the first case confirmation on March 13, 2020, the government of Ethiopia officially announced the closure of schools, including Kindergarten to Higher Education, on March 16, 2020. The Ministry of Science and Higher Education (MoSHE) quickly shifted its focus to Virtual Learning Platforms (VLPs). The Ministry developed a concept note for the education sector's COVID-19 preparedness and response plan on April 3, 2020. The objective of the response plan was to ensure the continuity of learning at all levels while schools were closed. The strategies included using digital technology such as e-learning for secondary education and multi-media channels (e.g., radio and television) for primary schools. It was, however, evident that online learning was constrained by connectivity to the internet, access to electricity, skills in technology use, availability of devices (e.g., computers, radio, TV, laptops and mobile), monitoring of actual online learning, and poor quality of education. As a result, most private schools in urban localities found temporary solutions to continue teaching their students from a distance by uploading reading materials and assignments via Google Meet, Telegram, e-mail, and social media platforms.

SOCIAL PROTECTION MEASURES

The government instituted social protection measures to protect vulnerable social groups such as the elderly, migrants, refugees, homeless children, adults, people with disabilities, and poor people. For example, the Ministry of Labour and Social Affairs (MoLSA) in partnership with private individuals provided transitory shelters for urban destitute street children in partnership with private donors. MoH, MoLSA, and donors first identified the vulnerable groups based on their age, gender, socioeconomic status, and marginalisation. They also designated medical care and food for disabled people.

MoLSA's annual report showed that it supported 45,000 vulnerable people and out of these 24,003 were reunited with their families. About 21 136 Ethiopian returnees from various countries received support, including reintegration into their families and communities. MoLSA provided food, sanitation, and counselling support to 743,949 vulnerable people (e.g., old people, the disabled, the homeless, and prostitutes) across the country. Moreover, 1,285,134 urban and rural developmental safety net beneficiaries received a three-month advance payment. The Ethiopian Federation of National Associations of Persons with Disabilities mobilised 17 million Birr from development partners and provided food and sanitation assistance to 5000 people with disabilities. Ethiopia's Productive Safety Net Program covers over eight million beneficiaries. Due to the pandemic, the public works requirement was waived, and thus all beneficiaries received unconditional transfers. At the onset of the pandemic, beneficiaries also received three months of payments in advance. Besides the PSNP, several smaller-scale initiatives, such as food banks, were launched to support the vulnerable (Abate et al., 2020).

ECONOMIC POLICY RESPONSES

The Government of Ethiopia has launched various economic measures, including tax exemption, cancellation of tax debts and property tax, employment tax reduction, injecting liquidity to private and government banks, loan rescheduling and additional loans to their businesses, various stimulus packages, and employment measures.

The cancellation of tax debts was among economic measures to sustain livelihood and businesses after the pandemic. Debts cancellation was one of some of the economic stimulus packages. A 10% reduction was given to firms that pay debt upfront. Regional governments also cancelled employment tax for four months.

The Central Bank of Ethiopia injected 15 billion Birr (or 0.45% of GDP) to private banks to allow banks to reschedule debt payments and interest reduction to firms without making a loss. The government also provided 33 billion in additional liquidity to the Commercial Bank of Ethiopia (Goshu et al., 2020). In addition, the government injected the liquidity of 1.5 billion Birr to farmers cooperatives to maintain the supply chain after the outbreak. Furthermore, the Development Bank of Ethiopia established a unique window to dispense micro and small-scale enterprises (MSES) loans quickly. In addition, the National Bank of Ethiopia provided additional liquidities to microfinance institutions to avail credit to borrowers. The government also supported microfinance institutions, farmers cooperatives, and some selected sectors. For instance, Ethiopian Airlines have had to implement new cost-cutting measures to secure its cash flow and revise its strategy from growth to survival.

The government also forbade public and private companies to lay off workers under a state of emergency. The Ethiopian tripartite constituents namely labour confederations, employers, and the government signed an agreement on the COVID-19 workplace response protocol on measures to be taken against the anticipated challenges of the pandemic on the economy and labour relations. The MoLSA protocol was consistent with ILO guidelines on crisis response and managing natural and artificial disasters. MOLSA monitored private employers and public enterprises and petitions of workers from 366 organisations by opposing layoffs, denial of wages and pay cuts and reinstated 12,004 workers.

One of the measures that made the Ethiopian approach unconventional was the focus on transporting food commodities. The transport ministry identified critical commodities and ensured uninterrupted agricultural commodity exchanges—farmer-to-farmer exchange, primary (farm gate), and secondary and tertiary agricultural commodity aggregation and distribution systems. In addition, efforts were put in place to ensure uninterrupted supplies of chemical fertilisers, improved seeds, pesticides, herbicides, and livestock medicine.

The Role of Non-state Actors in COVID-19 Intervention

The role of non-state actors such as the private sector, membership organisations, non-governmental organisations, and international organisations was significant in Ethiopia and as diverse as the sectors and the regions of the country in its forms, scope, and reach. The Ethiopian private sector remains adaptive in its response to the crisis. However, the engagement of the private sector goes beyond corporate social responsibility (CIPE, 2020). For example, following the government's request to contribute to the National COVID-19 Response Fund, the private sector contributed cash and in-kind to control the outbreak's spread.

Some private businesses have also contributed to shifting their production line to COVID-19 intervention demand following the requests of MOE. The demand for certain products, such as hand sanitisers, face masks, personal protective equipment (PPE), and other goods, was urgently required. In addition, enterprises such as hotels and banks promoted and deployed online services. They also embarked on remote working arrangements and safety protocols at work.

With the global value chain disruption and a slowdown in international trade, many companies partially closed down their facilities. Some enterprises have decided to close their doors, sending staff on paid leave for an indefinite period. As aggregators of private sector interests and critical agencies of advocacy, Business Membership Organizations (BMOs) play an essential role in the fight against the COVID-19 pandemic. Business chambers and associations are taking on various roles in this regard. For more detailed roles of BMOs since the pandemic.

Many international and local NGOs have been involved in COVID-19 policy interventions in various ways. For example, HOPE, a US-based NGO, provided over 56,000 protective masks to Ethiopia and virtual training for healthcare workers on COVID-19. Another NGO closely working with the federal ministry of health in COVID-19 intervention is 'Lifebox', an NGO that has made two innovative contributions in Ethiopia namely N95 mask decontamination and medical equipment reuse and maintenance (Starr et al., 2020). Lifebox, Tegbareid Polytechnic College (PC), and Ethiopia COVID-19 Response Team (ECRT) consisting more than 1,800 professionals worked together in areas of patient monitoring systems. They also repaired existing medical devices in healthcare facilities in the country.

According to key informants, some regions and sectors have gotten relatively better support from NGOs, but others did not. Specifically, WHO and Africa CDC have contributed significantly to the Ethiopian health sector by donating COVID-19 lab testing equipment and providing Lab training. ILO supported BoLSA in awareness creation to manufacturing and textile industries in Hawassa and Mekelle, Refugee and hosting communities in Somalia and Tigray regions and Ethiopian migrant domestic workers in major destination countries in the Middle East. An Irish Emergency Alliance worked with Plan International to support the government in pandemic awareness creation. The World Bank, IMF, WFP, IOM, and UNICEF provided financial support, while the Jack Ma Foundation provided various health kits and PPE.

INCLUSIVENESS OF POLICY RESPONSES

Participants have contradicting views on the social inclusiveness of the policy measures in Ethiopia. MoLSA provided direct support to 45,000 street children, food, and sanitation support to 743,949 vulnerable people, 21 136 returnees to Ethiopia, and about 13,863 detainees to their homelands with the necessary logistics from abroad. BoLSA also provided counselling and support services to 29,654 people with various addictions and three-month advance payment support to 1,285,134 safety net beneficiaries, and food and hygiene support to 600,000 disabled people. However, reaching the needy was a big challenge due to resource capacity.

Regarding education sector strategies, delivery techniques used during school closures were not inclusive. The coverage of radio and TV instructions was not only limited but also interrupted by power cuts in small towns and rural areas. Access to the virtual learning platforms also depended on access to the technologies and gadgets which low-income families, households in rural areas, and disabled children in poor households do not always have. Student with vision impairment, and their parents reported that students could not take part in TV programmes involving practical activities. As a result, talking textbooks were provided to visually impaired students in the Tigray Region to address the problem of access to virtual learning materials. Participants in key informant interviews confirmed that due to the COVID-19 pandemic school closures, there was significant learning loss and huge inequalities against disadvantaged segments of the population. There were already pre-COVID-19 inequalities in access to quality education between children in urban and rural localities and children from various socioeconomic backgrounds. The primary purpose of the instruction methods designed during school closure was not to give access to students but to reduce anxieties and to send students who were not ignored back to school when the spread of the virus has reduced.

The pandemic also had health effects on non-pandemic patients. In some regions, home deliveries increased as expectant mothers could not easily access health facilities due to restriction mandates. The pandemic also decreased the number of people visiting hospitals for diagnosis. For example, diagnosis of malaria, measles, and other frequently occurring diseases decreased as resources were dedicated to the pandemic. The regional health Bureaus established the COVID-19 diagnosis team and other diseases team to address the inequity. Some regions deployed quarantine at home, but later experts noted that the strategy was not feasible for larger family size households, particularly the poor with insufficient room numbers. However, poor room households were transferred to public quarantines to address the challenge.

ECONOMIC INCLUSIVENESS

In terms of economic inclusiveness, the economic policy measures were inclusive, according to the key informants. All economic sectors were targeted, but the policy emphasised airlines, industrial parks, health, education, and hospitality sectors. Interview participants argued that in collaboration with the transport sector, efforts were made to ensure that agricultural inputs were not disrupted and productivity was not affected. Menistu et al. (2020) explained that export-oriented firms were more likely to report receiving government support than domestic market-oriented firms. Goshu et al. (2020) found that agricultural operations were less adversely affected by the pandemic than non-agricultural businesses.

POLITICAL INCLUSIVENESS

According to the participants, COVID-19 policies were inclusive because the government involved all political parties. Nevertheless, some parties, including Tigray Peoples Liberation Front (TPLF), refused to work with the ruling party for political reasons. For instance, parliament postponed the national election because of the outbreak. Other opposition parties hindered the government's efforts to reduce the pandemic's spread. Most of those who opposed the intervention thought they had lost their power due to the current political reforms in the country. Therefore, they saw COVID-19 as a political agenda of the governing party. The political differences gradually reached a level of war between TPLF in Tigray and the federal government of Ethiopia. Despite these differences, however, the majority was cooperative in every aspect including compliance of pandemic protocols, resource mobilisation, and altruistic support for the vulnerable.

EQUITY IMPACT OF COVID-19 POLICY RESPONSES

Compliance with COVID-19 protocols was high among the population. For instance, over 99% of men and women-headed households reported washing hands more often since the outbreak. In addition, over 96% of all households abstained from handshakes, while 86% avoided crowds and gatherings since the outbreak. Compliance was also high in the regions such as Addis Ababa and Dire Dawa (99%) and Amhara (92%).

Policy responses to the pandemic affected social groups differently. Although people with disabilities knew the outbreak and mitigation measures, they faced difficulties adhering to social distance measures. For example, visually impaired persons and wheelchair users in need of community assistance did not often get people to help them due to fear of infection. In addition, some visually impaired people felt isolated because of the protocols. For example, a visually impaired man lost hope in his community in Dire Dawa town because he felt isolated. As a result, he committed suicide by burning himself (Emirie et al., 2020).

Moreover, income constraints and disabilities differently affected compliance with the policy measures. For example, a physically disabled 19-year-old girl in Bahir Dar explained that she shared a toilet with others and was worried that if she got infected, she was sure her body would not cope. Moreover, disabled migrants live in very low-cost housing in Addis Ababa without private piped water and toilet and are therefore more exposed to the pandemic (Emirie et al., 2020). In general, compliance was high during the first stage of the pandemic and relaxed during the second stage.

EQUITY OF ACCESS TO NECESSITIES

The pandemic had deleterious effects on access to services, but this was differentiated by sex. More male-headed households were more likely to report that there were unable to buy medication during the first stage of the pandemic. During the second stage, it was the reverse, where more women reported they were unable to buy medication. The factors contributing to respondents' inability to access necessities include shortages in shops, closure of markets, transportation challenges, restrictions on movement, increased prices, and a decline in regular income. The pandemic also caused rural–urban differences in access to necessities. For example, rural dwellers who could not buy medicine were 48%, while only 12% of urban people reported the same during the first stage of the pandemic. Similarly, 44% of the rural population compared to 17% of urban people surveyed were unable to buy sufficient 'injera', the local staple food (see Fig. 8.1). The results implied that although rural people are mainly in agricultural production, they were disproportionately affected with COVID-19 induced food insecurity.

Regarding regional disparities, respondents in the Somali region reported more difficulties accessing teff and wheat during the first and second rounds of the survey.

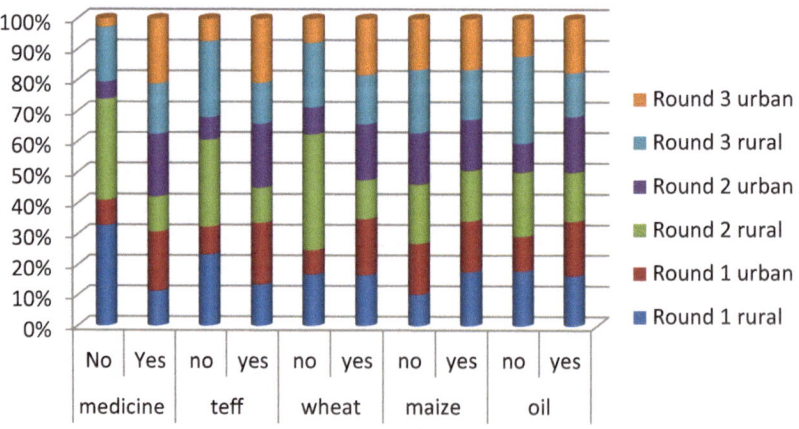

Fig. 8.1 Access to basic necessities by location and crop. *Note* 'yes' for access while 'no' for do not have access in both periods

EQUITY IN EDUCATION

School closures affected many school-going children, and over 47,000 schools were affected (MoE, 2020). The World Bank survey showed that out-of-school-age children did not engage in any learning during the period. The first-round survey showed that 65% of children in female-headed households and 68% in male-headed households were affected. Moreover, some children did not return to school when schools reopened.

The pandemic responses deepened the urban–rural education access inequity. In rural areas, 86% of out-of-school children did not engage in any learning during the pandemic. The figure for their urban counterparts was 57%. In addition, the second-round survey showed that rural children who stopped attending school after the pandemic were significantly higher than urban children who gave up school. Moreover, early marriage and child migration increased (Emirie et al., 2020).

Furthermore, the pandemic interventions had an unequal outcome on children's education across nine regional states in Ethiopia. Out of children in school before the pandemic, children engaged in learning activities after the outbreak was the highest in Tigray (61%) than in other regions except in Addis Ababa city administration (66%) in the first round. Other regions were within the range of 1% to 36% during the first round of the survey. In round two, the number increased in Tigray (77%), Addis Ababa (67%), and Dire Dawa (59%). The figures increased in subsequent periods in the other regions.

The pandemic generally affects school children from poorer and female-headed households and those in poor regions. Interventions to mitigate the disruptions in education (MoE, 2020) were more accessible to male-headed households and positively affected school children in those households. Most of the interventions increased the access of children in male-headed households to education compared to children in female-headed households. Children in female-headed households accessed lessons on mobile learning apps more in the first and second rounds of the survey. Similarly, urban school children accessed virtual learning platforms more than their rural counterparts.

EQUITY OF HEALTH SERVICE ACCESS

During the survey period, 17% and 18% of female and male-headed households reported needing medical attention. The figures increased to 23% for both household types in the second round. However, in the third round, it decreased to 18% and 20% for female and male-headed households, respectively. Regarding location, 19% of urban and 14% of rural households surveyed reported needing medical treatment. During the second round, the corresponding figures were 24% for urban and 22% for rural households. In the third round, 20% of urban and 18% of rural households surveyed needed medical treatment. The households reported they could not access medical care because of the pandemic. Figure 8.2 shows that while households in the upper and middle quintiles reported needing medical attention, the poor did not have access to medical care.

Regarding location, all respondents in the Somali region (100 per cent) had access to medical care, while Amhara (85%) had the least access. During the third round, however, Afar regions surveyed respondents had the highest (100%) access to medical care while Southern Ethiopia had the least 82%.

Urban youth in Ethiopia with disability faced difficulties accessing sexual and reproductive health services after the pandemic. Key informants explained that the outbreak interfered with essential health service delivery. Also, service delivery was affected by infections by health service

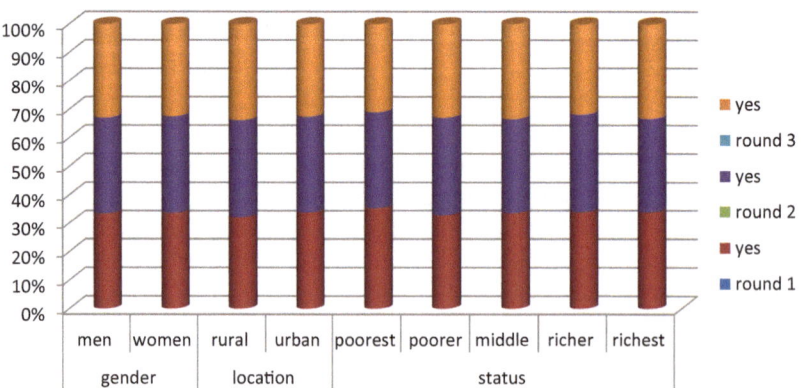

Fig. 8.2 Medical care need by location, social status, and sex

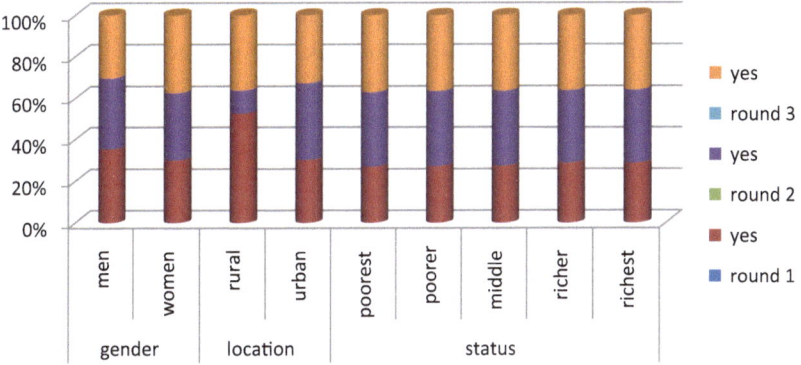

Fig. 8.3 Business closure-related job losses

workers. Some health service workers were deployed to attend to people in critical need of the services.

EMPLOYMENT EQUITY

Job losses were rampant during the pandemic period due to the closure of businesses and other factors. Job losses in urban areas attributed to business closure were significant compared to job losses in rural areas. The survey also showed that the pandemic-related business closure resulted in more job losses for the poor than for the rich (Fig. 8.3).

It is important to note that due to government directives to employers not to lay off workers, job losses were experienced more in the informal sector. Nevertheless, some organisations continued to work in various modalities. For example, some universities provided education via online platforms, and some sectors continued working with utmost care and halted employment reduction.

INCOME EQUITY

The COVID-19 policy responses have impacted income and living costs. Women headed households who earned agricultural income had more income reduction in all three rounds of the survey. However, meanwhile, men encountered significantly more agricultural total income loss than women in all survey periods. Moreover, rural farm income was more affected than urban income in all periods except total income losses.

Farm income loss disparities also existed across regions. The total income loss of 79% was highest in the Harar region, followed by 71% in Addis Ababa in the first round. Most urbanised regions in Ethiopia faced high farm income losses because of the pandemic. The highest farm income reduction of 99% and 94% in the first and second rounds occurred in the Somali region.

In terms of wage employment, more men experienced a reduction than women. The pandemic reduced urban wage-employment income more than rural income. Private schoolteachers also experienced income losses more than their public counterparts. Regarding regional differences, 47% wage-employment income reduction was reported in the Somali region and 24% in the Dire Dawa region. With a 20% total income loss in the same period Somali region was more hit by the pandemic.

The pandemic also resulted in a total income decline in Ethiopia. More men than women had total income decline. For example, while men's incomes were reduced to 72%, that of women was 28% (Fig. 8.4). In addition, the total incomes of urban people saw more decline than that of their rural counterparts.

Total income loss discrepancies occurred across regional states, with 94% total income reduction in the Somali region, 58% in Tigray, and 57% in the Oromia region in round one. The income losses were between 40

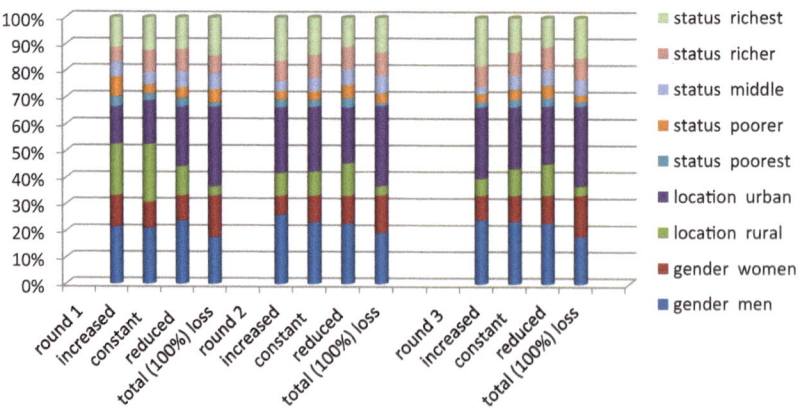

Fig. 8.4 Total income losses by sex and social status

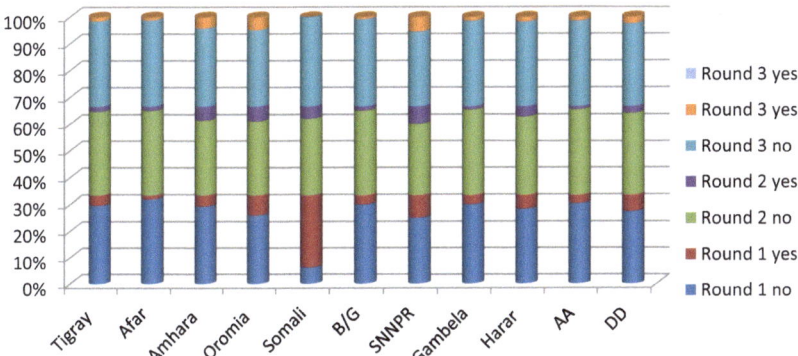

Fig. 8.5 Food insecurity by region

and 50% for all other regions. The income losses in the Somali region did not change in the third round. However, the status of income reduction in all other regions was still significant and ranged from 19 to 42%.

Food insecurity was also unevenly distributed. Twenty per cent of households surveyed ran out of food within 30 days of the pandemic, but food insecurity was more acute for female-headed households. On average, urban residents were more food insecure than rural households. While food insecurity affected the poor more than wealthier households. Ten per cent of wealthy households reported running out of food compared to 25% of their poorer counterparts. More female-headed and rural households reported that they had gone to bed without food than their male counterparts. In the first round, 57% of poor households and 36% of wealthier households reported going hungry.

Food security differences were also observed in regions with 64%, 40%, and 28%, respectively, in households in Somali, Afar, and Tigray regions having ran out of food in the last 30 days. The corresponding figure for other regions ranged between 8 and 24%. The figures, however, changed in the second and third rounds (see Fig. 8.5).

DISTRIBUTION OF WELFARE BENEFITS AND CORRUPTION

The key informant interview participants had insufficient information regarding the incidence of corruption during the COVID-19 intervention. As some argue, a state of emergency with strict control by the security sector may reduce rent-seeking. However, an interviewee from MoH explained that in some areas, including the ministry, there were some unsuccessful attempts. In some areas, youth groups took yellow t-shirts from health bureaus and collected money for personal use. In SNNPR, although there was a strong involvement of volunteers and follow-up mechanisms, some minor rent-seeking behaviours were still noticed. In SNNPR, the state of the emergency proclamation halved the size of the passengers and doubled prices, but service providers doubled prices but did not halve the number of passengers.

An expert working for MoE also expected that massive resource mobilisation to fight the pandemic might increase rent-seeking and corruption incidences. However, the organisations encountered incidences of corruption because of a lack of attention and preoccupation with national security problems. Most key informant interview experts from regional bureaus asserted that they had not encountered any misbehaviour related to corruption and rent-seeking as people engaged in supporting the vulnerable with altruistic motives.

Structural Change and Innovativeness of Policy Responses

The policy response led to structural changes and innovation. For example, an report of MoE explained that students developed self-learning, decreased dependence, and spoon-feeding and confronted various challenges that led to more practical learning. The use of technologies like telegram, mobile apps for education, and online education increased but was accessible to those with resources. In some regions, teamwork, access to laboratory equipment, a multisectoral approach to address health challenges, and increased attention and support to health sectors by authorities were deployed. Moreover, the number of hospital beds and inputs of disinfectants increased contrary to pre-COVID-19 period. Authorities gave more attention to health sector by allocating sufficient budget. Universities research and other support collaborations with health centres and hospitals also increased. Virtual meetings such as Zoom meetings since the outbreak created an opportunity to discuss with the large population at a time, including higher government officials which reduced the costs of travelling and hall renting for meetings. However, internet and power cut problems constrained the deployment of the e-technologies for meetings.

CONCLUSION AND RECOMMENDATION

The Ethiopian government implemented a step-by-step COVID-19 response plan considering the country's economic and social conditions. The country declared five months state of emergency and implemented a partial lockdown. The policy intervention maintained the balance between reducing the health effect of COVID-19 and its economic impact. The government emphasised preventive measures while maintaining some economic activities in the industry, service, and agriculture to satisfy the economic needs and prevent its devastating impact. The integrated role of the government, NGOs (local and international), the private sector, CBOs, and the community was significant in the intervention, particularly in awareness creation, resource mobilisation, and supporting the vulnerable. As a result, the overall effect of COVID-19 in Ethiopia is relatively low compared to other countries worldwide. However, the poor health system and inadequate preventive facilities (such as PPE and treatment equipment, among others); inadequate social services (e.g., water and sanitation), political turmoil and conflict, dependency on the informal economy, high unemployment rate, debt distress, high inflation rate, and low level of domestic resource mobilisation were the challenges in the fight against COVID-19. The equity impact was also significant in terms of income, employment, food security, and reaching the disabled, socially marginalised groups and others living with other chronic diseases. The equity difference was significantly based on age, gender, income status, and geographic location. It is fair to conclude that COVID-19 in Ethiopia was not only a curse but also an opportunity to improve health infrastructure and promote technological innovation in the health, education, and economic sectors. It is also an opportunity to prepare for future similar health crises.

The Ethiopian case shows that the government and non-state actors participated in the implementation of public and social, economic, and governance lockdown policy responses to reduce the spread of COVID-19. Unlike some countries in the region, the lockdown in Ethiopia was partial with selected restrictions. A prevention-focused health sector strategy also guided the overall intervention effort, and the government tried to balance a health crises and its socioeconomic fallouts.

The federal and regional governments adopted significant economic policy responses, including liquidity injection, to allow banks to reduce interest rates and extended debt payment mandates. About leadership and governance, various committees were established to make proactive non-routine decisions to address the challenges of the pandemic. However, resource allocations to control the pandemic competed for limited health facilities and health workers available to provide essential health services. Although the state-enforced social distancing through the state of emergency, shortage of rooms to quarantine and water for hand washing in some parts of the country and power and internet cuts to work from home were among the challenges that hindered the implementation.

Although the government and non-government actors supported vulnerable social groups, the inclusiveness of policy measures was questioned. School closure was implemented while the virtual platform and other modalities used to continue education were affected by various setbacks and resulted in huge inequity. Lessons taught using TV and radio programmes and online excluded the poor and the disabled more. Children in big cities benefited from the interventions than their rural counterparts. Also, innovations practised reducing physical contacts discriminated against the disabled. Home quarantines were impossible for the poor that lacked sufficient rooms. The emphasis on the pandemic compromised essential health services and decreased the number of patients visiting hospitals and maternal care.

Moreover, the lockdowns increased women's domestic violence, sexual assault, early marriage, and school dropout rates. The lockdown measures disproportionately impacted the informal income, aviation, and entertainment sectors. Efforts to reduce the transmission of the outbreak concentrated in urban areas, and in effect, protective measures were less practised in the countryside.

The case analysis demonstrated that Ethiopia's policy responses had equity impacts. Policy responses to the pandemic unequally affected the vulnerable social groups in Ethiopia. The partial lockdowns in Ethiopia affected urban food and medicine access more than rural ones and resulted in regional variations but were not gendered. The outbreak responses also led to differences in rural–urban, income class, and regional education access. Urban people in need of medical treatment were not only more significant. However, they had more access to medical treatment than rural people in all survey periods after the pandemic. The rich have had more need for medical treatment and accessed the medical treatment more than the poor. Despite the regional inequities across regions, people needing medical treatment and who had accessed it after the pandemic was significant.

The outbreak resulted in more job losses for men, as the survey has shown. Business closures affected the poor and urban jobs more significantly. Informal sector jobs were more affected than formal sector jobs. During the three survey periods, policy responses affected total agricultural and waged employment income losses for men more than women.

The policy responses significantly impacted food security in Ethiopia. Female-headed households were more food insecure than men, and the poor were more food insecure than the rich. However, a significant proportion of the rich were food insecure. Rural people were more food insecure, but there were still instances of urban people being more food insecure than rural people.

Recommendations

- Given the differential impacts of the pandemic and its policy responses on diverse groups, the government must make efforts to reach targeted groups with specific interventions. Proper targeting can be achieved with structural changes in the economy and deployment of innovative tools.
- The government must strengthen and institutionalise existing social protection programmes in rural and urban areas to reach large-scale vulnerable groups such as the elderly, disabled, women, and children so that they will be protected from future health and socioeconomic shocks.
- There is the need for an expansion in education, health, and water and sanitation infrastructure in rural and poor urban neighbourhoods to enhance access for the poor.

References

Abate, G. T., de Brauw, A., & Hirvonen, K. 2020. *Food and nutrition security in Addis Ababa, Ethiopia during COVID-19 pandemic: June 2020 report*, Intl Food Policy Res Inst.

ADB. (2020). Afr can Development Bank Group. Afr can Economic Outlook 2020: Africa's economy forecast to grow despite external shocks. Disponible en:https://www.afdb.org/en/news-and-events/press-releases/african-eco nomic-outlook-2020-africas-economy-forecast-grow-despite-external-shocks-33839.

Central Statistical Agency. (2016). Ethiopia. In the world factbook. https://www.cia.gov/library/publications/resources/the-world-factbook/geos/et.html

CIPE. (2020). Responding to the COVID-19 Pandemic in Ethiopia: The Private Sector Experience.

Degye, G., Mengistu, K., Getachew, D., & Tadele, F. (2020). Assessment of COVID-19 effects and response measures in Ethiopia: Livelihoods and welfare implications. In E. E. Association (Ed.). Add s Ababa

Deressa, T. T. (2007). *Measuring the economic impact of climate change on Ethiopian agriculture*, World Bank Publications.

Emirie, G., Iyasu, A., Gezahegne, K., Jones, N., Presler-Marshall, E., Tilahun, K., Workneh, F., & Yadete, W. (2020). Experiences of vulnerable urban youth under covid-19: the case of youth with disabilities. *Policy brief: COVID-19 Series, Ethiopia, London: Gender and Adolescence: Global Evidence (GAGE).*

FAO, IFAD, UNICEF, WFP and WHO. (2019). The State of Food Security and Nutrition in the World 2019. Safeguarding against economic slowdowns and downturns. FAO.

Geopoll 2020. The financial impacts of Coronavirus in Sub-Saharan Africa

Getaneh, Y., Yizengaw, A., Adane, S., Zealiyas, K., Abate, Z., Leulseged, S., Desalegn, H., Yimer, G., & Abate, E. (2020). Global lessons and potential strategies in combating COVID-19 pandemic in Ethiopia: Systematic review. *Med xiv.*

Goshu, D., Ketema, M., Diriba, G., & Ferede, T. (2020). Assessment of COVID-19 effects and response measures in Ethiopia: Livelihoods and Welfare Implications.

Hai, W., Zhao, Z., Wang, J., & Hou, Z.-G. (2004). The short-term impact of SARS on the Chinese economy. *Asian Econ, 3*, 57–61.

ILO. (2020). Employment by sex and age—ILO modelled estimates. ILOSTAT. Accessed 14–02–2020. https://ilostat.ilo.org/data. In ILO (Ed.).

MOE. (2020). Ministry of education concept note for education sector COVID-19-preparedness and response plan. In 1 (ed.).

NBE. (2019). Ann al Report of 2018/2019. Add s Ababa National Bank of Ethiopia.

OECD. (2020). OEC country policy tracker. Retrieved from https://www.oecd.org/coronavirus/en/

Proclamation No 3/320 State of Emergency Proclamation Enacted to Counter and Control the Spread of COVID-19 and Mitigate Its Impact Proclamation No. 3/2020.

Starr, N., Panda, N., Johansen, E., Forrester, J., Wayessa, E., Rebollo, D., August, A., Fernandez, K., Bitew, S., & Mammo, T. N. (2020). The Lifebox surgical headlight project: Engineering, testing, and field assessment in a resource-constrained setting. *British Journal of Surgery, 107*, 1751–1761.

Statista. (2020a). Ethiopia: Total population from 2009 to 2019, by gender. In H. Plecher (Ed.).

Statista. (2020b). Ethiopia: Unemployment rate from 1999 to 2020. In H. Plecher (Ed.).

Taddesse, L. (2020). Solidarity, agility and continuity: Three cornerstones of Ethiopia's COVID-19 response.

United Nations. (2019). Department of Economic and Social Affairs, Population Division (2019). World Population Prospects 2019: Online Edition. In U. Nations (Ed.).

WHO. (2020a). Coronavirus disease 2019 (COVID-19): Situation report, 72.

WHO. (2020b). https://www.afro.who.int/news/over-10-000-health-workers-africa-infected-covid-19 (Accessed July 26 2020)

WHO. (2020c). Pas the message: Five steps to kicking out coronavirus. *World Health Organization (WHO)*.

World Bank. (2019). World Development Indicators. In W. Bank (Ed.).

Worldometer. (2021). Countries in the world by population (2020)- Worldometer[Internet]. Worldometers. Info. 202.

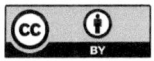

CHAPTER 9

Kenya

Laura Ferguson, Krishni Satchi, Irene Kizito, and Shiphrah Kuria

INTRODUCTION

The Covid-19 pandemic across the world has raised many debates about the implications of structural inequalities and Covid-19 responses on vulnerable populations. In Kenya, these debates present an opportunity to examine the existing structures that posed severe ramifications for both response and mitigation measures. According to the 2019 Kenya Population and Housing Census, young people constitute the largest segment of the population of 47.5 million in Kenya. 19.5 million of the population are classified as poor, with 14 million, 1.3 million, and 4.2 million living in rural areas, peri-urban and core-urban and informal settlements,

L. Ferguson · K. Satchi
Institute on Inequalities in Global Health, University of Southern California, Los Angeles, CA, USA
e-mail: Laura.Ferguson@med.usc.edu

I. Kizito · S. Kuria (✉)
Amref Health Africa, Nairobi, Kenya
e-mail: Shiphrah.Kuria@amref.org

© The Author(s) 2024
A. Altaf et al. (eds.), *EQUITY IN COVID-19*, EADI Global Development Series, https://doi.org/10.1007/978-3-031-58588-3_9

199

respectively.[1] Poverty is also feminized. The 2015/2016 Kenya Integrated Household Budget Survey (KIHBS) results show that 30.2% of female-headed households are poor compared to 26.0% of their male counterparts.[2]

Kenya's Gini coefficient of 44.540 is above the 2013 Sub-Saharan African average of 43.841, indicating higher than average wealth inequalities in Kenya. The latest KIHBS results show that nationally, more than half (59.4%) of total expenditure is controlled by the top quintile, while the bottom quintile controls a mere 3.6% of expenditure. Pre-pandemic, the KNBS estimated that unemployment stood at 14.2% among youth aged 20–24. Women comprise 70% of low-wage earners. Most are employed in the informal sector or run micro and small enterprises. Daily wages characterize this sector, with limited social protection measures or savings, making women particularly vulnerable.[3]

Covid-19 hit Kenya with an already weak health system with frequent health worker strikes and unequal distribution of health facilities. The country also had very low health worker-to-population ratios. Regarding critical care facilities, only 22 of the 47 counties had at least one intensive care unit. There were 537 ICU beds, three-quarters of which were in Nairobi or Mombasa, and only 58% of hospital beds nationally were in hospitals with an oxygen supply.[4] The cost of health care is also prohibitive. Although the National Hospital Insurance Fund (NHIF) was introduced in 2004 to facilitate cheaper access to services, in 2019, the Ministry of Health reported that this scheme covered only 11% of Kenyans. Furthermore, with 70% of the Kenyan workforce working in the informal sector, most are ineligible for the NHIF or unable to afford its premiums. Most Kenyans pay out of pocket to access health services, which means that they delay care-seeking, if possible, which, in the context of Covid-19, has dire consequences.[5]

All of this raised concerns about the ability to mount an effective biomedical response to the pandemic, and the fear that necessary public health measures such as physical distancing, handwashing, and wearing

[1] Kenya National Bureau of Statistics (2019).

[2] Kenya National Bureau of Statistics (2018).

[3] Kenya National Bureau of Statistics (2018).

[4] Barasa et al. (2020)

[5] Ouma et al. (2020).

facemasks might also be challenging to implement, particularly among specific populations, including the poorest of the poor. This chapter explores Kenya's national legal and policy response to Covid-19 with particular attention to human rights and equity. It encompasses issues such as civil society participation in the response and the unequal impact of the response on different populations. This work has been guided by a socio-ecological framework whereby individuals' experiences are shaped by a range of nested, interrelated factors around them, from seemingly 'distant' factors such as laws and policies down to more 'proximal' factors such as their immediate living situation. The interplay of these factors, mainly the range of laws, policies, and regulations relevant to Covid-19 and how they impact different populations, is explored.

METHODOLOGY

This mixed-methods study includes policy, quantitative and qualitative research, and a joint analysis to combine all these different data types. We reviewed web-based search engines such as Google and Google Scholar for the legal and policy analysis. Searches were limited by date range of publication and were restricted to the year 2020. Data were assessed for relevance and systematically extracted based on their direct or indirect implications for vulnerable communities. The data were organized thematically and categorized according to date, issuing body, and type of measure issued to create a timeline of the national response. In addition, we relied on secondary literature sources on the theme. The study also used media reports compiled during the period. The data generated were tabulated, indicating the date, the main issue, and reference. Organizations actively engaged in the Covid-19 response in Kenya were identified from the media analysis, including UN organizations such as the WHO, UNDP, UNICEF, WFP, FAO, UN Women, as well as civil society organizations including Amref Health Africa, The Red Cross, the Population Council, KELIN Kenya, and Amnesty International. Their latest reports on areas of interest were reviewed, and data relevant to answering the study's research questions were systematically extracted. The information was drawn from their research findings, programmatic reports, and experiences of the realities encountered in their programme implementation.

Key informant interviews were conducted with ten participants using a semi-structured interview guide. This included four representatives of government (governance, health, education and gender, and culture), three parastatal organizations, and three civil society organizations (working across health, law, and inequalities). These interviews took place at the national and county levels in Homa Bay County as an example of how the Covid-19 response has been implemented sub-nationally. Interviews were recorded and transcribed verbatim for analysis. Ethical approvals were secured through the Amref Ethics Review Committee and the University of Southern California Institutional Review Board.

Mapping the Evolution of the Pandemic in the Context of Policy Response

On February 28, 2020, as a response to the looming threat of coronavirus, President Kenyatta issued the first executive order addressing Covid-19, in which he called attention to the necessity of bolstering health systems. He called for completing a national isolation and treatment facility at Mbagathi Hospital in Nairobi and establishing a National Emergency Response Committee (NERC) on coronavirus. The NERC entailed a Covid-19 Task Force, composed of the Ministry of Health, other government agencies, United Nations agency representatives, development partners, NGOs, and civil society, which plays an advisory role to the committee.[6] Noticeably missing from the task force was representation from religious leaders, youth, women and women's organizations in civil society, marginalized communities such as refugees, and the private sector. The primary role of NERC, which was 81% male, was to advise the President and coordinate preparedness, prevention, and response to the threat of Covid-19.[7]

On March 24, 2020, the Ministry of Health issued guidelines for the promotion of preventive measures, such as physical distancing and handwashing, and ensuring the continuity of antiretroviral treatment for the 1 million people living with HIV, among other essential services. The next day, the government announced that it would put aside Ksh 1 billion to recruit medical personnel. The Cabinet Secretary for Health followed these guidelines with the issuance on April 3 of the Public Health Act

---

[6] Thinkwell. *COVID-19 summary update for Kenya.* Accessed April 23, 2021. https://thinkwell.global/wpcontent/uploads/2020/05/COVID-19-Kenya-Update-22-May-2020.pdf.

[7] Barasa et al. (2020).

on Covid-19, which consisted of general guidelines for medical officers about Covid-19 patients and people potentially exposed to the coronavirus. Later in April, a guideline was issued to support the continuity of reproductive, maternal, newborn, and family planning services.

The Kenyan government launched significant health system measures on June 10 in response to data showing that 78% of infected persons admitted to hospitals were either asymptomatic or mildly symptomatic. These protocols included advice on home-based isolation and care, especially as asymptomatic Covid-19 positive cases were discharged from health centres. Protocol implementation was designed to start immediately. However, according to the protocols, if positive cases could not afford to be isolated at home due to spatial concerns, facilities within the community that met specific recommendations were available to provide care.

The Nairobi Hospital formed a strategic partnership with the United Nations on July 21 to manage diplomatic personnel and all dependents with suspected or confirmed cases of Covid-19. The agreement included the construction of an Ksh 1.1 billion health facility with an Intensive Care Unit consisting of 25 beds and an additional 50 in the High Dependency Unit. The facility was intended to serve over 20,000 United Nations staff based in Kenya and East Africa, along with locals in the vicinity. In addition, during a September 10 meeting overseen by President Kenyatta, the Cabinet approved a comprehensive insurance plan to cover all health workers on the frontline of the pandemic. They also announced an Inter-Agency Programme to prevent and respond to gender-based violence, which had increased because of Covid-19.

At the county level, Homa Bay County had enacted a County Health Act less than a month before the Covid-19 pandemic, which included guidance on addressing emergencies such as pandemics and was therefore valuable in guiding the local response.[8]

Other policy measures included travel restrictions, quarantining and closing public places and schools, and scaling down the work of the judiciary. These restrictions began on March 15, 2020, and gradually expanded with intensity and geography. Some of these included suspensions of flights, quarantining of passengers, and imposition of a 7 pm–5 am curfew, among others.

---

[8] Kenya News (n.d.).

It appears that compliance with government response measures varied widely. Some people chose not to comply, mainly if the regulation did not make biomedical sense (e.g. wearing a mask while driving alone in a car); some people did not want to comply, and some people could not comply due to more urgent competing needs (e.g. they could not afford a face mask). Of those who complied, many believed in the public health measures, while some were simply trying to avoid arrest.[9]

MITIGATION MEASURES

Kenya implemented a range of fiscal measures to counter the negative economic impact of the pandemic on individuals and businesses. This began on March 12, 2020, when the Ministry of Tourism and Wildlife announced that it had set aside the US$5 million to support the tourism sector for a post-Covid-19 recovery plan.

On March 15, Safaricom and the Central Bank announced that charges on mobile money transactions would be dropped to limit the use of cash. Then on March 24, the Central Bank lowered its policy rate to 7.25% (which was then lowered to 7% on April 29), lowered banks' cash reserve ratio to 4.25%, increased the maximum tenor of repurchase agreements from 28 to 91 days, and announced flexibility to banks on loan classification and provisioning for loans that were performing on March 2 but were restructured due to the pandemic.

Immediately after this, on March 25, President Kenyatta outlined tax interventions the government would make to protect the country against the economic effects of Covid-19. This included the government's decision to earmark funds for expediting payments of existing obligations to maintain business cash flow during the crisis. The President also declared that resident corporate income tax would be reduced from 30 to 25% and that the turnover tax rate would be reduced for Micro, Small, and medium enterprises from 3 to 1%. In addition, the plan included 100% tax relief for anyone in the low-income earner's category. In addition, the Ministry of Labour and Social Protection planned to allocate Ksh 10 billion (about €76m) to the elderly, orphans, and other vulnerable groups through cash transfers to cushion them against the effects of Covid-19.

---

[9] Key informant interview 5.

On April 15, 2020, the Central Bank suspended for six months the listing of adverse credit information for borrowers whose loans became non-performing after April 1, setting a new minimum threshold of $10 for negative credit information submitted to credit reference bureaus.

The Head of Public Service announced a voluntary government pay cut programme which started in April and aimed to cover lower cadre civil servants. With savings towards funding the Covid-19 response, voluntary pay cuts of 80% for the President and his deputy, 30% for cabinet secretaries, and 20% for chief administrative were announced.

The President announced the National Hygiene Program on April 25, designed to create youth employment while addressing health promotion. Phase 1 of the programme launched on April 29 and targeted 26,000 youth in 23 informal settlements most affected by the pandemic. Also, in April, the government earmarked Ksh 40 billion (about 350m USD) for the following additional health expenditures: surveillance, laboratory services, isolation units, equipment, supplies, and communication; social protection and cash transfers; food relief; and funds for expediting payments of existing obligations to maintain cash flow for businesses during the crisis.

On May 23, President Kenyatta showcased a new 8-Point Economic Stimulus Programme, which totalled Ksh 53.7 Billion. The programme focused on (1) infrastructure, including the hiring of local labour to fix roads and bridges, (2) education, including the hiring of 10,000 teachers and ICT interns to support digital learning, (3) fast-track payment of outstanding VAT refunds and other pending payments to small and medium enterprises, (4) health care, including 5,000 healthcare workers and the expansion of bed capacity in public hospitals, (5) agriculture, including e-vouchers for 200,000 small-scale farmers, (6) soft loans to support the tourism industry, (7) the environment, including the rehabilitation of wells, water pans, and underground tanks, and (8) manufacturing, such as the investment to purchase locally manufactured vehicles under the "Buy Kenya Build Kenya" policy.

Kenya's National Treasury announced on May 1 that they would create a fund of close to Ksh 100 billion to protect micro, small, and medium enterprises against the effects of Covid-19. Additionally, on August 8, the Education Cabinet Secretary stated that the Ministry would provide Ksh 7 billion concessionary loans to struggling private schools. Finally, on September 10, the government approved establishing a Credit Guarantee Scheme to support the businesses mentioned above.

SOCIAL PROTECTION AND CASH TRANSFER PROGRAMMES

The Ministry of Labour and Social Protection is responsible for social protection and cash transfer programmes. They used pre-existing cash transfer programmes to reach "the most vulnerable" (elderly, orphans, people with disabilities) with cash transfers.[10] At the time of writing, the reach and impact of these programmes had not yet been documented, but the absence of poverty status as an inclusion criterion is striking.

The government social protection programmes are complemented by programmes implemented by non-State actors. These are described below in turn.

The government has implemented four main cash transfer programmes (see Table 9.1).

That all the government programmes pre-dated, the pandemic suggests that stakeholders key to the Covid-19 response were not included in the design of these programmes, nor were they tailored to the realities of the Covid-19 pandemic.

Under the Covid-19 Emergency Response Fund, Kenya's private sector stepped in to try to help fill the gap between the government's limited response and those in need, establishing a Board led by the CEOs of the biggest companies, which worked with a consortium of NGOs to disburse money via M-Pesa.[11] Under the Inua Jamii programme, KShs 13 billion was disbursed by the government to cover January to June 2020 Government to Persons (G2P) payments and cushioned recipients from Covid-19 shocks.[12] The Ministry of Labour and Social Protection was instrumental in successfully transforming this programme's payment delivery mechanism from a manual system to a fully digital solution that

---

[10] Key informant 1.

[11] *The new humanitarian: A Kenyan Covid-19 notebook: The 'Mama Mbogas' and the path to recovery.* Accessed February 4, 2021. https://www.thenewhumanitarian.org/news-feature/2020/08/06/Kenya-coronavirusinformal-economy-mama-mbogas.

[12] *Kenya enhances its cash transfer programmes in response to the Covid-19 pandemic.* Financial Sector Deepening Kenya. Accessed February 4, 2021. https://www.fsdkenya.org/blog/kenya-enhances-its-cash-transferprogrammes-in-response-to-the-covid-19-pandemic/.

Table 9.1 Summary of cash transfer programmes in Kenya

Programme	Target group	Target numbers	Budget allocation	Amount disbursed	Mode of payment
Covid-19 emergency response fund	Nairobi's most vulnerable communities & hotspot towns	Not known. KShs 2000 weekly payment	KShs 500m on cash transfers (out of the total 2.8 billion in the general fund)	Ongoing	M-Pesa
Additional cash transfers	Expansion of the existing cash transfer programmes across the country for the elderly, orphans, vulnerable children and people with disabilities	669,000 households across the country to be paid KShs 1,000 weekly	KShs 10 billion ($100m)	Between May and August: 341,958 households. Due to dwindling funds, it was expected to end by October 2020	M-Pesa
Kazi Mtaani	Public works programmes across the country aimed at engaging youth in restoring public hygiene standards and urban civil works and providing them with cash relief	200,000 youth in 23 informal settlements among them; Mathare, Mukuru, and Kibera	KShs 10 billion	Ongoing with a pilot of 26,000 youth in Nairobi informal settlements	M-Pesa
Inua Jamii	Across the country	1.1m beneficiaries paid, KShs 4,000 every two months	KShs 13 billion	KShs 13 billion	Inua Jamii payment system—bank accounts

Sources Authors' compilation based on key informant interviews and media reports

offered choice, convenience, and greater dignity to the recipients.[13] No literature was found documenting (potential) beneficiaries' experiences of the programme. Key informants suggested that government-run cash transfer programmes did not reach all intended beneficiaries and that, for those in the programme, long delays were experienced. They intimated that there were some problems with corruption, but they could not be specific regarding the extent to which the different cash transfer programmes were affected.[14]

The governmental cash transfer programs were complemented by various additional programmes implemented by multilateral agencies and NGOs. For example, the European Union (EU) partnered with several other organizations and foundations aiming to provide cash transfers to 20,000 households in Nairobi informal settlements for three months starting in June 2020. The EU also provided Ksh 606 million earmarked to be distributed to 80,000 households in informal settlements through M-Pesa.[15] Aiming to reach 120,000 people, Oxfam Kenya, with other NGO partners, distributed cash transfers through M-Pesa to Nairobi urban settlers and women and girls at risk of gender-based violence in Mombasa and Nairobi.

Despite all these programmes being documented, many studies reported participants stating that they had not received any support of this nature. There were also complaints that the transfer amounts were insufficient, delays in payments were a challenge, some people were overlooked, and others told they were ineligible. People noted that registration processes were not transparent, and people did not have information about how to access these cash transfers. Caregivers were omitted even if they were unable to work due to their care duties: the transfer was designed to be sufficient only for the vulnerable individual targeted.[16] Evaluation of these cash transfer programmes is needed.

---

[13] *Kenya enhances its cash transfer programmes in response to the Covid-19 pandemic.* Financial Sector Deepening Kenya. Accessed February 4, 2021. https://www.fsdkenya. org/blog/kenya-enhances-its-cash-transferprogrammes-in-response-to-the-covid-19-pandemic/.

[14] Key informant 1.

[15] *Covid-19: 80,000 slum households to receive Sh 5,000 monthly.* The Standard. Accessed February 4, 2021, https://www.standardmedia.co.ke/nairobi/article/2001374784/covid-19-80000-slumhouseholds-to-receive-sh5000-monthly.

[16] Obulutsa (2020).

A final note on the cash transfer dilemma hinges on unease about privacy concerns. A key informant explained that individuals were concerned about what the government might do with personal data about them and therefore were unwilling to share the type of information that might better underpin cash transfer and other social safety net programmes.[17]

In September 2020, Kenya introduced the Covid-19 Country Socio-economic Re-engineering and Recovery Strategies (CCSERS). As part of these strategies, Kenya planned to protect health services and systems, scale-up social protections and essential services, protect jobs and support small and medium-sized enterprises (including the most vulnerable productive actors), enhance social cohesion and community resilience, and provide 'green' recovery strategies that embraced technology. As a subset of these measures, initiatives were introduced to enhance access to affordable credit for microenterprises, financial literacy programs were promoted, frameworks were introduced for microleasing, and access to a credit guarantee scheme was enhanced. Kenya also introduced plans to provide material and non-material resources to help build business capacity. Among these resources were support to improve market access, physical infrastructure, and designated worksites for creating and selling goods and services.[18]

On December 22, Kenya's parliament voted to end all Covid-19 tax relief schemes, noting that this would help plug gaps in government revenue even as others warned of a negative impact on individuals. The only tax relief measure that was maintained was that Kenyans earning less than KShs 24,000 ($220) would still be granted 100% tax relief.[19]

INCLUSIVITY OF MITIGATION MEASURES AND POLICY RESPONSES

Many civil society organizations raised the issue of participatory Covid-19 management, noting the lack of inclusivity in initial responses. Many key informants interviewed felt that the level of inclusion of vulnerable

---

[17] Key informant interview 2.

[18] *Resident rep remarks at launching the county Covid-19 social-economic reengineering and recovery strategy, 2020/21–2022/23.* UNDP in Kenya. Accessed April 23, 2021.

[19] Obulutsa (2020).

communities in policy development was insufficient; therefore, the policy did not cover them. Even where they were considered, such as for cash transfer programmes which targeted the elderly, people with disabilities, orphans, and vulnerable children, these groups were not involved in developing or implementing the programmes. Also, there was a lack of clarity about beneficiary selection. Moreover, many vulnerable people were unaware of the programmes.[20]

The unforeseen negative impacts of the curfew on pregnant women who needed to access health facilities for deliveries at night were attributed to the minimal participation of women in the design of the policy.[21] One key informant noted a significant class differential in the impact of the Covid-19 response, noting that the 'political elite', which includes those involved in policy-making, was least affected while the low-income earners, the people who rely entirely on the informal economy and survive on daily income, were most affected.[22] This suggests that the elite designed a policy response with minimal participation of less advantaged groups and little consideration of how these policies might work for and affect them.

Over time, there were some efforts to become more inclusive, such as Ministry of Health officials advocating for the inclusion of sex workers in the national response and setting up communication platforms for government partners to exchange inclusive strategies.[23] In addition, in an initiative in Siaya, efforts were made to include adolescent girls in Covid-19 prevention efforts.[24]

Within the education sector, in the guidelines and training for safe return to school, there were considerations of children with disabilities. Some of the areas in the guidelines included how to help children with autism wear masks appropriately; ensuring that children in wheelchairs can reach handwashing facilities and adapting materials for students or teachers with visual or hearing impairments. There were some sensitization efforts with duty bearers to highlight the needs of people with visual or hearing impairments, particularly in the context of required face

---

[20] Key informant interview 10.

[21] Key informant interview 10.

[22] Key informant interview 8.

[23] Kelin (2020).

[24] Mbogo (2020).

masks.[25] Some efforts were also made to distribute learning materials to students in hard-to-reach areas during the time that schools were closed. Although efforts were made to teach online and to broadcast educational programmes on the radio, the coverage remained low, and it was the most vulnerable students who could not access these programmes.[26]

There were also concerns about the plans for using the private sector to roll out vaccines, which would likely disadvantage those of lower socioeconomic status who might struggle to access these services.[27]

IMPACTS OF THE COVID-19 RESPONSE MEASURES

The Covid-19 response measures had many impacts on a range of vulnerable groups and health workers. One of the challenges that existed from the outset, from a civil society perspective, was the definition of 'vulnerable' in the context of Covid-19. The government focused on older people and people with underlying medical conditions. They defined vulnerability biomedically. This overlooked the social and economic vulnerability that is so prevalent in Kenya. The government reportedly gave very little attention to addressing poverty in the context of the pandemic, including trying to understand the potential impacts of mitigation measures on people living in poverty, which undermined the success of these efforts. The lack of attention to people living in informal urban settlements and people living on the street was a particularly striking shortcoming of the national response.[28,29] A member of the national Covid-19 Response Taskforce explained that the government wanted to reach the most vulnerable, but due to the inadequacy in the identification and classification of the very poor and the near-poor population, this might not have happened as intended.[85] Relatively early in the pandemic response, members of the national task force visited different counties to document the situation and capacity to respond across the country.[30] Later on, the Presidential Policy & Strategy Unit, Executive Office of the

---

[25] Key informant interview 3.

[26] Key informant interview 7.

[27] Key informant interview 8.

[28] Key informant 1.

[29] Key informant interview 2.

[30] Key informant interview 10.

President, working with partners, carried out a study to document the impact Covid-19 had had on adolescent girls in particular around school dropout, teenage pregnancy, and early marriage; and how these short-term effects translated into longer-term economic disadvantages, poorer health outcomes, and increased violence for women.

The primary 'vulnerable groups' covered in the literature include people living in urban informal settlements, informal sector workers, boda boda (motorcycle taxi) riders, individuals in poverty, youth, and women. In addition, the literature documents lessons learned about what was and was not working for vulnerable groups across different areas of the response, as explored below.

The health sector itself was hit immensely by Covid-19 measures. There was insufficient support and protection for health risks for health workers and caregivers throughout Kenya. They complained about a lack of personal protective equipment (PPE), including N95 masks and surgical gloves.[31,32,33] Clinics reported shortages of hand sanitizer even though they had been recommended to use sanitizer between client visits when water was not accessible. Furthermore, smaller clinics could not follow 1.5 metre separation guidelines due to their small rooms. Community health workers were not provided protection and had to buy and bring their sanitizing products and/or water containers before visiting households. In addition, their transportation costs to carry out their work were not covered. Also, healthcare providers and community health workers reported lack of training on Covid-19. Some healthcare providers even fled from patients with Covid-19-like symptoms. Poor quality PPE was linked to Covid-19 infections in healthcare workers.[34]

The Covid-19 response reduced the affordability of healthcare services (due to lost income) and the quantity and speed of services available due to pandemic restrictions. It also affected access to essential drugs such as antiretrovirals, reduced antenatal attendance, and caused shortages in contraceptives among many other commodities. It is of concern that Caesarean-section rates increased during the pandemic to

---

[31] Wangamati and Sundby (2020).

[32] Lagat et al. (2020).

[33] Noor (2020).

[34] Dahir (2020).

beyond the WHO recommendation of 10–15%.[35] In addition, maternal health resources, including health workers, were being reallocated for Covid-19 patients, slowing down maternal health services.[36] In neonatal care, health providers were under increased burden because regulations mandated that Covid-19-positive mothers should be separated from their babies and that both should be cared for separately. In addition to the health system strain, mandating the separation of Covid-19-positive mothers from their infants was more harmful than helpful, particularly as it can cause physiological stress for both mothers and children.

Overall, Covid-19 was characterized by mass unemployment, loss of income, and increased dependents. Labour participation fell due to the pandemic from 75% in 2019 to 56.8% in April 2020.[37] At least one million people lost their jobs or were placed on unpaid leave in both formal and informal sectors as of June. This is in part because curfews and restrictions that made jobs redundant. According to a survey published in August, 69% of Kenyans reported reduced earnings and 43% reported a complete loss of income. Many upper/middle-class Kenyans let go of their domestic workers due to fears of contracting Covid-19, exacerbating unemployment among the lower class.[38]

Economic insecurity caused by reduced earnings and job cuts made it difficult for vulnerable individuals to pay rent, with 30.5% of Kenyans reporting that they could not pay rent in April and only 41.7% of tenants reporting that they paid their rent on time.[39] However, only 8.7% of landlords waived rent in April, while others resorted to ending contracts, locking tenants out, and cutting essential services.

According to one survey, 92% of Nairobi County's low-income residents had suffered reduced income by May 2020.[40] A study by the Population Council revealed that 80% of individuals living in Nairobi's most significant urban informal settlements had experienced a decline in income, increase in expenditures, and increase in food prices. Most respondents had not received government support. In general, there was

---

[35] Shikuku et al. (2020).

[36] Kimani et al. (2020b).

[37] Kenya National Bureau of Statistics (2020).

[38] Kenya National Bureau of Statistics (2020).

[39] Kenya National Commission on Human Rights (2020).

[40] Wendy et al. (2020).

a lack of social support systems that could provide adequate resources for sustenance. Individuals who worked from home often experienced internet problems, including low connectivity and affordability of internet services. This restricted the ability to work from home, forcing some back to workplaces where they could not socially distance themselves.

According to one key informant, it appeared that the guidelines influencing the fiscal response were 'copy/pasted' from well-established economies that had substantial stimulus packages that Kenya did not have. In doing this the response did not accurately consider the challenge of supporting vulnerable groups.[41] Another key informant pointed to the gaps in mitigation measures for vulnerable groups, noting that the extent of their consideration was not very reflective in the issuance of guidelines. Had the government focused its attention on specific populations, the language would have been less generalized across policies.[42]

Research suggests that attempts to create policies and plans mitigating the impact of the lockdown did not take into consideration the specific needs of women, and as a result, the lockdown measures also disproportionately impacted the livelihoods of women.[43] More women worked in jobs that were vulnerable to disruption, including the service and manufacturing industries. Women also tend to operate businesses associated with traditional gender roles and therefore require face-to-face interactions. Single mothers who contracted Covid-19 or could not work due to pandemic measures risked bringing the household into economic insecurity more so than in two-parent households. In addition, fewer women work in formal employment and thus did not benefit from tax reliefs to the same extent as men.[44]

Women comprise more than 60% of informal businesses. The partial lockdown disproportionately impacted informal sector workers, who survive on daily wages and work in casual labour or petty trade and

---

[41] Wangila (2020).

[42] Key informant interview 10.

[43] Saks et al. (2020).

[44] Key informant interview 10.

often lack access to the financial resources, social protection, or employment benefits necessary to survive financial shocks.[45,46] In addition to the impact of travel restrictions, the imposition of a curfew limited their income and put them in danger of poverty.[47] Due to the lack of a regional response to Covid-19, trade declined by more than 50% in the early months of the pandemic and impacted cross-border traders, most of whom were women.[48,49] Finally, significantly more women than men reported increases in household expenses.[50]

Many fiscal policies designed to provide financial reliefs focused on those with a steady income, leaving out all of those in the informal sector (which comprises 85% of the urban population). These exclusionary policies included tax relief for low-income individuals, relief funds, suspension of listing with the Credit Reference Bureau, and a Covid-19 support stipend to target poor communities.[51,52] Social protection relief measures came into effect after people had lost their income, and logistical challenges impeded implementation in many cases, leading to minimal relief.[53,54] One study proposed that direct cash transfers and utility fee waivers could have been more beneficial for informal sector workers. Tax relief programmes did not reach those who did not pay taxes, such as those in the informal sector who live most 'hand to mouth'. Further, the tax relief benefit was repealed even as the curfew remained, still limiting

---

[45] Kenya's informal workers struggle under lockdown. *African Business*. Accessed February 4, 2021. https://african.business/2020/05/economy/nairobis-informal-workers-struggle-under-lockdown/.

[46] *Impact of Covid-19 on livelihoods*. Food Security and Nutrition in East Africa. Accessed February 4, 2021. https://unhabitat.org/sites/default/files/2020/08/wfp-000 0118161_1.pdf.

[47] Wangila (2020).

[48] Phillip (2020).

[49] *African women bear bigger brunt of the pandemic*. Accessed February 4, 2021. https://www.theafricareport.com/29306/coronavirus-african-women-bear-bigger-brunt-of-the-pandemic/.

[50] Karijo et al. (2020).

[51] Nderitu and Kamaara (2020).

[52] Muigua (2020).

[53] Kansiime et al. (2021).

[54] Shumba et al. (2020).

the hours people could work, making it hard for them to earn enough money to start paying taxes again and supporting their families.

Eligibility for cash transfers was determined by pre-existing government registers, which are widely recognized to be incomplete. Key informants noted that there was a 'poverty of data' to help identify the most vulnerable and that the few data that existed were under-utilized for appropriate targeting. A key informant explained that the cash transfer programme, which pre-dated the pandemic, "has been based on a single registry, but this single registry has a blind spot-on poverty", which seems like a significant shortcoming for such a programme.[55] Referring to the cash transfers, another key informant described them as "basically seeping out of the pipes that are supposed to deliver them to the recipients"[56] suggesting that, through corruption or inefficiencies, they did not reach their intended beneficiaries.

A key informant noted that had the government considered the number of people in Kenya who are small-scale traders or women or youths living in informal settlements or even in rural communities and had brought populations such as these to the decision-making table; the economy may not have been as affected as it was. The absence of trade unions, including for street hawkers, 'matatu' drivers, and other informal business sectors, from policy development processes created blind spots that exacerbated the economic impact of the response.[57]

For young children, alongside the vulnerability of caregivers to morbidity and mortality, the restricted access to social protection services or psychosocial support may have prevented caregivers from providing effective nurturing care to their children.[58] When caregivers succumbed to Covid-19 or indirect health impacts of Covid-19, children were orphaned.[59] Moreover, when caregivers experienced financial hardship or became ill during the pandemic, children were forced to beg for food and engage in hazardous work, and they also became vulnerable to violence

---

[55] Key informant interview 10.

[56] Key informant 9.

[57] Key informant interview 8.

[58] Shumba et al. (2020).

[59] Shumba et al. (2020).

and exploitation.[60] To supplement the family income, children participated in a variety of labour activities, including khat plucking, fetching
firewood, tea picking, coffee harvesting, working as part-time house help,
running farming errands, household chores for employers, selling water
at kiosks, and babysitting, all of which prevents them from engaging in
learning.

Young people were disproportionately affected as they were primarily
employed in the informal sector.[61] Youth reported income loss, increased
expenses, increased food costs, and loss of jobs. As a result, they were
forced to engage in income-generating activities to support their families.[62] An economic stimulus plan included a particular focus on youth
to reach large segments of informal workers and invest in long-term
economic success; it will be important to evaluate its implementation and
impact.[63]

Sex workers, whose income was essentially wiped out by curfew
measures, were noted to lack alternative sources of income, and yet some
were openly criticized for breaking physical distancing rules in crowded
informal settlements. Some sex workers produced and sold personal
protective equipment (masks, sanitizer) to generate alternative forms of
income.[64]

Released prisoners face a range of challenges, including vulnerability
to criminality, difficulties reintegrating into the community due to insufficient re-entry preparation and a lack of counselling, lack of access to
income-generating activities, and, for those living with HIV, particularly the elderly, a potential lack of support. Offenders on probation
would have challenges meeting with probation officers due to Covid-
19 measures.[65] The pandemic measures exacerbated challenges faced by

---

[60] *Save the children—Our response to COVID-19—Kenya*. Accessed February 4, 2021.
https://kenya.savethechildren.net/what-we-do/our-response-covid-19.

[61] *Kenya: Rising unemployment leads people to line for dirty jobs*. Accessed February 4,
2021, https://www.aa.com.tr/en/africa/kenya-rising-unemployment-leads-people-to-line-
for-dirty-jobs/1965212.

[62] Huho (2020).

[63] *5 countries that took proactive action on Covid-19—one*. Accessed February 4, 2021.
https://www.one.org/international/blog/proactive-action-countries-covid-19-response/.

[64] Kimani et al. (2020a).

[65] Langat et al. (2020).

refugees trying to be economically productive and resulted in greater economic instability among this population.[66]

The most common coping strategy was to change dietary patterns and rely on savings. Other strategies included reduced gifts/remittances, lending less money, postponed loan repayments, depositing less new savings, increased support from family and friends, and selling assets. As economic strain increased, there was a reported increase in dependence on relatives and friends for food, remittance, masks, sanitizers, and medicine. Coping through savings was more associated with the ability to withstand income shocks and remain food secure than coping through social protection schemes.[67],[68] Two groups of people reported financial gains from the pandemic: boda boda riders who indicated that sneaking individuals past road barriers was financially rewarding due to their increased rates, and those who were eligible for full or partial tax relief.

GDP growth of about 6% was forecast prior to the pandemic, but this was not realized, subsequently affecting the financial sector. The effects of this contraction were widespread and had significant implications on the government's ability to raise taxes and carry out necessary functions. One key informant pointed out that the debt level rose as Kenya had to take on additional debt from the World Bank, among others, for the emergency response.

Small businesses were negatively impacted, with permanent closures and an enormous loss of savings. Businesses experienced decreased production, a shortage of goods, and disruption within the supply chain. The worst-hit sectors were tourism, transport, horticulture, communications, and education. Changes in burial traditions due to Covid-19 had a spiralling impact on multiple different groups of people, including catering service groups, photographers, small traders selling things outside funerals, music providers, motorcycle operators transporting mourners to funerals, loitering groups who preyed on food at funerals, and illicit brew sellers. The closure of bars, restaurants, and schools pushed employers to terminate contracts, sometimes in a manner contrary to their employment contracts.

---

[66] *Two refugees explain how Covid-19 is changing their lives.* World Economic Forum. Accessed February 4, 2021. https://www.weforum.org/agenda/2020/04/covid-19-poses-its-own-set-of-challenges-for-refugees/.

[67] Wendy et al. (2020).

[68] Kansiime et al. (2021).

Curfews and other restrictions reduced the number of hours of work available per week in almost all sectors of the economy, especially in education and the hotel sector, causing reduced revenue and job losses. In addition, while Kenya reduced VAT from 16 to 14%, this did not help the business community because their sales volume had decreased dramatically. One study suggested that to aid businesses, it would have been helpful for the government to remove payroll costs. Some businesses benefited from the pandemic response; 12 companies were awarded Ksh 3 billion contracts with KEMSA to provide items not covered by the government budget.[69]

The pandemic measures specifically impacted the fishing industry, causing a decline in fishing trips. Market closures made it hard for fisherfolk to sell their fish and farmers to sell their cattle. Farmers were more likely to suffer income shocks compared to salary and wage earners because they reported difficulties accessing their farms, accessing farming inputs, and transporting their produce to markets due to the lockdown. Some wage earners, although by no means all, could work from home and earn an income. Kenyan farms also reduced exports to 50%, placing them in danger of downsizing and closure, which would increase poverty, insecurity, and hunger.[70] Lack of manufacturing from neighbouring countries caused a halt in the production of the dairy meal and unaffordable hay, leading to reductions in milk yield for farmers and an increase in milk prices. Rather than relying on savings as a coping strategy as salary-earning workers do, farmers and low-wage earners are more likely to cope by changing dietary patterns.

Though there was the intention to reach the most vulnerable, including the poor, through the different measures, it appears that this was unsuccessful due to two main factors: first, the government appears not to have anticipated the impact the mitigation policies would have, particularly on the vulnerable and therefore failed to consider this when structuring the pandemic mitigation as well as the social protection measures. Secondly, the system in place to implement the social protection measures such as cash transfers and tax relief was blind to poverty

---

[69] *Traders who made millions from Covid supplies.* Nation.

[70] Horticulture industry losing sh100m. *Daily Nation.* Accessed February 4, 2021, https://nation.africa/kenya/lifeand-style/smart-company/horticulture-industry-losing-sh100m-daily-1316172.

and the informal sector[71] hence it further disadvantaged the poorest and the near-poor who were sliding back into poverty. The need to update the register through various means was clearly articulated by most key informants who were not from the government sector.

There were reported rises in sexual offences, domestic violence, intimate partner violence, gender-based violence, and violations of the rights of children during the pandemic.[72] Financial pressure due to Covid-19 stimulated violence against individuals, some of whom were thrown out of their homes during the pandemic without financial support. A survey revealed that 10% of Kenyans reported being worried about GBV and 21% reported being worried about domestic violence during the pandemic.[73]

Covid-19-related isolation and economic anxiety amplified the mental health crisis in Kenya: isolation, cessation of movement, and loss of jobs due to the pandemic caused fear, anger, loneliness, stress, and anxiety in most Kenyans, particularly those of low income. As a result, about 75% of Kenyans reported worry, stress, and anxiety; suicides were also reported.[74] The inability to attend social gatherings contributed to these feelings of fear, uncertainty, and stress. The mental and psychological stress could partially be attributed to lack of health insurance and fear of loss of livelihood, both of which disproportionately affect those of lower socioeconomic status.[75]

Accessibility to food was reduced due to food shortages, income loss, increases in food prices, bans on outdoor markets, and diversion of funding from nutrition services to the Covid-19 response.[76,77] The pandemic was reported to have worsened an already bad food crisis; many individuals limited food consumption and a majority of Kenyans worried about food insecurity. Three-quarters of individuals reported eating less or skipping meals and that their most significant unmet need

---

[71] Key informant interview 10.

[72] Huho (2020).

[73] *Job losses and violence top list of Covid impact.* The Standard. Accessed February 4, 2021. https://www.standardmedia.co.ke/business/business-news/article/2001393199/job-losses-and-violence-top-list-ofcovid-impact.

[74] Wenzel Geissler and Prince (2020).

[75] Ouma et al. (2020).

[76] Kansiime et al. (2021).

[77] Saks et al. (2020).

was food.[78,79,80] 86% of Kenyans overall were worried about having food.[81] Families incurred debts from vendors, neighbours, and landlords and reported sacrificing their nutrition to provide adequate food for children.[82]

COVID-19 RESPONSES: INCLUSION AND ACCOUNTABILITY

Many stakeholders were active in the Covid-19 response but seemingly working independently rather than seeking involvement in the national response. The main role of these non-state actors seems to have been to provide financial support for vulnerable communities and direct funds for Covid-19-related relief programmes and innovation. Global and international organizations, as well as the private sector, collaborated to provide support to Kenya through money, food assistance, and other essential resources. The national private sector institutions involved in these efforts appear to represent large-scale, well-established companies. Representatives of the informal economy, on which most Kenyans rely, were not included in advisory committees nor the management and distribution of Covid-19-related relief funds.

Civil society was more proactive in pushing for inclusion in the governmental response and demanding government accountability for the response. National-level civil society actors tried to help shape the legal and policy environment from the very beginning of the response, informing the government about things it would be essential to consider. However, one key informant described this as "an exercise in futility" as the government did not heed this advice. In some instances, they only provided 1–2 days for civil society input, making comprehensive consultation impossible; in most cases, none of the recommendations were taken on board. The minimal room for public input into the regulations, which limited public and parliamentary scrutiny of the response, was challenged in Court.

---

[78] Kenya National Bureau of Statistics (2020).

[79] Kansiime et al. (2021).

[80] Abuya et al. (2020).

[81] Saks et al. (2020).

[82] Kenya National Bureau of Statistics (2020).

There was disappointment among civil society actors with the measures that the government introduced, with one key informant highlighting the stigmatizing language used in some regulations and the negative impacts that many of the regulations have had. Furthermore, the top-down approach led to inappropriate measures with unintended negative consequences that might have been better foreseen had civil society, including representatives of vulnerable and marginalized populations, been active participants in designing the response.[83]

There were challenges to ensuring accountability for the national Covid-19 response. Ostensibly, the Kenyan Judicial system was an accountability mechanism to ensure that all laws enforced during the pandemic did not infringe upon citizens' civil, political, economic, or social rights. In some cases, this worked well. For example, when Kenya Airways tried to amend workers' contracts due to economic hardships during the pandemic without consulting unions, the Court ruled against this. They specifically protected the workers' rights and prevented the company from making decisions that could have consequences for employees, regardless of the pandemic.[84] However, in other cases, perceived impunity persisted. For example, one key informant shared reports that parliamentarians were involved in the 'disappearance' of PPE, yet no action was taken to investigate this. Responsibility for the health worker strike fell between the national and county governments, with nobody assuming ultimate responsibility for its cause or resolution.[85] Civil society organizations took the lead in pressuring the government to implement Covid-19 measures and address accounts of police brutality and corruption. In Homa Bay County and Siaya County, lobby groups and civil society contacted the police and released statements urging police to not act with force.[86]

Overall, the responses and reactions to Covid-19 in Kenya may endure and exacerbate inequalities, worsening health conditions of the most vulnerable due to resource allocation and other measures.

---

[83] Key informant 1.

[84] Onyano (2020).

[85] Key informant 1.

[86] Uproar over police brutality during virus curfew in Kenya. *Nation*. Accessed February 3, 2021. https://nation.africa/counties/Uproar-greets-Kenya-coronavirus-cur few/1107872-550734012qc9qy/index.html.

CONCLUSION AND RECOMMENDATIONS

The pandemic exposed societal inequalities and lack of emergency preparedness, which must now be addressed. Fighting poverty and addressing inequalities should be prioritized. The importance of a targeted approach that considers people's differing vulnerabilities and resilience has been emphasized. This might best have been achieved by ensuring that all appropriate stakeholders were represented in the design and governance of the Covid-19 response. While this might not have been possible in the initial stages of the response, at the later stages, membership of advisory committees and other governance structures might usefully have been revisited. It would have been essential to improve coordination between national and county governments and governments at all levels and civil society. Transparency in decision-making would have been essential to allow people to understand how trade-offs among competing needs were being made and to provide avenues for accountability as necessary.

While fully recognising the government's need to move quickly in the face of a crisis, adopting a participatory approach that included broader inclusion of stakeholders from different parts of the private sector as well as civil society might have helped identify potential shortcomings and allowed for more appropriate options to be put forward. Young people constitute a large proportion of the total population; they are embedded in communities and often committed to effecting positive change. This is a demography whose involvement in the response should have been considered.

Although key informants' views on government receptivity to criticism varied, civil society representatives working on health noted that the government was open to criticism and magnanimous even in accepting that criticism. Instead of ignoring feedback, the government listened and showed some degree of openness to the media too. Furthermore, as the pandemic progressed, the government appeared to react more responsibly and responsively to people's needs.

The people's trust in their government is critical during a crisis such as Covid-19 when the government must ask people to make sacrifices and follow public health directives. Mired in a long history of corruption allegations, the government was not well-positioned in this regard going into the Covid-19 pandemic. It should not wait for the next disaster to try to build this trust. A conscious effort to rebuild trust in government structures, institutions, and leaders is urgently needed. As noted by one interview participant, community trust in government is critical, and two immediate opportunities for helping to rebuild this trust include ensuring an efficient and equitable vaccine rollout programme and building a robust health system to support the achievement of Universal Health Coverage.

It would be helpful to create emergency structures that can be mobilized as the need arises to tackle pandemic. This would include multi-stakeholder planning groups that would allow for government responses to be informed by a broad range of civil society and private sector actors and representatives of different sectors, including public health, economy, education, labour and justice, to help ensure a coherent, comprehensive response. In addition, understanding and better documenting the synergies between different stakeholders' work in the response would help allay competition concerns and identify how each organization or constituency can best play to its strengths in a collaborative and coordinated response.

All restrictions can have economic consequences. That is not to say that epidemic response is a trade-off between health and the economy. Rather that if restrictions are warranted from a public health perspective, the economic impacts on different groups of people must be foreseen and mitigated. Given that there will be more infectious disease outbreaks, it will be helpful for the government to plan how they might financially support a large proportion of the population in order that they might be able to follow the necessary directives. For any response to succeed, it must be pro-poor. This is another area where attention to committee membership is critical: those with a seat at the table can lobby for their constituents' interests; those excluded from the committees have no voice in these policy discussions.

References

Abuya, T., Austrian, K., Isaac, A., Kagwana, B., Mbushi, F., & Muluve, E. (2020). *Covid-19-related-knowledge-attitudes-and-practices-in-urban-slums-in-Nairobi, Kenya*. Harvard Dataverse, V1. https://doi.org/10.7910/DVN/VO7SUO

Barasa, E. W., Ouma, P. O., & Okiro, E. A. (2020). Assessing the hospital surge capacity of the Kenyan health system in the face of the COVID-19

pandemic. *PLoS One, 15*(7), e0236308. https://doi.org/10.1371/journal.
pone.0236308

Dahir, L. A. (2020, September 15). Kenya's health workers, unprotected and
falling ill, walk off job. *The New York Times.* https://www.nytimes.com/
2020/08/21/world/africa/kenya-doctors-strike-coronavirus.html

Huho, J. M. (2020, August). The two sides of Covid-19 in Kenya: Getting
a closer look. *International Journal of Scientific and Research Publications,
10*(8), 478. https://doi.org/10.29322/IJSRP.10.08.2020.p10459

Kansiime, K. M., Tambo, J. A., Mugambi, I., Mbundi, M., Kara, A., & Owuor,
C. (2021, January 1). *Covid-19 implications on household income and food
security in Kenya and Uganda: Findings from a rapid assessment.* World
Development 137. https://doi.org/10.1016/j.worlddev.2020.105199.

Karijo, E., Wamugi, S., Lemanyishoe, S., Njuki, N., Boit, F., Karanja, S., &
Abuya, T. (2020, June). *Knowledge, attitudes, practices, and the effects of
COVID-19 on health seeking behaviors among young people in Kenya.* https://
doi.org/10.21203/rs.3.rs-34861/v1

Kelin. (2020, March). *Kelin convenes a multi-stakeholder rights-based response to
curbing Covid-19.* https://www.kelinkenya.org/wp-content/uploads/2020/
03/for-immediate-release.pdf

Kenya National Bureau of Statistics. (2018). *Kenya integrated household budget
survey 2015–2016.* https://new.knbs.or.ke/wp-content/uploads/2023/09/
2015-2016-Kenya-Integrated-Household-Budget-Survey-Highlights.pdf

Kenya National Bureau of Statistics. (2019). *Kenya population and housing census:
Volume III.* https://housingfinanceafrica.org/app/uploads/VOLUME-III-
KPHC-2019.pdf

Kenya National Bureau of Statistics. (2020). *Economic survey 2020.* The
Elephant. Accessed February 4, 2021. https://www.theelephant.info/doc
uments/kenya-national-bureau-of-statistics-economic-survey-2020

Kenya National Commission on Human Rights. (2020). *Situational report no. 1
of 2020.* www.intercode.co.ke.

Kenya News. (n.d.). *Ministry launches COVID-19 national education response
committee.* https://www.kenyanews.go.ke/ministry-launches-of-covid-19-nat
ional-education-response-committee/

Kimani, J., Adhiambo, J., Kasiba, R., Mwangi, P., Were, V., & Mathenge, J.
(2020a, May). The effects of Covid-19 on the health and socio-economic
security of sex workers in Nairobi, Kenya: Emerging intersections with
HIV. *Global Public Health, 5*(2), 1–10. https://doi.org/10.1080/17441692.
2020.1770831

Kimani, W. R., Maina, R., Shumba, C., & Shaibu, S. (2020b). Maternal and
newborn care during the Covid-19 pandemic in Kenya: Re-contextualising the
community midwifery model. *Human Resoures for Health, 18*, 75. https://
doi.org/10.1186/s12960-020-00518-3

Lagat, H., Sharma, M., Kariithi, E., Otieno, G., Katz, D., & Masyuko, S. (2020). Impact of the Covid-19 pandemic on HIV testing and assisted partner notification services, Western Kenya. *AIDS and Behavior, 24*(1234), 3010–3013, https://doi.org/10.1007/s10461-020-02938-7

Langat, K. C., Melly, J., & Nyawira, M. (2020). Impact of Covid-19 on incarcerated offenders and community reintegration challenges in Kenya prisons. *American Research Journal of Humanities & Social Science, 3*(6), 55–62. https://edition.cnn.com/2020/04/02/africa/kenya-courts-onskype/index.html

Mbogo, W. R. (2020, August 10). Leadership roles in managing education in crises: The case of Kenya during Covid-19 pandemic. *European Journal of Education Studies, 7*(9), 19. https://doi.org/10.46827/ejes.v7i9.3250

Muigua, K. (2020). *Redefining development in Kenya-reflections and lessons from the coronavirus disease (COVID-19).* Redefining Development in Kenya. https://www.the-star.co.ke/authors/alex-awiti

Nderitu, D., & Kamaara, E. (2020). Gambling with covid-19 makes more sense: Ethical and practical challenges in Covid-19 responses in communalistic resource-limited Africa. *Journal of Bioethical Inquiry, 17*, 607–611. https://doi.org/10.1007/s11673-020-10002-1

Noor, F. A. (2020). Effect of Covid-19 on loan repayment of small businesses in Kenya: A case study of eastleigh business community. *European Journal of Business and Strategic Management, 5*(2), 1–14. https://doi.org/10.47604/ejbsm.1122

Obulutsa, G. (2020). *Kenyan parliament halts Covid-19 related tax relief.* Reuters. https://www.reuters.com/article/health-coronavirus-kenya-economy/kenyan-parliament-halts-covid-19-related-taxrelief-idUSL8N2J12LX

Onyano, O. K., (2020, October 13). Non-performance: The impact of Covid-19 on contractual obligations in Kenya. *SSRN Electronic Journal.* https://doi.org/10.2139/ssrn.3707988

Ouma, P. N., Masai, N. A., & Nyaburi, N. I. (2020). Health coverage and what Kenya can learn from the Covid-19 pandemic. *Journal of Global Health, 10.* https://doi.org/10.7189/jogh.10.020362

Phillip, X. (2020, August 19). *Uganda/Kenya: Women traders hit hard by 'Covid-19 nationalism.* Accessed February 4, 2021. https://www.theafricareport.com/38015/uganda-kenya-women-traders-hit-hard-by-covid-19-nationalism/#:~:text=East%20African%20Community%20women%20traders,the%20region's%20major%20trade%20routes

Saks, A., Ajisola, M., Azeem, K., Bakibinga, P., Chen, Y. F., & Choudhury, N. N. (2020). Improving health in slums collaborative: Impact of the societal response to Covid-19 on access to healthcare for non-COVID-19 health issues in slum communities of Bangladesh, Kenya, Nigeria and Pakistan: Results of pre-Covid and Covid-19 lockdown stakeholder engagements. *BMJ*

Global Health, 5(8), e003042. https://doi.org/10.1136/bmjgh-2020-003 042.PMID:32819917;PMCID:PMC7443197

Shikuku, D., Nyaoke, I., Gichuru, S., Maina, O., Eyinda, M., & Godia, P. (2020). *Early indirect impact of Covid-19 pandemic on utilization and outcomes of reproductive, maternal, newborn, child and adolescent health services in Kenya*. https://doi.org/10.1101/2020.09.09.20191247

Shumba, C., Maina, R., Mbuthia, G., Kimani, R., Mbugua, S., & Shah, S. (2020). Reorienting nurturing care for early childhood development during the Covid-19 pandemic in Kenya: A review. *International Journal of Environmental Research and Public Health, 17*(7028), 1–19. https://ecommons. aku.edu/eastafrica_fhs_sonam/293

Wangamati, K., & Sundby, J. (2020, September). The ramifications of Covid-19 on maternal health in Kenya, sexual and reproductive health matters. *Sexual and Reproductive Health Matters, 28*(1), 1804716. https://doi.org/ 10.1080/26410397.2020.1804716

Wangila, B. (2020). *Who speaks for women in the informal sector in Kenya during the coronavirus pandemic?* https://www.africanwomeninlaw.com/post/who-speaks-for-women-in-the-informal-sector-in-kenya-during-the-coronavirus-pandemic

Wendy, J., Menno, P. P., de Groot, R., Estelle, S., Hermann, D., & Amanuel, A. (2020, July 1). *The short-term economic effects of Covid-19 and risk-coping strategies of low-income households in Kenya: A rapid analysis using weekly financial household data* (Tinbergen Institute Disucssion Paper 2020–040/ V). Available at SSRN https://ssrn.com/abstract=3640340

Wenzel Geissler, P., & Prince, J. R. (2020, April 5). Frontline: Primary health care and Covid-19 in Kenya. *Somatosphere.* https://somatosphere.com/for umpost/primary-health-care-covid-19-kenya/

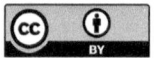

CHAPTER 10

Mozambique

Adriano Nuvunga, Angela Collet, and Dimas Sinoia

INTRODUCTION

The socioeconomic shocks caused by the COVID-19 pandemic have brought the debate on income distribution/redistribution and social protection to the centre of the public agenda. In Mozambique, this topic is especially relevant because of the cyclical and structural context, which is characterised by multiple crises, including poverty[1] and economic, social, gender, and regional inequalities; food insecurity and chronic malnutrition; lack of confidence on the part of development cooperation partners (including as a result of the 'hidden debts'[2] Scandal and lack of progress in good governance); the unsustainable level of

---

[1] An estimated 41–46% of the population, or between 10.5 and 11.3 million people, live in absolute poverty (Santos & Savucci, 2016).

A. Nuvunga (✉) · A. Collet
Centre for Democracy and Human Rights (CDD), Maputo, Mozambique
e-mail: Adriano.nuvunga@cddmoz.org

D. Sinoia
Fórum de Monitoria Do Orçamento, Maputo, Mozambique

[2] Mozambique's biggest corruption scandal. State guarantees of USD 2.2 Billion were issued in secret, without parliamentary approval (CDD, 2020b).

© The Author(s) 2024
A. Altaf et al. (eds.), *EQUITY IN COVID-19*, EADI Global
Development Series, https://doi.org/10.1007/978-3-031-58588-3_10

external public debt, which has led to a sharp depreciation of the national currency (Mozambique metical) against the US dollar (CDD, 2020b); and political-military instability in the central region of the country and the insurgency (including violent extremists) in the province of Cabo Delgado (Presidência da República, 2020). In addition, the crisis generated by the COVID-19 pandemic, mixed with these structural crises, weakens the government's ability to respond to the socioeconomic shocks caused by the COVID-19 pandemic (CDD, 2020a), which has led to the partial paralysis of many economic activities, leading to the closure of companies, increased unemployment, and increased cost of living.

Data from the National Statistics Institute (2020) for April to June 2020 revealed that, because of the measures adopted to curb the COVID-19 pandemic, 62,700 workers were affected by the suspension of contracts. Another 77,489 workers were affected by the termination of contracts, and 43,579 by the closure of companies. In addition, an inquiry made by the Association of Trade, Industry and Services (Associação de Comércio, Indústria e Serviços, ACIS) found that Mozambican companies had registered a 60% drop in sales due to the impact of COVID-19 (República de Moçambique, n.d.). As a result, the Government of Mozambique was called upon to establish a long-term approach to tackling the pandemic. The mitigation strategies should enable structural changes in the economy in the long term.

The study's main objective was to analyse Mozambique's national COVID-19 response in terms of policy coherence from an equity perspective, focusing on policies/measures that formally target the most vulnerable groups.

Mozambique's COVID-19 Situation

This case study addresses two 'waves' of the COVID-19 pandemic in Mozambique: the first covering nine months from March to November 2020 and the second from late December 2020 to the time of writing (February 2021). It is essential to remember that Mozambique is currently facing a State-citizen crisis, in which part of the population lack trust in the central Government for various reasons, including the 'hidden debt' scandal, which is an important context to consider in the analysis. Considering this, before December 2020, the existence of COVID-19 was unclear to most of the population. During the first wave, individual prevention practices relied mainly on the population's limited trust in the information shared by the Government and their willingness to follow the government's state of emergency/calamity decrees. On top of this, fake news spread through informal channels and social media posts made some people believe that COVID-19 would not spread in Mozambique.

The analysis notes that the worsening of the COVID-19 pandemic in Mozambique has been associated with two phenomena (Tibana, 2021): the relaxation of prevention measures announced by the Government on December 17, 2020, and the penetration of the South African strain of the virus in November 2020, which is considered more infectious and lethal. As a result, as illustrated in Fig. 10.1, the number of COVID-19 cases has increased significantly from December 2020 to February 2021.

The increase in cases preoccupied the national health system, as health facilities are not equipped to deal with the volume of people needing treatment, as noted in the President's speech on February 4, 2021, (Presidência da República, 2021). Since March 2020, debates have intensified about the dilemma faced by the Government, namely, the need to implement a 'total lockdown' to contain the spread of COVID-19 and relieve the pressure on the health system versus the need to keep the economy running to some extent. Some actors have argued that while it is crucial to ensure economic stability, saving human lives and caring for the most vulnerable sectors of the population should also be a priority. However, the debate as to whether a lockdown should be applied is not unanimous. In addition, civil society has no formal channel to

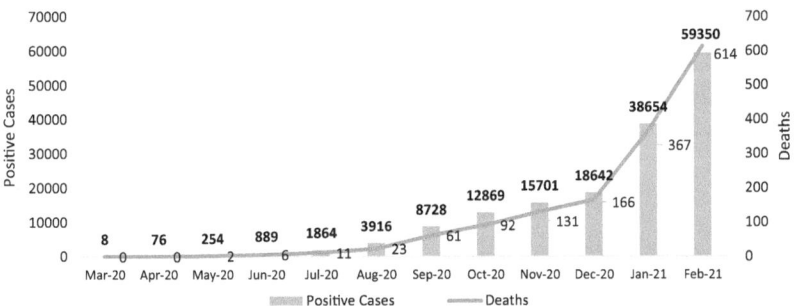

Fig. 10.1 Cumulative COVID-19 cases in Mozambique (March 2020 to February 2021). *Source* Based on Worldometer (https://www.worldometers. info/coronavirus/country/mozambique/); and Mozambican National Institute of Health)

be involved in such debates and decisions related to COVID-19 policies. It was due to this situation that many civil society organisations (CSOs), such as the Budget Monitoring Forum (FMO), Mozambican Civil Society Platform for Social Protection (PSCM-PS), women's organisations and non-governmental organisations (NGOs), prioritised monitoring the implementation of COVID-19 policies. They also conducted equity-related advocacy campaigns and research, arguing that the main focus of efforts should be to protect the most vulnerable population groups.

COVID-19 Mitigation in the Provinces

COVID-19 exacerbated existing crises. For instance, since 2017, the province of Cabo Delgado, where Pemba is located, has faced violent extremism, which has resulted in an estimated 530,000[3] internally displaced persons (IDPs) fled to cities where people were already facing multiple crises (i.e., low food supply, unemployment, climate change and others). Sofala province, where the City of Beira is located, was one of the regions most affected by Cyclone Idai in March 2019, which destroyed houses, infrastructure, and production units, thus increasing the number of vulnerable citizens in need of support from government social protection programmes. Although, so far, the epicentre of the COVID-19 pandemic has been Maputo, the capital of Mozambique (Presidência da República, 2021), transmission has been increasing in other parts of the country. As a result, health facilities specially equipped to treat people with COVID-19 have been built/repurposed in provincial capitals. However, if the recent rapid rise in cases (second wave) seen in the capital carries over to the provinces, health facilities are unlikely to be able to cope with the demand for COVID-19 treatment services.

National Social Protection System

On March 30, 2020, a State of Emergency was declared throughout Mozambique (Presidential Decree No. 11/2020) to allow the Government to implement measures to combat the spread of COVID-19. The

---

[3] Numbers include IDPs located in the provinces of Cabo Delgado, Nampula, and Niassa (UNHCR, 2021).

Minister for Gender, Children, and Social Action—MGCAS (2020a)[4], advised the INAS (National Institute of Social Action) and the Provincial Social Affairs Services to implement a sectorial plan at the national level to mitigate the negative socioeconomic impacts on the most vulnerable population groups in Mozambique, because of the measures taken to control the spread of the virus (UNICEF & ILO, 2020).

Basic Social Security is provided by INAS through the following programmes (República de Moçambique—Sistema de Protecção Social, 2019a):

- Basic Social Subsidy Programme (PSSB) and Productive Social Action Programme (PASP)—cash transfers;
- Direct Social Support Programme (PASD)—food vouchers, in-kind transfers, service payments;
- Social Action Social Services Programme (PSSAS)—assistance in social units and social services.

For the COVID-19 pandemic, however, non-contributory social protection is primarily covered by external funds (MGCAS, 2020a), as it is assumed that State funds for emergency purposes are unavailable.

METHODOLOGY AND ANALYTICAL FRAMEWORK

The case study used the data triangulation technique, based on a combination of methods as illustrated in Fig. 10.2 and Table 10.1.

Data analysis was based on qualitative techniques, as the surveys used an exploratory approach to COVID-19 pandemic policies and their effectiveness in the field. As for sampling, because this was a qualitative study,

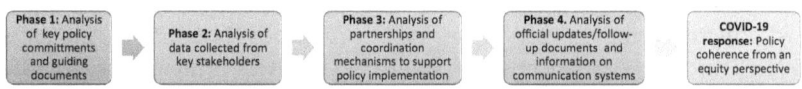

Fig. 10.2 Four phase methodology

---

[4] Article 36 of Decree No. 12/2020, April 2.

Table 10.1   Data collection methods and techniques applied in each phase

Phase	Data collection methods and techniques
Phase 1	• Review of key documents: on the planning/implementation of the national response plan to COVID-19, focusing on non-contributory social protection policies
Phase 2	• Surveys were submitted via electronic channels to (1) The Government of Mozambique and The Assembly of the Republic to collect information on the suggested topics (ToRs—INCLUDE case study); (2) Civil society organisations to collect good practices and challenges (support/advocacy actions); and (3) The Confederation of Economic Associations to collect examples of the impact of social protection actions targeting formal workers
Phase 3	• Literature review: according to predetermined thematically relevant criteria and document analysis with a focus on good practices in the context of the response to the COVID-19 pandemic • Workshops (2): with community-based organisations, in the cities of Pemba and Beira, with a total of 38 participating institutions • Email interviews (3), online survey and Internet search: on best practices of CSOs concerning actions for monitoring the COVID-19 response
Phase 4	• Literature review and Internet search: on official COVID-19 policy updates/follow-up documents and social protection information and communication systems

techniques such as convenience sampling were used to identify respondents. The primary data collection process ended in November 2020, and COVID-19 statistics were updated until the end of February 2021.

ANALYTICAL FRAMEWORK

The analytical framework for this study is an adaptation of the 'policy' coherence for development—PCD (Cadernos de Estudos Africanos, 2017) through a perspective of 'equity'. The PCD principle helps assess to what extent specific policies (in this case, the COVID-19 response) contribute to the broader policy objectives of the National Development Strategy of Mozambique, namely combating poverty and promoting inclusive development. The applied policy coherence approach relates directly to the Government's Five-Year Plan (approved by the Assembly of the Republic and annually transformed into the social, economic plan and state budget) and to the way society organises its power structures to solve development challenges and the State organises itself to protect vulnerable groups. Considering that exclusion and human rights violations become more severe in times of crisis, addressing this question is even more relevant during the COVID-19 pandemic.

The perspective of equity is a lens that pays attention to social justice.[5] Whereas 'equity' has been chiefly applied to public policies on gender, it needs to be better understood as an inclusive policy approach to guarantee social justice. The Social Action Policy and its Implementation Strategy (Resolution 46/2017, November 2) include 'Social Justice' as a principle. Therefore, when the Government designed the COVID-19 Response Plan for social protection, there was an implied commitment to formulating equitable policies.

Policy coherence, combined with an equity lens, is also about questioning the centralisation of budget resources and focusing on justice in the distribution of resources. These lenses look at how public policies are formulated—to what extent they are participatory and based on context evidence and data gathered by trusted and independent entities. Effective participation is a crucial indicator of equity, related to the presence (or lack) of social justice and opportunities for the most vulnerable groups to access information and participate in decision-making processes. This approach can also benefit from a search for transparent mechanisms for sharing information and implementing monitoring and evaluation systems.

MEASURES: PLANNED RESPONSE TO COVID-19, BUDGET, AND ALLOCATION TO SOCIAL PROTECTION

COVID-19 Response Plan (PRC19).

The Government of Mozambique had taken a series of measures to combat the pandemic since mid-March when the first case was recorded. One of the most significant was the declaration of a State of Emergency (MEF, 2020a). In parallel, and to respond to the direct and indirect (potential) impacts of COVID-19, the Government recognised the need to support different sectors (health, social protection, and the private sector) and State revenue, among other things (MEF, 2020b).

---

[5] Social justice is highlighted in Article 1 of the Constitution of the Republic of Mozambique, which states that Mozambique is an 'Independent, Sovereign, Democratic and Socially Just State'.

PUBLIC BUDGET

The Ministry of Economy and Finance estimated that the activities and actions under the COVID-19 Response Plan (PRC19) would cost around USD 700 million (about 5% of Mozambique's GDP, compared to a world average of 3.7%) (BBC, 2020). The Government's budget for the PRC19 is set out in Table 10.2.

An equity lens notes that around a third of the total PRC19 budget (approximately USD 240 million) was allocated to 'Transfers to families, to guarantee social protection to the most vulnerable households during the pandemic'. Hence, this appears to be the highest priority in allocating funds (34% of funds). 'Micro businesses' are also targeted (with 23% of funds). The budget allocated to the health sector (14% of funds) also impacts the most vulnerable groups, who rely on the national health system.

Due to the budget deficit, which is mainly the high debt servicing required because of the unsustainability of Mozambique's internal and external public debt (CDD, 2020c), and what happened when the country was hit by cyclones Idai and Kenneth in 2019, the Government requested USD 700 million to finance the plan from development cooperation partners. However, the lack of confidence of development partners in the Government, caused by the 'hidden debt' scandal and the lack of progress in good governance, particularly in combating corruption and promoting transparency and accountability, hampered the Government's ability to obtain financial support. However, despite this, the Government managed to mobilise significant resources through loans and grants. For example, through its USD 309 million credit approval document to contribute to the PRC19 budget, the International Monetary Fund (IMF) expressed a desire to see its financing (as a conditional loan) not

Table 10.2 The government budget for COVID-19 Response Plan (USD)

Areas prioritised	Requested amount
Prevention and treatment	100,000,000
Loss of revenue	200,000,000
Transfers to families	**240,000,000**
Micro businesses	160,000,000
Total	**700,000,000**

Source: *Status of Commitments under COVID-19* (MEF, 2020b, November)

only help Mozambique in the fight against COVID-19 but also to have a catalytic effect on Mozambique's other development partners (IMF, 2020). For this reason, the IMF incorporated transparency and accountability mechanisms into the agreement, including the publication of large public procurement contracts and the carrying out and publication of audits.

COMPLEMENTARY FUNDS

From the perspective of transparency in policy coherence, it is essential to recall that the PRC19, provided by the Government in its Status of Commitments under COVID-19 (MEF, 2020b), does not explicitly mention other types of support, such as programmes (i) financed by the private sector and operated by the Government; (ii) financed by external funds and operated by the Government (not directly included in the state budget); (iii) financed and operated by development cooperation partners and coordinated by the Government; (iv) financed, operated, and coordinated by development cooperation partners; or (v) financed and operated by civil society and the private sector. In addition, other programmes were implemented in coordination with the Government. Some of these were not included in the PRC19 mentioned above.

SOCIAL PROTECTION RESPONSE

A sectoral budget analysis of the Social Action sector (which includes a specific chapter on the Social Protection Response Plan to COVID-19—PRC19-PS) states that 'The ambitious Social Protection Response Plan to COVID-19 in Mozambique, if implemented in its entirety (…) would imply an unprecedented extension of the social protection system coverage, both at the national level and in the sub-Saharan Africa region, adding, even if temporarily, almost 1 million new vulnerable beneficiaries not yet included in the non-contributory system managed by INAS' (UNICEF & ILO, 2020, p. 15). The brochure *COVID-19 Response Plan—Social Protection* (June 2020) also highlights the ambitious nature of this plan and notes that to ensure its implementation, the Ministry of

Gender, Children, and Social Action was coordinating efforts with various Government partners (see MGCAS, 2020b for details).[6]

In general terms, the PRC19-PS is anchored in the current framework of the National Basic Social Security Strategy II (ENSSB II), which allows social protection programmes to be activated in 'emergency scenarios' (MGCAS, 2020b). However, the plan also encompasses actions considered 'innovative', including an objective selection of programme implementation sites, information management system; digitalised payments to beneficiaries; comprehensive programme coverage; and identification of new beneficiaries.

CASH TRANSFERS

A core strategy of the Social Protection Response is to adapt the current Basic Social Security programmes managed by INAS to make cash transfers available. Accordingly, the Ministry of Gender, Children, and Social Action clarified this measure as non-contributory social protection implemented through external funds and that, in addition to making cash transfers available to new beneficiaries (for six months), three-month cash transfers were also forecasted for current beneficiaries of the PSSB (Basic Social Subsidy Programme) and PASP (Productive Social Action Programme) (MGCAS, 2020b).

The criteria defined by the MGCAS (October 2020) for receiving cash transfers are households in situations of poverty and vulnerability and households living in urban, peri-urban and border areas, with priority given to households headed by: older people, people with chronic and degenerative diseases, people with disabilities, children, pregnant women without a source of income, and women with six or more dependents. In addition, households that host internally displaced persons are also given priority.

In addition to the criteria for households, the following socioeconomic categories were identified as priorities for pandemic response measures/policies: internally displaced people/refugees; disabled people; children under challenging situations; older people in absolute poverty; disabled people in absolute poverty; people with chronic and degenerative diseases; people benefiting from Basic Social Security programmes;

---

[6] See also the United Nations Multi-Sector Response Plan to COVID-19 for Mozambique—ONU Moçambique, 2020a, 2020b.

women/women heads of households; and people living on the streets (MGCAS, 2020a).

In-kind Social Protection Measures

The Ministry of Gender, Children, and Social Action foresees the allocation of a food basket corresponding to three months of food to existing beneficiaries through the PASD (Direct Social Support Programme) for 18,438 current beneficiaries. In addition, other in-kind benefits are related to providing hygiene and personal protection equipment to vulnerable people, technicians, and employees, totalling 600,000 beneficiaries (provision of hygiene material) and 1.6 million beneficiaries (provision of individual protection material such as masks). These are also non-contributory social protection programmes implemented through external funds (MGCAS, 2020a).

Credit for Small and Medium Enterprises

The Government created a credit line to support small and medium enterprises (SMEs).[7] On July 1, 2020, the National Investment Bank (BNI), the Mozambican bank for development, proceeded with the launch of two special credit lines with 100% state capital: (i) the 'Gov. COVID-19 Credit Line', with USD 15 million funded by the IMF through the state budget, and (ii) the 'BNI COVID-19 Credit Line', with USD 9 million funded by the INSS. The BNI created the Special Credit and Evaluation Committee to approve proposals for financing, with a total of 900 proposals received and 151 approved worth USD 18,975,000.

Although there is a need for a more in-depth analysis of selected SMEs (i.e., in terms of the equity of the selection criteria), the Government's focus on SMEs is justified by the fact that they absorb the most significant part of the active workforce, represented mainly by low-income young people with a low level of academic and technical-professional training. Financial support for SMEs in this context can be an indirect way of protecting vulnerable groups who are dependent on employment by SMEs. The government initiative to protect SMEs supported the Confederation of Economic Associations (the largest association in the

---

[7] See Presidential Decree no. 37/2020, of June 2, 2020.

Mozambican private sector). However, the challenges identified include adequately reaching vulnerable groups, as the implementation of these plans is still deficient.[8]

SUPPORT FOR THE INFORMAL SECTOR

Another issue that has hampered the efficient implementation of social protection programmes in the context of COVID-19 is the high level of informality in the economy. In this regard, support was provided to low-income self-employed workers by promoting their affiliation with the INSS (ILO, 2020). In addition, ILO also conducted A *Rapid Assessment of the Impact of COVID-19 on the Informal Economy in Mozambique* (ILO, 2020) with recommendations to mitigate the negative socioeconomic impacts of COVID-19 on workers in the informal economy.

The Social Protection Response does not explicitly include measures to subsidise the cost of electricity, gas, water, or public transport (MGCAS, 2020a). Although it is known that some of these measures are being implemented, it is not clear the source of the funds (private and/or public) or which sector is accountable for such interventions. In addition, it should be noted that policies in the health and education sectors, implemented in response to the COVID-19 pandemic, despite not being included in social protection actions, also benefit the most vulnerable groups in the population.

POLICY COHERENCE AND EQUITY OF SOCIAL PROTECTION RESPONSE TO COVID-19

As shown in Table 10.2, in requesting financial assistance from the international community, social protection was the top priority of the Government of Mozambique in its plan to mitigate the effects of COVID-19. Table 10.3 provides an update, up until December 2020, showing that out of a total of USD 700 million, development partners had disbursed approximately USD 662 million.

---

[8] Survey questionnaire answered by Non-State actors for the Case Study INCLUDE Equity COVID-19.

Table 10.3 The government budget for COVID-19 response (USD) up to December 2020

Sector	Type of planned activity	Requested amount	Disbursed amount	Amounts channelled to sectors	Expenditure up to December 2020
Health	Prevention and treatment	100,000,000	111,412,785	111,412,785	111,412,785
State budget 2020	Loss of revenue	200,000,000	496,137,974	285,027,174	285,027,174
MGCAS/ INAS	Transfers to families	240,000,000	38,999,185	31,140,385	29,368,183
BNI	Micro business line of credit	160,000,000	15,000,000	15,000,000	24,000,000
	Total	700,000,000	661,549,943	450,439,144	449,808,142

Note MGCAS = Ministry of Gender, Children and Social Action; Source: MEF (2021, January)

In the follow-up report, *Status of Commitments under COVID-19—Maputo (December 2020)*, two inconsistencies can be identified, which require further attention:

- Although the periodic dissemination of information was acknowledged as a good practice, the updates report only on the funds received by the Government to implement its response plan to COVID-19. They did not report on every fund applied in response to COVID-19 in the country. The response to COVID-19 in Mozambique included interventions by development cooperation partners, whose actions have the same objective.
- The shift in budget prioritisation weakens the original focus on targeting vulnerable groups—it is concerning to see (through the comparative data on budget allocation per sector in 2020) an apparent decrease in the budget funds for social protection targeting vulnerable groups (funds allocated to transfers to households).

By comparing the initial plan and the most updated data (December 2020), we see that the initial allocation to the social protection sector

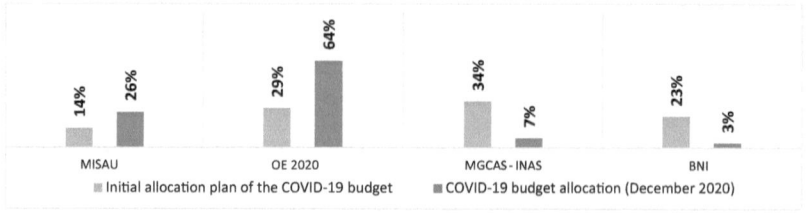

Fig. 10.3 The relative deviation between the planned and actual allocation of funds. *Note* MGCAS = Ministry of Gender, Children and Social Action; OE = State budget; BNI = National Investment Bank. *Source* MEF (2020c, December)

was the highest priority, with a relative weight of around 34% (USD 240 million) of the total financing volume. However, of the total amount disbursed to date (USD 661.5 million), only 7% (USD 38.9 million) has been channelled to social protection (Fig. 10.3).

The budget signals a change in the Government's understanding of the allocation priorities for COVID-19, which has sacrificed the funding provided to protect vulnerable households from financing the state budget above what was initially planned. However, explanations for this shift were not provided in the analysed reports. As the social protection benefits refer to cash and in-kind transfers, not prevention or treatment, the fact that the number of cases (by December 2020) had not been as high as initially expected cannot be a reason for the diminished support to vulnerable households, most of which were highly affected by the economic impact of the COVID-19 pandemic.

Inappropriate Use of Funds

Since August 2020, the Budget Monitoring Forum has been assessing the policy coherence of the Government's interventions under the COVID-19 Response Plan, including monitoring the procurement processes carried out and tracking expenditure. Below are the core findings and recommendations from FMO for better public finance management, particularly within the response to COVID-19 (FMO, 2020):

The key findings showed that not all work carried out by the Ministry of Public Works, Housing and Water Resources was submitted for the inspection process, and about 99.97% of the funds allocated to the

Ministry were spent in the form of direct adjustments.[9] There seems to be excessive use of the funds by the Ministry through the direct award method, even in cases where it was possible to purchase goods and services in good time.

In the health sector[10] out of the total funds allocated to the Ministry of Health, about 67.1% were allocated to the central level, 31.4% to the provinces, 0.8% to the National Institute of Health, and 0.7 to Maputo Central Hospital. About 84% of the funds allocated to the Ministry of Health to prevent and combat COVID-19 at the provincial level were spent on food and accommodation expenses for health professionals in hotels in the provinces of Nampula and Maputo (MZN 25 million and MZN 10.8 million, respectively).

The transport sector (investment in public transport) does not appear in any plan/budget for the mitigation of the impacts of COVID-19. However, for individuals who depend on overloaded public transport to go to and from work (formal or informal), transport presents a significant risk of contracting COVID-19. This daily risk makes the other individual prevention measures less effective (FMO, 2020). Through an equity lens, the findings of FMO bring to light, among other things, the fact that:

- Establishing fair criteria based on the evidence of the needs of the most vulnerable groups should be at the core of an equity-oriented planning process.
- Rationality in the use of resources is crucial to guarantee equitable policies. Conscience about budget expenditure is a core ethical value of social justice, as funds allocated to social areas can substantially contribute to people's lives.
- The decentralisation of expenditure execution is key to inclusion, the equitable distribution of resources, and the reduction of regional/urban–rural inequalities.

---

[9] Data shared with the FMO for accountability about the PCR-19 by the Ministry of Public Works, Housing and Water Resources.

[10] Data was shared with the FMO for accountability about the PCR-19 by the Ministry of Health.

Equity in Budget and Implementation

An analysis of the equity of the budget for the Social Action sector reminds us that (UNICEF & ILO, 2020):

- As social protection programmes target poor and vulnerable populations,[11] the most critical allocations from the sector should be directed to the provinces with a higher percentage of poor and vulnerable households. However, while allocations from social protection programmes to the most disadvantaged provinces have increased nominal, per-capita allocations are not yet equitable.
- The country's poorest provinces[12] continue to receive the highest nominal allocations from the INAS social protection programmes. However, allocations to provinces with the country's highest poverty rates are still insufficient to meet the enormous needs of their vulnerable populations. As for geographical equity, in terms of per-capita allocation among the poor population, the three poorest provinces receive the lowest allocation.[13]

The analysis of local actors and community-based organisations (CBOs), based on their concrete experiences, also points to significant structural challenges that prevent policies from effectively reaching the most vulnerable groups in all parts of the country. The following examples are based on the data collected from CBOs in the Beira and Pemba:

- Difficulties in accessing and disseminating correct and inclusive information (e.g. on people with disabilities) to communities and beneficiaries;

[11] The definition of a poor and vulnerable population is based on the poverty line, which is defined in Mozambique as USD 1.90 per day (MEF, 2017).

[12] The provinces of Nampula and Zambézia were attributed MZN 1.125 billion and MZN 0.87 billion, respectively. On the other hand, Maputo City and Maputo province received the lowest budget for INAS programmes: MZN 138 million and MZN 145 million, respectively (UNICEF & ILO, 2020, p. 16).

[13] Although the national average allocation per poor person is approximately MZN 464 per year, the allocation for the poor was only MZN 327 in Niassa and MZN 375 in Nampula, while in Maputo, it was MZN 959 per year. This points to a gap in the distribution of sector resources per capita among those below the poverty line (UNICEF & ILO 2020, p. 17).

- Weak knowledge on the part of local leaders about the population, especially vulnerable communities;
- Current practices of corruption, sexual harassment, and poor policy transparency;
- Poor dissemination of information on social protection benefit packages to beneficiaries;
- Poor understanding by beneficiaries of their rights and responsibilities;
- Lack of inclusion of representatives of vulnerable groups in monitoring mechanisms;
- Poor coordination between Government and CBOs;
- Instability due to violent conflict.

Justice and Transparency in Targeting Criteria

Given that the COVID-19 pandemic context has restricted access to resources and exacerbated historical and structural socioeconomic inequalities, the definition of criteria for prioritising social protection policies has become a vital issue. The task of prioritising certain groups of beneficiaries over others (who may also be vulnerable) or focusing on measures targeting the 'poorest of the poor has proved to be ethically complex, requiring focused attention'. As addressed above, the Government has identified a list of vulnerable groups but has not clarified the criteria for prioritising the 'most vulnerable groups in its response to the pandemic'. Also missing was an intersectionality approach (to look at multiple inequalities and discriminations) to identify persons/groups that belong to more than one social category or have more than one condition that creates barriers to access to resources and services. Examples based on the Pemba, Beira, and Maputo contexts include the importance of paying specific attention to:

- People with disabilities who, in addition to tending to be economically vulnerable, may encounter barriers to access to information and services.[14]

---

[14] INCLUDE Equity COVID-19 Case Study Workshop data collection with community-based organisations (CBOs) Beira-City (interview by CDD) Beira City, Mozambique, 2020.

- Internally displaced persons (IDPs) who, in addition to typically facing severe economic vulnerability, may also suffer from inclusion barriers linked to gender, religion, ethnicity, age, disability, chronic illness, or other inequalities, as well as IDP women who may have specific needs (e.g., access to sexual and reproductive health services).[15]
- Women heads of households can be more vulnerable to sexual violence (domestic or in public spaces), which adds to their economic vulnerability, and can have other vulnerabilities linked to gender inequalities.

Hence, beneficiaries can be identified using diverse factors. For example, *economic condition* (serves as a defining criterion for the choice of households in poverty, although the definition of poverty does not consider only family income), *geographical locality* (households/population living in urban, peri-urban and border areas), *social inequality* (based on gender, ethnicity/race, age, women-headed household, elderly, children), and/ or *health/biological conditions* (chronic diseases and disabilities among others). Conditions of emergency, whether due to violent conflict or climate crises, can result in the creation of new categories of beneficiaries, such as internally displaced persons.

EQUITY WITH REGARD TO HEALTH

Another gap identified relates to equity regarding the budget for health and the identification of target groups in terms of health. As noted through the shared experience of the Citizen Observatory for Health (Observatório Cidadão para a Saúde), there is a need to enhance strategies to reach out to vulnerable groups with chronic diseases or others who may depend on domestic medical support during the pandemic.[16] With regard to the expenditure by the Ministry of Health, analysis shows that the distribution of funds among provinces has been uneven, and

[15] INCLUDE Equity COVID-19 Case Study Workshop data collection with community-based organisations (CBOs)Pemba-City (interview by CDD) Pemba City, Mozambique, 2020.

[16] Individual questionnaires were answered by civil society organisations for this case study. These findings are indicative only, requiring further study with a targeted and more comprehensive sample.

government follow-up reports have not explained the criteria used to determine the amounts to be allocated to each province or the criteria used to allocate 67.1% to the central level and 31.4% to the provinces (FMO, 2020). Noteworthy, although the pandemic can potentially affect anyone, its impact is also determined by inequalities. The definition of criteria becomes a core mechanism for decisions, including prioritisation during the vaccination process.

EXPANSION OF COVERAGE
AND DECREASE IN PLANNED INVESTMENT

As already pointed out, although the PRC19-PS was considered 'ambitious' (in terms of its expansive coverage), there have been decreased financial resources necessary to fulfil the desired goals. Still, even when funds are available, an equity lens calls attention to the need to expand the spectrum from a narrow perspective focused on quantitative goals to the broader aim of pursuing the goal of social justice and qualitative impacts.

Collected data also reinforced that the Government has limited capacity to protect its vulnerable population.[17] In social protection policies, numbers refer to human beings; therefore, quantitative and qualitative results should go together. If the Government sets a plan that is ambitious in terms of the number of beneficiaries, qualitative equity measured by indicators (i.e., equitable distribution of resources, justice in the definition of policy criteria, affirmative action defined according to evidence-based data, multiple inequalities and discriminations, inclusive and transparent governance mechanisms, among other things) is also necessary.

---

[17] Civil society organisations answered individual questionnaires for this case study. These findings are indicative only, requiring further study with a targeted and more comprehensive sample.

GENDER INEQUALITY AND VULNERABILITY OF WOMEN AND GIRLS

One of the principles of the Social Action Policy is gender equality and equity (República de Moçambique, 2017). However, research[18] carried out by Women and Law in Southern Africa (WLSA), called attention to key gender equity challenges, including in relation to women' access to health and informal labour market, in the context of the COVID-19 (WLSA, 2020).

The Women's Forum has also prepared a 'Positioning of Women and Girls' (Mulher, 2020a) at the beginning of the COVID-19 pandemic (April 7, 2020). Recommendations included; circulating relevant information (disseminated in several national languages and through various means), validated by the scientific community, on the risks posed by the COVID-19 pandemic and the preventive measures that individuals, in particular girls and women, can and should take; to create an emergency telephone number to report or call for help in cases of violence; to establish (legal and social) rules for the protection of employment, among others.

ROLE OF CSOS AND CBOS IN MONITORING OF NATIONAL RESPONSE

The present analysis has identified the absence of participation by civil society organisations in the multi-sectoral Technical and Scientific Commission created to advise the Government on the COVID-19 response policies and measures. The fact that the role of civil society is not understood and/or valued deserves further reflection, as this sector has vast knowledge about the needs of the most vulnerable groups and can play a crucial role in providing support to ensure the equity of COVID-19 policies and plans.

However, in theory, the Government recognises the crucial role of CSOs in monitoring and identifying potential beneficiaries to be enrolled in the PASD-PE 'COVID-19', as well as channelling complaints and

---

[18] Entitled: *'Desigualdades e resistência em tempos de pandemia. Impactos da Covid-19 nas mulheres do mercado informal em Maputo'. Authours: Conceição Osório, Ana Loforte and Sérgio Vilanculos. Available at:* https://www.wlsa.org.mz/lancamento-de-um-relato rio-de-pesquisa-sobre-mulheres-e-covid/

claims by beneficiaries (MGCAS, 2020b, p. 2). At the meeting on 'The Role of CSOs in the consolidation of the Social Protection Response Plan to COVID-19 in Mozambique', it was also noted the preeminent role of civil society in mapping, identifying, and registering people eligible for post-emergency social support as well as the advance submission of lists of potential beneficiaries to the INAS.[19]

Specific roles of CSOs mentioned included: advocacy and policy influence, accountability, denouncing, proposing, and supporting government action for prevention and awareness raising and translating and ensuring that reliable information reaches communities.[20]

When assessing their role, CSOs and CBOs at the provincial level (both in Beira and in Pemba) stressed that they face several challenges in fulfilling their role. The main barrier highlighted is the lack of access to information about the Government's COVID-19 Response Plan and its benefits for vulnerable groups. Access to this information was noted as essential for monitoring and channelling complaints. It identified various civil society actions that carried out actions and research-oriented monitoring and accountability. For instance, the Mozambican Budget Monitoring Forum (FMO)[21] advocates for transparency and accountability in public finances, particularly on the issue of public debt. FMO implemented the initiative 'Response to COVID-19 with Right Accounts' to ensure that the resources to mitigate the effects of the COVID-19 pandemic are being effectively applied and that the response is coherent and compelling. Other CSOs such as the Centre for Democracy and Development (CDD), the Rural Observatory (OMR), Center for Public Integrity, the Institute of Social and Economic Studies(IESE), and the Independent Community Monitoring (MCI) project played roles in the

---

[19] Facebook page of PSC-PS: https://www.facebook.com/pscmps/

[20] Ibid.

[21] FMO members are: Centro para Democracia e Desenvolvimento (CDD), Nwete, Grupo Moçambicano da divida (GMD), Centro de Integridade Pública (CIP), Centro de aprendizagem e capacitação (CESC), Fundo para desenvolvimento da Comunidade (FDC), Observatorio Cidadão para Saúde (OCS), Forum Mulher, JOINT, Mozambican Civil Society Platform for Social Protection (PSCM-PS), Observatório do Meio Rural (OMR), ROSC, Helvetas Swiss Intercooporations, Instituto de Estudos Sociais e Económicos (IESE), Water Aid, Associação Mulher, Lei e Desenvolvimento (Muleide), Mept Moçambique, Fórum Nacional de Rádios Comunitárias (Forcom), Actionaid, Open Society Initiative for Southern Africa (OSISA), and Swiss Embassy in Mozambique.

research, monitoring and advisories on issues to do with social protection for the vulnerable among others.

Conclusion and Recommendations

The chapter presents an analysis of the COVID-19 response by the Government of Mozambique in terms of policy coherence and equity. The analysis has highlighted many areas that need attention to protect vulnerable citizens. This chapter draws conclusions and makes recommendations, including areas for further study.

Suitability of Measures and Proportionality of Response

Based on an assessment in terms of the planning and allocation of resources, it can be concluded that the government measures in response to COVID-19 have, up until December 2020, failed to strongly prioritise social protection, as committed to by the Government in the original budget plan. Given that the state budget deficit was a reality (which could not be solved in the short term), the decision to ask for external aid or loans was appropriate. However, as analysed by FMO, how the funds were used was not appropriate, especially since the misuse and/or inefficient use of funds has had a direct negative impact on the most vulnerable groups to which the funds could have been channelled.

On the impact of social protection policies, it is recommended that further follow-up/evaluation be conducted on the following:

- Government budget planning and updates have so far failed to explain the criteria (and data/evidence underpinning such criteria) used for decision-making about areas to prioritise and the amount of funds to allocate. There is a need to evaluate to what extent the decision to adapt the existing policies to the context of COVID-19 has led to the support of the groups most vulnerable during the pandemic.
- As noted by CBOs (in Beira and Pemba), the lack of information provided to CBOs and beneficiaries about the planned social protection benefits under the Government's PRC19 indicates the need for an assessment of the extent to which the transfers to families were

effective in reaching the groups most impacted by COVID-19. In other words, whether the policy decision to reach out to a more significant number of beneficiaries has enabled the support to those groups most affected.

• The economic measures taken during the early stages of the COVID-19 pandemic (when the Government declared a State of Emergency when there were only a few imported cases of COVID-19 and no community transmission) need to be adequately evaluated in terms of their appropriateness and proportionality, especially as these measures had significant negative impacts on the economy, which is now almost at the point of collapse, while at the same time the cases of COVID-19 are increasing.

Inclusiveness of Policies/Measures, Planning, and Implementation

The original demand for external funds (aid or loan) was inclusive, as the request strongly prioritised social protection (based on the assumption that the country would need to protect vulnerable groups if it entered lockdown). However, at the time of allocating these funds, social protection became secondary. Hence, implementing policies is at significant risk of not being inclusive in prioritising the protection of vulnerable groups.

This lack of inclusion is also noted in the weak, unequal, and inefficient allocation of funds to the provinces, with priority given to the central level. Therefore, an equity-accountability assessment of the COVID-19 budget plan should be conducted concerning the allocation of funds to the provinces because, historically, the central level has not prioritised allocating funds to promote inclusion and reduce urban–rural or province-central structural inequalities.

Inclusive policies that promote a better understanding of the State-citizen relationship were also relevant. The rationale behind the public debate, in which the public was partially blamed for the substantial increase in COVID-19 cases, needs to be further understood and clarified, especially in terms of the State's role in formulating policies to ensure that the population can exercise their right to health. For instance, the fact that public transportation investments were not prioritised in the Government's budget for the COVID-19 Response Plan weakens the responsibility of poor/low-income workers, who do not have any other option than to take an overloaded bus to work every day.

As pointed out above, the lack of inclusion is also present in the shift of priorities, from social protection policies to other areas, which did not aim to directly benefit the poor or tackle the specific needs of vulnerable groups.

An inclusive approach also needs adequate and transparent mechanisms for decision-making regarding the criteria for the prioritisation of vaccines. As noted by the CDD (CDD, 2021b), as the first batch of vaccines arrived in Maputo, the Ministry of Health is called on to disseminate the vaccination plan to inform public debate openly.

Participatory Mechanisms of Communication and Consultation

The Government's decision-making mechanisms about the COVID-19 pandemic failed to include civil society stakeholders and lacked official consultation mechanisms, including a CSO representative in the COVID-19 Technical-Scientific Committee. This Committee did not establish a formal communication channel with the public, CSOs or CBOs, nor did it conduct press conferences, as expected. It was established without the composition or structure to be robustly inclusive in terms of representation, and it lacked a participatory mechanism to generate the lessons that the Government would need to be able to enhance knowledge based on the local context, which is necessary to deal with the current COVID-19 pandemic, as well as future crises. With an overall and detailed content that still requires further analysis, the letter of resignation of Professor Helder Martins from the role of a member of the Scientific Technical Commission for Prevention and Response to the COVID-19 pandemic on February 16, 2021, (Martins, 2021) (Res. of the Council of Ministers no 20/2020, of March 25th) reinforces, among other things, that politicians cannot manage an epidemic and that the opening of the Commission to society and the media could have helped to prevent fake news, circulated on social networks, causing panic in the population.

In terms of effective participation, CSOs expected that the Government would have learnt from past experiences (i.e., Agenda 2025) and established a Committee to connect diverse sectors, from national to local stakeholders, including channels for shared information and data gathering on the needs and context-specific impact of COVID-19 on the most vulnerable populations. On the contrary, the CBOs consulted lacked access to information on the planned social protection policies, which prevented them from exercising their role and supporting the Government in implementing local level actions to prevent and mitigation of the impacts of COVID-19.

This case study showed that analysing the policy coherence and equity of the COVID-19 response in Mozambique goes far beyond the current pandemic context and concerns the country's ability to deal with crises in general. During the current crisis, civil society organisations have been active and willing to engage in inclusive governance, which requires efforts from all sectors. Likewise, international cooperation and private sector actors have supported government policies, despite the lack of confidence generated by the 'hidden debts' scandal.

REFERENCES

BBC. (2020, May 19). *Coronavírus: os 10 países que mais gastaram para enfrentar a pandemia de covid-19* [Coronavirus: the 10 countries that have spent the most to tackle the covid-19 pandemi. BBC NEWS, Brasil]. https://www.bbc.com/portuguese/internacional-52721417

Budget Monitoring Forum (FMO). (2020). *Análise do procurement público no âmbito do combate à COVID-19: Obras Públicas e Sector da Saúde* [Analysis of public procurement in the fight against COVID-19: Public Works and the Health Sector]. Fórum de Monitoria do Orçamento.

Cadernos de Estudos Africanos. (2017). *Desenvolvimento e a coerência das políticas* [Development and policy coherence]. Posted on 29 December 2017, updated 19 September 2020. http://journals.openedition.org/cea/2261; https://doi.org/10.4000/cea.2261. Excerpt from: "Desenvolvimento e a Coerência das Políticas", Apple Books.

Centro para Democracia e Desenvolvimento (CDD). (2020a, May 4). *Os desafios do CONSAN para garantir segurança alimentar e nutricional num contexto de "crise na crise"* [The challenges of CONSAN to guarantee food and nutrition security in a context of 'crisis in the crisis']. *Especial Covid-19.* https://cddmoz.org/wp-content/uploads/2020/05/COVID-19-E-INSURG%C3%8ANCIA-EM-CABO-DELGADO-_Os-desafios-do-COSAN-para-garantir-seguran%C3%A7a-alimentar-e-nutricional-num-contexto-de-%E2%80%9Ccrise-na-crise%E2%80%9D.pdf

Centro para Democracia e Desenvolvimento (CDD). (2020b, April 26). *Alguns exemplos do fracasso das primeiras medidas de política económica contra a covid-19 em Moçambique* [Some examples of the failure of the first economic policy measures against covid-19 in Mozambique]. *Especial Covid-19.*

https://cddmoz.org/wp-content/uploads/2020/04/Depreciac%CC%A7a%CC%83o-do-Metical-e-%E2%80%9Ceclosa%CC%83o-de-bolsas-de-fome%E2%80%9D-Alguns-exemplos-do-fracasso-das-primeiras-medidas-de-poli%CC%81tica-econo%CC%81mica-contra-a-covid-19-em-Moc%CC%A7ambique

Centro para Democracia e Desenvolvimento (CDD). (2020c, November 23). *Excessivo endividamento público continua a aumentar o custo de vida dos moçambicanos* [Excessive public debt continues to increase the cost of living for Mozambicans]. *Desenvolvimento Review*. https://cddmoz.org/wp-content/uploads/2020/11/%E2%80%9CExcessivo-endividamento-p%C3%BAblico-continua-a-aumentar-o-custo-de-vida-dos-mo%C3%A7ambicanos%E2%80%9D.pdf

Centro para Democracia e Desenvolvimento (CDD). (2021a, January 19). *Chega de Institucionalizar o Roubo! – estado deve indemnizar comerciantes cujos produtos foram apreendidos ilegalmente pela polícia* [No more institutionalising theft! – the state must compensate traders whose products were illegally seized by the police]. Boletim Sobre Direitos Humanos. https://cddmoz.org/wp-content/uploads/2021/01/CHEGA-DE-INSTITUCIONALIZAR-O-ROUBO-Estado-deve-indemnizar-comerciantes-cujos-produtos-foram-apreendidos-ilegalmente-pela-PolA%CC%83-cia.pdf

Centro para Democracia e Desenvolvimento (CDD). (2021b, February 25). *MISAU deve divulgar urgentemente o plano de vacinação contra COVID-19 para permitir um debate público informado* [MISAU must urgently publicise COVID-19 vaccination plan to allow informed public debate]. *Política Moçambique*. https://cddmoz.org/wp-content/uploads/2021/02/PRIMEIRO-LOTE-DE-DOSES-JA-ESTA-EM-MAPUTO_-MISAU-deve-divulgar-urgentemente-o-plano-de-vacinacao-contra-Covid-19-para-permitir-um-debate-publico-informado.pdf

CIP. (2020). *COVID-19: Resources allocated for social protection may not reach all beneficiaries.* Public Finances, Center for Public Integrity. https://cipmoz.org/2020/09/22/covid-19-recursos-alocados-para-proteccao-social-podem-nao-chegar-na-totalidade-aos-beneficiarios/

FMO. (2020). *Análise do procurement público no âmbito do combate à COVID-19: Obras Públicas e Sector da Saúde* [Analysis of public procurement in the fight against COVID-19: Public Works and the Health Sector]. Fórum de Monitoria do Orçamento (Budget Monitoring Forum).

ILO. (2020). *Rapid assessment of the impact of COVID-19 on the informal economy in Mozambique.* International Labour Organization. https://www.ilo.org/africa/countries-covered/mozambique/WCMS_755922/lang--en/index.htm

IMF. (2020), *IMF Executive Board Approves US$309 Million in Emergency Assistance to Mozambique to Address the COVID-19 pandemic.* International Monetary Fund. https://www.imf.org/en/News/Articles/2020/04/24/pr20190-mozambique-imf-executive-board-approves-emergency-assistance-to-address-covid-19

Martins, H. (2021). *Extracto duma Carta a SExa Presidente da República e Chefe do Governo* [Extract of a Letter to the President of the Republic and Head of Government]. Press Release. https://macua.blogs.com/files/carta-a-sexa-pre sidente-da-repu%CC%81blica-extracto-pu%CC%81blico_heldermartins.pdf

Ministry of Economy and Finance (MEF). (2017). *Quarta avaliação nacional de pobreza* [Fourth national poverty assessment]. Ministério de Economia e Finanças. http://www.mef.gov.mz

Ministry of Economy and Finance (MEF). (2019). *FinScope consumer survey.* FSDMOC. http://fsdmoc.com/

Ministry of Economy and Finance (MEF). (2020a, August 25). *Ponto de situação dos compromissos no âmbito da COVID-19* [Status of Covid-19 commitments]. Ministério da Economia e Finanças. https://www.mef.gov.mz/index.php/covid-19/927--229/file

Ministry of Economy and Finance (MEF). (2020b, November 2). *Ponto de situação dos compromissos no âmbito da COVID-19* [Status of Covid-19 commitments]. Ministério da Economia e Finanças.

Ministry of Economy and Finance (MEF). (2020c, December). *Ponto de situação dos compromissos no âmbito da Covid-19* [Status of Covid-19 commitments]. Ministério da Economia e Finanças.

Ministry of Economy and Finance (MEF). (2021, January). *Ponto de situação dos compromissos no âmbito da Covid-19* [Status of commitments under Covid-19]. Ministério da Economia e Finanças. https://www.mef.gov.mz/index.php/covid-19/927--229/file

Ministry of Economy and Finance (MEF). (n.d). *Estimativas e perfil da pobreza em Moçambique: uma analise baseada no inquérito sobre Orçamento Familiar* [Poverty estimates and profile in Mozambique: an analysis based on the Family Budget Survey]. Direcção de Estudos Económicos e Financeiros. Ministry of Economy and Finance/DEEF. https://www.mef.gov.mz/index.php/docume ntos/estudos/artigos/752--150/file

Ministry of Gender, Children and Social Action (MGCAS). (2018). *Programa Conjunto das Nações Unidas para a Protecção 2017–2020* [Joint United Nations Programme for Protection 2017–2020]. UNICEF. https://www.uni cef.org/mozambique/sites/unicef.org.mozambique/files/2018-08/03-Pro grama-Conjunto-Proteccao-Social-2017-2020.pdf

Ministry of Gender, Children and Social Action (MGCAS). (2020a, October 14). INCLUDE equity COVID-19 case study questionnaire. (CDD, Inter-viewer) https://www.surveymonkey.com/r/Preview/?sm=u3L3sj0ZNWxV ZFBw99EBpQ5cH_2B_2FXC0UE0eAj8OlKA5TT3YpxGXl_2FyOZZnlVS cZic

Ministry of Gender, Children and Social Action (MGCAS). (2020b). *Plano de Resposta à COVID-19 em Moçambique – Protecção Social* [Response Plan to COVID-19 in Mozambique – Social Protection]. Ministério do Género, Criança e Acção Social.

Ministry of Health (MISAU). (2020, March). *Plano Nacional de Preparação e Resposta a Pandemia do COVID-19* [National COVID-19 Pandemic Preparedness and Response Plan]. Ministério da Saúde.

Ministry of Interior (MINT). (2010). *Atendimento da M. e Criança—Estatistica* [Mother and Child Care—Statistics]. Ministry of Interior. https://196.3.96.161/mint.gov.mz/index.php?option=com_content& view=article&id=55&Itemid=89&limitstart=6.

Mulher, F. (2020a, April 7). *Impacto da COVID-19 na vida das mulheres e Raparigas em Moçambique* [Impact of COVID-19 on the lives of women and girls in Mozambique]. Fórum Mulher

Mulher, F. (2020b, April 7). *As dimensões de género da COVID-19 em Moçambique* [The gender dimensions of COVID-19 in Mozambique]. Fórum Mulher. http://forumulher.org.mz/project/impacto-do-covid-19-na-vida-das-mulheres/

National Statistics Institute. (2020). *Resultados do inquérito sobre o impacto da COVID-19 nas empresas* [Survey results on the impact of COVID-19 on businesses]. Maputo: Instituto Nacional de Estatística. http://www.ine.gov.mz/estatisticas/estatisticas-sectoriais/resultados-do-inquerito-sobre-impacto-da-covid-19-nas-empresas.pdf

ONU Moçambique. (2020). *Plano de Resposta Multissectorial à COVID-19* [Multisectoral Response Plan to COVID-19]. Maputo: Organização das Nações Unidas.

Presidência da República. (2020). *Comunicado de imprensa do conselho* [Council press release]. Gabinete de Imprensa. https://www.presidencia.gov.mz/por/ Actualidade/PR-dirige-Segunda-Reuniao-Ordinaria-do-CNDS

Presidência da República. (2021, February 4). *Balanço da implementação das medidas decretadas no contexto da declaração da situação de calamidade pública, no âmbito da pandemia do corona vírus—COVID-19* [*Review of the implementation of the measures decreed in the context of the declaration of a situation of public calamity in the context of the coronavirus-COVID-19 pandemic*]. Comunicação à Nação de Sua Excelência Filipe Jacinto Nyusi, Presidente da República de Moçambique. https://www.presidencia.gov.mz/ por/Media/Files/100-Comunicacao-a-Nacao-0402021

PSCM-PS. (2020a, December 3). *Plataforma da Sociedade Civil Moç. para Protecção Social* [Moz. Civil Society Platform for Social Protection]. Social Protection Platform of Civil Society. https://web.facebook.com/pscmps/ posts/3761031570593892?_rdc=1&_rdr

PSCM-PS. (2020b) *Monitoria comunitária independente. relatório, 2019* [Independent community monitoring—report, 2019]. *Plataforma da Sociedade Civil Moçambicana para a Protecção Social*. https://www.social-protection. org/gimi/ShowRessource.action;jsessionid=01Az4DEhxStaIVd8ScBJ-BWH K7CpT-6OAGYIpMIIXHAgvaFByKt7!445242879?id=56938&lang=RU

PSCM-PS. (2020c). *Monitoria comunitária independente relatório—Ano 2019* [Independent community monitoring report-Year 2019. Social Protection Platform of Civil Society]. https://www.social-protection.org/gimi/Ressou rcePDF.action;jsessionid=2BHutP0MGJlunN4w0p-xzIj4H8Vxty_E41PzDi8e Efr4urk_Hcx8!539423187?id=56938

Rádio de Moçambique. (2020, March 23). *Governo estima em USD700 milhões o impacto negativo do COVID-19 no país* [Government estimates $700 million negative impact of COVID-19 on the country]. Rádio de Moçambique. https://www.rm.co.mz/rm.co.mz/index.php/sobre/item/10088-governo-estima-em-usd700-milhoes-o-impacto-negativo-do-covid-19-no-pais.html

República de Moçambique. (2017, November 2). *Política de Acção Social e Estratégia de Implementação* [Social Action Policy and Implementation Strategy]. Boletim da República (I Série–Número 171). Government of Mozambique.

República de Moçambique. (2018, August). *Política de Género e Estratégia de Implementação* [Gender Policy and Implementation Strategy]. Government of Mozambique.

República de Moçambique. (n.d.). *Empresários nacionais procuram alternativas para o impacto de COVID-19* [National entrepreneurs seek alternatives to the impact of COVID-1]. Portal do Governo de Moçambique. https://www.portaldogoverno.gov.mz/por/Imprensa/Noticias/Emp resarios-nacionais-procuram-alternativas-para-o-impacto-de-covid-19

República de Moçambique—Comité de Conselheiros. (2003). *Agenda 2025: visão e estratégias da nação* [Agenda 2025: the nation's vision and strategies]. Maputo: Conselho Nacional da Agenda. https://www.mef.gov.mz/index. php/documentos/instrumentos-de-gestao/agenda-2025/83-agenda-2025/ file

República de Moçambique—Sistema de Protecção Social. (2019a). *1º Boletim Estatístico sobre Protecção Social* [1st Statistical Bulletin on Social Protection]. Government of Mozambique. http://www.mitess.gov.mz/node/631

República de Moçambique—Sistema de Protecção Social. (2019b). *2º Boletim Estatístico sobre Protecção Social* [2nd Statistical Bulletin on Social Protection]. Government of Mozambique. http://www.mitess.gov.mz/node/630

Santos, R., & Salvucci, V. (2016). *Poverty in Mozambique: significant progress but challenges remain.* Policy Brief. UNU Wider.

The survey, non-State actors. (2020). Questionnaire answered by Non-State Authors for the Case Study INCLUDE Equity COVID19.

Tibana, R. J. (2021, February). *A dinâmica da pandemia da COVID-19. Destaque Rural nº 115* [A dinâmica da pandemia da COVID-19. Rural Highlight no. 115]. https://omrmz.org/omrweb/wp-content/uploads/ DR-115-A-din%C3%A2mica-da-pandemia-da-COVID-19-em-Mo%C3%A7a mbique.pdf

UNHCR. (2021). UNHCR Mozambique update: Cabo Delgado situation, December 15th 2020, to January 15th 2021. https://data2.unhcr.org/en/documents/details/84513

UNICEF. (2018, March 1). *Joint programme on social protection launched in Mozambique*. UNICEF Mozambique. https://www.unicef.org/mozambique/en/press-releases/joint-programme-social-protection-launched-mozambique

UNICEF & ILO. (2020). *Informe orçamental 2020 do sector da acção social* [2020 budget report for the social action sector]. United Nations Children's Fund. https://www.unicef.org/mozambique/media/2936/file/Budget%20Brief%202020:%20Social%20Action.pdf

WLSA. (2020, November 24). *Campanha dos 16 dias contra a violência de género—2020* [16 days against gender-based violence-2020 campaign]. WLSA. https://www.wlsa.org.mz/campanha-dos-16-dias-contra-a-violencia-de-genero-2020/#more-14754

World Bank. (2011). *Demographic and Health Survey*. World Bank. https://datacatalog.worldbank.org/dataset/mozambique-demographic-and-health-survey-2011

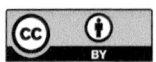

CHAPTER 11

Rwanda

Martin Luther Munu and Zjos Vlaminck

INTRODUCTION

The Covid-19 pandemic experience and policies in Rwanda are situated in a climate of developmental ambivalences which determined the nature of policies and their impact on different social groups. Rwanda is a small country in East Africa with a turbulent political climate since independence, culminating in the 1994 genocide. Since then, the country has been under the stable leadership of the Rwanda Patriotic Front (RPF), with Paul Kagame as president since 2000. As a result, Rwanda has been hailed as a success story in sub-Sahara Africa with persistent growth rates, stability and progress in human development, such as increased school enrolment and universal social protection (Crisafulli & Redmond, 2012; Vlaminck et al., 2014). On the other hand, some argue that Rwandans have been negatively affected by the country's chosen developmental path and that macro-economic progress has gone at the cost of civil liberties,

M. L. Munu (✉)
Department of International and European Law, Maastricht University, Maastricht, The Netherlands
e-mail: m.munu@maastrichtuniversity.nl

Z. Vlaminck
Cobquecura, Chile

© The Author(s) 2024
A. Altaf et al. (eds.), *EQUITY IN COVID-19*, EADI Global Development Series, https://doi.org/10.1007/978-3-031-58588-3_11

259

food security and the well-being of Rwandans, especially the rural populations (Ansoms, 2020; Ansoms et al., 2017; Dawson, 2018; Verpoorten, 2014).

Rwanda has experienced high levels of economic growth (approx. 9% GDP growth in 2019), alongside improving Rwandans' living standards (World Bank, 2020) consistently. For example, there has been a two-thirds drop in child mortality and near-universal primary school enrolment (Laterite, 2017). The impressive indicators have been attributed to homegrown policies (World Bank, 2020). For example, the World Bank and other donors supported Rwanda in 2009 to develop and implement social protection programme known as the Vision 2020 Umurenge Program (VUP), which has been expanding to benefit more than a million people, with women constituting half of the beneficiaries (Gatzinsi et al., 2019).

Rwanda's sizeable agricultural sector contributes 29% of the Gross Domestic Product (GDP), constitutes 80% of the country's foreign exchange and employs two-thirds of the total population. More than 80% of the population survives on subsistence farming. The sector accounts for 78% of Rwanda's informal sector workers (ILO, 2018). Rwanda's green revolution, initiated in 2007–2008, has not have positive effect on rural areas. With rural farmers embedded in market-oriented agriculture, food insecurity increased as they have little control over their bargaining power (Ansoms, 2020).

Industry contributes 16.2% of GDP and 9% of employment, while the services sector contributes about 47.8% of GDP (NODEA, 2020). Kigali, the capital city, doubles as the economic hub for the country, while the rest is mainly rural. The country has a large informal sector which accounts for over 94% of total employment, driven by rural–urban migration (Munu, 2019). An estimated 97.2% of Rwanda's urban employment is informal (ILO, 2018, p. 91). The high incidence of informality raises questions regarding decent work standards, including the bargaining power of Rwanda's workforce. In the context of Covid-19, where responses have severely impacted people's jobs and livelihood strategies, the issue of workers' bargaining power is crucial because it is related to the leverage and voice workers can have in the formulation of Covid-19 responses. Furthermore, the increasing food insecurity in rural areas raises questions about the resilience of farmers in the face of Covid-19, mainly as government support has only targeted urban areas.

The chapter systematically reconstructed, documented and analysed how state and non-state actors in Rwanda take equity into account in the formulation and implementation of policy responses and interventions during the Covid-19 pandemic and how they have had an impact on material, relational, subjective and collective well-being of Rwanda's poor and marginalised.

METHODOLOGICAL APPROACHES

The research was conducted in line with existing Covid-19 restrictions and protocols. Therefore, the research was primarily based on desk research (including a literature review and document analysis) and key stakeholder interviews conducted over skype or phone and through email questionnaires. We have also conducted face-to-face interviews with vulnerable groups to shed light on the perceptions of the poor.

We identified the vulnerable groups through triangulating existing quantitative and qualitative studies on poverty in Rwanda and insights from key stakeholder interviews. The final selection was based on the following criteria: gender, age, and location. Male and female-dominated sectors, as well as young and older, were included. We included rural areas to understand the equity dimensions of responses. We selected Kigali and Iburengerazuba (Western) provinces based on their higher Covid-19 infection rates and prolonged lockdown period. We interviewed older people in the Western Province, market women in Kigali, taxi-velo and taxi-moto drivers. Within these groups, we investigated short-term effects on people's well-being, the long-term structural impacts, and how Covid-19 has affected existing inequalities.

THEORETICAL FRAMEWORK

There has been a rise in scholarship and policy attention on inclusive development and the importance of addressing poverty and inequality (Bourguignon, 2015; OECD, 2014; Piketty, 2014). However, the concept of equity in secular philosophy dates to ancient Greece with Plato, who pointed out the dangers of inequality for political stability (Attinc et al., 2005, p. 76). Since the 1970s, the understanding of equity has been shaped by the idea of creating equality in liberties (Rawls, 1971), opportunities (Roemer, 1998; Dworkin, 1981 cited in Attinc et al., 2005, p. 77) and capabilities (Sen, 1995 cited in Attinc et al., 2005, p. 77).

In a nutshell, social equity based on Rawls, Sen, Dworkin and Roemer's theories roughly entails an equal starting point or set of opportunities or capabilities. However, creating a level playing field or equal opportunities still does not always result in more equal societies. Firstly, by taking the gaze away from the result, equality of opportunity theories has been used to justify inequality. It has been argued that inequality results from differences in individual effort or merit or lack thereof (Natasnon, 2016). Secondly, when translated into policies, focusing on equality of opportunities often implies creating "universal" essential services such as public healthcare or free primary education. Although egalitarian in theory, such programmes often overlook structural inequalities that deprive certain people of accessing essential public goods. Lastly, and this is especially relevant in the case of Rwanda, the urge to reach universal coverage might come at the cost of the fairness of the measures adopted to get there.[1]

Therefore, to understand the extent to which Covid-19 response and mitigation measures have taken equity into account, it is necessary to re-centre the result in the analysis. More precisely, we focused on the impact on the well-being of the poor. The conceptualisation of well-being is drawn from McGregor and Pouw (2017). They portray well-being as a multidimensional concept consisting of material, relational, subjective and collective well-being (Fig. 11.1). It allows for the analysis of the impact of Covid-19 and related state and non-state responses on:

- work and income as well as access to essential services (material well-being);
- social relations, social capital and social safety nets and support networks (relational well-being);
- individual perceptions of the impact on one's quality of life (prior to and post Covid-19) (subjective well-being);
- political empowerment (collective well-being).

The analysis is guided by intersectionality, which allows us to capture the differentiated nature of vulnerability and resilience of people in the current health crisis (Chaplin et al., 2019).

---

[1] Egalitarian approaches here mean that all citizens are targeted equally and are (in theory) beneficiaries of a particular policy or program.

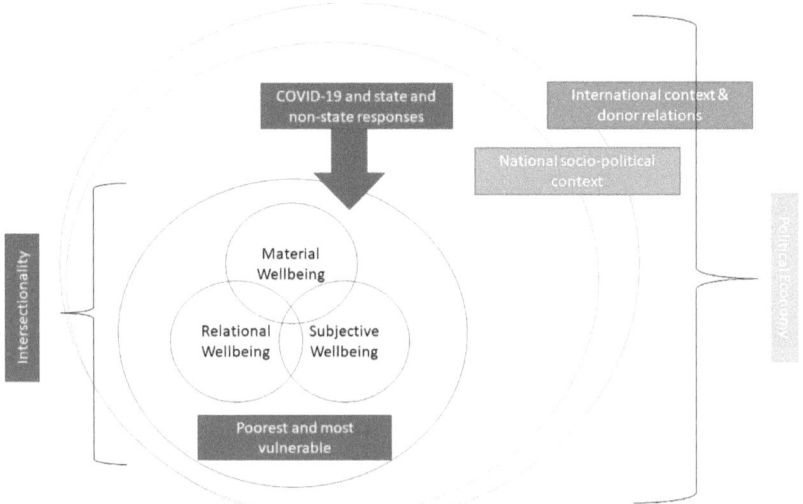

Fig. 11.1 Analytical framework of Covid-19 responses and well-being (*Source* Developed by authors based on McGregor and Pouw [2017])

SITUATIONAL SKETCH OF COVID-19 IN RWANDA

Covid-19 was confirmed on March 14, 2020, in Rwanda with the first patient coming from India. The patient was quarantined, and contact tracing started. Kigali was placed under lockdown as a result. However, soon, other cases emerged through border transit zones and truck drivers, leading to the decision of a nationwide lockdown with restrictions on movement between regions. Kirehe and Bugesera districts, which accounted for the highest number of coronavirus infections, are transit routes for cross-border truck drivers and hosted the Covid-19 isolation centres (Byishimo, 2020). In terms of vulnerability, the Western Province of Iburengerazuba was, according to the Africa Covid-19 Community Vulnerability Index (CCVI)[2] vulnerable due to the high refugee populations, food insecurity, lower socioeconomic status and high elderly population (Africa CCVI, 2020). Kigali city districts of Gasabo, Kicukiro and Nyarugenge were also areas of high infection (Byishimo, 2020).

---

[2] https://precisionforcovid.org/africa

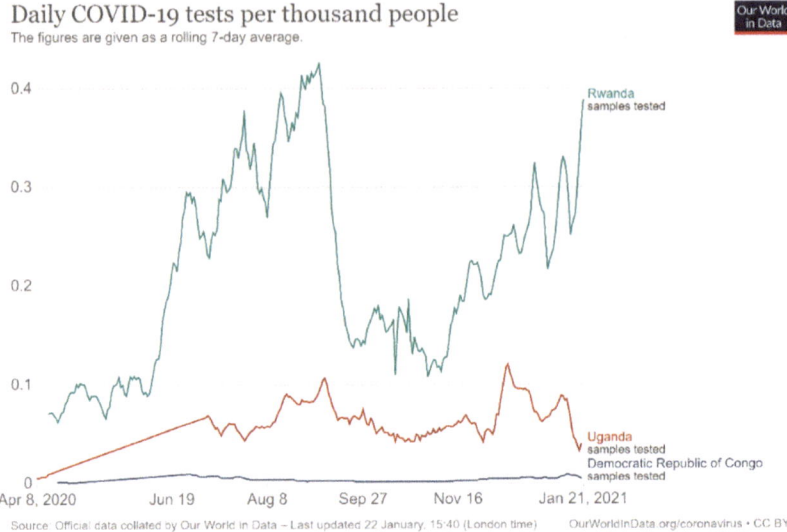

Fig. 11.2 Daily Covid-19 tests/1000 people (*Source* Our World in Data [2020])

Rwanda's Covid-19 testing rates were higher than the Democratic Republic of Congo, Uganda and others in the region. The pandemic management used a decentralised approach through laboratories at district levels and pool-testing, which increased efficiency and testing capacity. The Rwanda Biomedical Center coordinated testing, and by mid-July, over 200,000 samples had been tested for Covid-19 (Government of Rwanda, 2020). Rwanda has been largely successful in containing the first wave of the virus, but the second wave, which began in December 2020, was more challenging to curb (Broulard, 2021) and therefore led to the imposition of more stringent measures. See Fig. 11.2 for testing information (see Fig. 11.2).

RWANDA'S COVID-19 POLICY FORMULATION PROCESS

Even before Covid-19 was confirmed in Rwanda, the country was on high alert. The government directed ministries in charge of local government and health to take measures to prevent the importation of the virus by dispatching health officials with fever scanners to all border posts and installing handwashing systems in Kigali bus stations (Edwards, 2020). After the first case was reported on March 14, 2020, President Kagame called for calm but also solidarity and discipline to curb the spread (WHO, 2020a, 2020b). Subsequently, the cabinet held bi-weekly meetings to review and adopt policy measures accordingly. Different ministries and local government entities then implemented the cabinet decisions according to their respective mandates.[3] Local village leaders have, for instance, been activated to compile lists of vulnerable people for targeting food distribution. Communication was done through addresses by the prime minister, occasional presidential addresses or communiqués by the Ministry of Health (MoH), as well as through broadcast, print media and transmitted via WhatsApp.[4]

This approach, namely, central decision-making, disseminated and implemented through decentralised local government entities, is characteristic of Rwanda's governance style and has both strengths and weaknesses (see Table 11.1) in line with those found in existing literature (Chemouni, 2018 and Gaynor, 2014).[5]

The government has not consulted CSOs in the formulation of the Covid-19 containment measures.[6] Development partners such as UNDP have, on the contrary, worked closely with the government, raising questions regarding downward versus upward accountability and the embeddedness of the government's response in local realities. The UNDP emphasised its involvement stating that,

In addition to providing technical inputs and advice in the formulation of the plans, UNDP has been working closely with the Ministry of Finance on the planning for Social-Economic Impact Assessment jointly with UNECA, the World Bank, and the IMF. UNDP and the World Bank have been designated to co-lead the COVID19 Socio-Economic

---

[3] Interview with a representative of local CSOs.

[4] Interview with a representative of local CSOs.

[5] Legally, it is based on article 6 of Rwanda's Constitution of 2003, revised in 2015, which stipulates that public powers are decentralised at local administrative entities per law provisions.

[6] Interview with a representative of local CSOs.

Table 11.1   Strengths and weaknesses of a decentralised Covid-19 response in Rwanda

Strengths	Weaknesses
Efficient targeting of the poor and vulnerable through the village or *umudugudu* leaders who, based on their experience with Ubudehe participatory poverty assessment exercises and monthly community meetings (prior to Covid-19), identify the vulnerable people. Village-level data is then centrally gathered by LODA (Local Administrative Entities Development Agency)	Village leaders have a monopoly over the targeting process as monthly community meetings were suspended during the lockdown. Village leaders overlook those with non-permanent housing situations (who often have precarious, flexible working situations obliging them to move between places)
LODA serves as a central source of data for targeting the poor and vulnerable	Due to centralisation, the government has monopolised targeting. So, when people are excluded, they are excluded by the government, NGOs, or other development partners
Efficient service delivery through the lowest decentralised level (village or *umudugudu*) of government-linked to results-oriented governance	Results-oriented governance could lead to policies being rapidly implemented but not necessarily effective in equity
Increased solidarity between village members. Village leaders, via WhatsApp, asked village members to give what they could to support the most vulnerable in the village. As a result, resources have been mobilised to support the poor	Some of the most vulnerable do not belong to one village but move between various locations depending on job opportunities
Strict coordination of social protection measures at the district level decreased the incidence of duplication of interventions by government and development actors	A high level of government control restricts the implementation of solidarity initiatives by individuals and CSOs (e.g., journalists who wanted to give support in an informal settlement were been arrested)

Source Authors' compilation from literature review and key stakeholder interviews

Sub-Group working with the Ministry of Finance. This sub-group will co-lead on the socioeconomic impact assessment of the COVID-19 (UNDP, 2020b).

The cabinet has also worked closely with WHO and CDC officials on health-related issues. Both organisations worked with the government during the Ebola outbreak. On issues related to education, UNICEF played an informative role. On a regional level, EAC developed the East

African Community Covid-19 response plan, which President Kagame signed, but close observers indicate that the regional response has been fragmented border issues dealt with through ad-hoc bilateral dialogue (EAC Secretariat, 2020; O'Reilly & Vaughan, 2020).

Trade unions and workers' associations such as taxi-moto or taxi-velo associations were consulted on effective enforcement of Covid-19. This structure confirms studies on CSOs in Rwanda, which argue that the CSOs are tolerated only when they play a constructive (non-critical) role. In the case of COTRAF, external mediation via Friedrich Ebert Stiftung (FES) was used to open conversations with MINALOC, trade unions and other CSOs. On another occasion, COTRAF also met with the Ministry of Public Works and Employment representatives of other trade unions and the private sector to discuss health and safety issues during the pandemic and how to decrease infection, for instance, through the payment of salaries through banks.[7] The farmer union, SYNATRAEL, mentioned they did not raise any concerns to the government as their sector fell under essential services and was, therefore, less affected by the government's containment measures.

Despite the limited social dialogue on the pandemic management, trade unions have made their views clear through research on the impact of Covid-19 on the workforce and various communiqués directed at the government. According to trade union representatives, the government implemented the private sector fund and loans for private school teachers[8] as a response to some concerns. However, their demands to make mitigation measures more inclusive to informal workers were left unanswered. The media has also played an essential role as leverage to influence Covid-19 policies. Despite this, containment measures restricted their movement. (HRW, 2020b). Taxi-moto associations also advocated for the lifting of the ban on their services.[9]

[7] Interview with a trade union representative.

[8] Interview with a trade union representative.

[9] Interview with a trade union representative.

Rwanda's Stringent Containment Measures and Its Economic Impact

Rwanda's Covid-19 response has been robust and rapid (Bower et al., 2020). It was the first country to impose a nationwide lockdown on March 21, 2020, in the region. Handwashing stations and ThermoScan-checks were installed (Edwards, 2020), and hundreds of volunteers were recruited for contract tracing. The processes were digitalised. It was not clear how people without mobile phone devices were monitored since 48% of the poorest quintile in Rwanda do not own a cell phone. While technological innovations, such as robot nurses have been touted as helping with the pandemic management, the approach forecloses issues of equity. The Covid-19 Community Vulnerability Index (CCVI) (CCVI, 2020) rated Rwanda as one of the least at vulnerable countries partly due to the stringent measures imposed. According to the Oxford Covid-19 Governance tracker, Rwanda had a stringency score of 75.93 (Ghana, e.g., had a score of 44.44) (University of Oxford, 2020). The high score is mainly due to the prolonged national lockdown, restriction on mobility and closure of schools. The following are some of the government directives from the government[10]:

- Social distancing.
- Ban on public gatherings, places of worship, schools, weddings and sports events.
- Thirty-day suspension of all commercial flights to and from Rwanda and indefinite suspension of domestic travel between cities and districts.
- Closure of all land borders except for Rwandan residents and essential businesses.
- Ban on public transport except for buses within provinces and ban on all public transport between provinces.
- Closure of all businesses except those providing essential services such as medical care, telecommunications, security and banking services.
- Mobile money and online banking service use encouraged

---

[10] Source: Compiled by authors based on government pronouncements and field interviews.

- National curfew from 9 pm to 5 am and later extended from 7 pm to 5 am.
- Nationwide lockdown two weeks starting on March 21, which was extended twice until May 4.

As infections surged in June, the government adopted punitive measures to increase compliance. Fines were imposed on people who flouted protocols and stadiums were used as "education" centres for Covid-19 regulation offenders. Offenders were forced to stay overnight to serve as an example to others. Among those brought to stadiums were various journalists and bloggers covering the impact of Covid-19 measures on citizens (Asala, 2020). The police also issued lists of offenders with names and number plates to increase responsibility through social naming and shaming campaign.[11] Due to the economic realities of the poor, offenders were more likely to be of lower social classes. Social distancing in informal settlements and restrictions on movement constrained the poor since their livelihoods depend on moving between the city (Kigali) and their villages in rural areas. A respondent, for example, mentioned "*some people walked for days, hiding from the authorities in the bush to travel back to their homes*".[12] The closures of land borders have also been devastating for many informal traders and market women. Informal traders account for the 59% exports to Rwanda's neighbouring countries. Already between 60 and 80% of the border dwellers live below the national poverty line. While cargo vehicles were allowed to pass, small-scale, informal traders (an estimated 80% of whom are women in East Africa) who trade on foot or by motorcycle taxis were excluded (Stuart, 2020; Klopp et al., 2020). On the border with the Democratic Republic of Congo, a specific crisis has unfolded as Goma relies on water brought by informal traders from Rwanda. With the closure of the borders, Goma ran dry, and the Rwandans who lived by supplying water were left to find alternative means of income (Mwasa, 2020).

The stringent containment measures and punitive enforcement have had a significant socioeconomic impact on the poor and vulnerable and the economy at large, which cannot be underestimated. Many business ventures and services in both public and private institutions have

---

[11] Interview with Amnesty International representative.

[12] Interview with T.U. representative.

either been closed or have had their operations drastically reduced. As a result, GDP growth dropped to 3.5% in 2020 from 10.1% in 2019 which is a deviation form 6.7% projected for 2021 (Bizoza & Sibomana, 2020). Unemployment reached 22.1% in May 2020 (NISR, 2020a) and was higher among young people (Matengo, 2020). The lockdown was expected to rate from 38.67% to 44.33% (UNDP, 2020a). The RECOVR survey also captured the increase in poverty and income insecurity. The result showed that 80% of the respondents have used their savings on basic needs.

In terms food security, 50% of the respondents had to decrease their food consumption, and 25% stated they had trouble buying food due to restrictions on mobility and market closures (IPA, 2020). Many Rwandans have relied on social and family networks for financial support as a coping strategy (IPA, 2020) rather than the state. Informal sector workers who are already in precarious conditions disproportionately affected by the measures. Without adequate social security and safety nets, many households were left without an income to cover food and other basic needs. Besides informal workers, SMEs have also suffered. A study by Business Professionals Network (BPN) and the University of Rwanda (UoR) shows that at least 57.5% of SMEs operating across different industries were forced to shut down between March and April due to Covid-19 (BPN & UoR, 2020). Many reduced their capacity and employees even when the lockdown measures were relaxed.

The educational sector also experiences its fair share of the pandemic fallouts. Due to school closures, about 80% of children in primary and secondary schools were forced to learn from home (Debenedetti et al., 2020). The remote learning programme did not cover all children because of differentiated access to the resources for the programmes. Poorer households relied more on radio lessons, which limited their access to education, while wealthier households got access to different platforms such as television, WhatsApp groups set up by the respective schools and internet-based learning programmes. In addition, school closure led to an increase in teenage pregnancy, particularly among poor and vulnerable girls (Nkurunziza, 2020).

RWANDA'S SOCIO-ECONOMIC
IMPACT MITIGATION MEASURES

The economic mitigation measures were mainly targeted at formal sector employees. Similarly, measures were biased towards urban citizens and companies and were justified by the saying in rural areas: "one always has something to eat" (Table 11.2). However, in the context of the decreasing food security of Rwandan farmers (Ansoms, 2020), this assumption is questionable. A survey conducted by IPA (2020) on the impact of Covid-19 debunked the myth of rural plentitude and found that rural citizens were more likely to have trouble buying food than urban dwellers. In the same survey, only 10% of the respondents stated they had accessed the government's food aid and utility subsidies (IPA, 2020). The figures could be lower is Kigali is taken out form the sample. Considering that 16% of the national population falls under the lowest poverty category or the extreme poor according to the Ubudehe assessment, the IPA survey estimates that approximately half of the extreme poor have received government support during Covid-19.

RESPONSES BY NON-STATE ACTORS
AND DEVELOPMENT PARTNERS

A wide range of non-state actors has rolled-out measures to mitigate Covid-19's negative impacts. These ranged from trade unions' awareness raising campaigns to solidarity between citizens at the village level and INGOs providing cash transfers. The Rwandan government, through its decentralised authorities, oversees these initiatives. The district-level government authorities approved each programme along the lines of its Covid-19 preparedness and response plan and targeting of the poor using the village-level data centralised by LODA.

Trade Unions and workers' associations have reached out to their members by implementing Covid-19 awareness raising campaigns, creating Covid-19 clubs in factories, lobbying companies to ensure safe workplaces and making agreements with companies fabricating sanitisers to give a lower price rate for taxi-moto drivers and paying out part of the savings to members in need. However, most union and association leaders said that their main objective was to support their members in fulfilling the government requirements. Both taxi-moto and taxi-velo associations in this regard mentioned they worked together with security guards to

Table 11.2 State socio-economic impact responses and equity considerations

Actor	Measures	Equity considerations
Central Government	Fixed prices for selected essential food products consumed by most people (e.g., maize, beans, bananas, sugar, rice, and cooking oil, among others)[13]	Fixed prices benefited everyone. Nonetheless, more than 50% of respondents of a RECOVR survey (2020) stated to have reduced food consumption due to decreased income
Central Government, through village leaders	Food distribution to support vulnerable families who had been affected by the lockdown. Food was sourced from the National Strategic Grain Reserve managed by the Ministry of Agriculture and Animal Resources. About 20,000 households targeted	The programme's coverage is uncertain; some respondents mentioned it was restricted to Kigali, while others said it was rolled out nationally.[14] Targeting was rapid but dependent on "being of the village", leading to the exclusion of people with non-permanent homes, such as day labourers in the construction sector. Moreover, no specific attention was given to gender as rations were handed out on the household level without considering intra-household inequalities and discrimination

[13] For example, the price of a 25 kg bag of rice was fixed at Rw18,000 and a kg between Rw750 and 800. On the other hand, a 25 kg bag of Pakistan rice was fixed at Rw20,500 or 900 a kilo. The kilo of sugar cost was between Rw850 and Rw1000 and Rw1500–2000 per litre for cooking oil.

[14] Interview representative CSO; interview representative CSO.

Actor	Measures	Equity considerations
Central Government	"Social-Economic Recovery plan to support activities affected by Covid-19". This provided a fund to support access to capital for small and medium enterprises (SMEs) with the reported plan to launch a targeted USD 200 million funds, including the IMF borrowed funds	The Recovery Plan is not accessible to informal businesses due to registration requirements
Rwanda Revenue Authority (RRA)	Extension of deadlines for businesses to file and pay income taxes from the end of March to the end of April and relaxed other administrative requirements	Informal businesses did not profit from these tax reliefs
National Bank of Rwanda (BNR)	Instruction to commercial banks to ease loan repayment conditions to borrowers and introduced an Extended Loan Facility to banks of RWF 50 billion	Informal businesses generally do not have loans with commercial banks and therefore did not benefit from this measure
Central Government	The government promised to inject Rwf 100 billion to start a coronavirus (Covid-19) exit process and counteract the impact of the pandemic on the economy. The funding would be used to support agriculture and livestock activities to enhance food security and agro exports. Other sectors to benefit from this fund include industry, tourism and hospitality, and water, electricity, and road infrastructure projects. Since tourism and hospitality are expected to be affected for much longer, special funding should be allocated to the sector	Focus on agribusinesses instead of small-scale farmers and formal sector businesses. Informal workers have been excluded

(continued)

Table 11.2 (continued)

Actor	Measures	Equity considerations
Ministry of Finance, Planning and Economic Development	Waived Pay as You Earn (PAYE) Taxes for six months, starting with April 2020, for private schools' teachers earning up to Rwf150, 000 net salaries. For those in the tourism industry, this waiver applied for three months (April-June) for employees of tourism and hotels earning Rwf150, 000 net salaries	These measures are only for formal sector workers
MINECOFIN	Value Added Tax (VAT) exemption was placed on all face masks made in Rwanda	Everybody could benefit from this measure
Central Bank	Lifting of transaction costs of mobile money for three months (March 18–June 2)	Use of mobile money increased by 450% in 4 months (moto-taxi association leaders were pleased with the measure)

Source Compiled by authors based on Broulard (2020), Bower et al. (2020), Edwards (2020), IPA (2020), Mwai (2020), Sabiiti (2020), Tabaro (2020), WHO (2020a, 2020b)

ensure compliance. The only support from government for this group is the fact that, they were allowed to operate.

It is difficult to access the success of programmes because of the time limit of the research. However, at first glance, most aid focuses on strengthening the health sector through in-kind contributions of equipment and PPEs as well as capacity building. Social protection programmes such as cash transfers were also implemented. Only one donor is supporting CSOs, which is the European Union. The other agencies seem to work through the government, explicitly supporting its Covid-19 preparedness and response programme. If programmes do not address existing barriers experienced by the poor in accessing essential services, the investments in healthcare infrastructure will generally not favour the poor. The inclusiveness of cash transfers will mainly rely on the transparency and efficiency of targeting. The former is the most challenging in the context of Rwanda.

Apart from the key development partners outlined already, Rwanda hosts many local and international NGOs. For example, Worldrelief works with local organisations, such as churches, while others are focused on education, yet others provide direct cash transfers to beneficiaries. GIVEDIRECTLY serves as an excellent example of the latter. By October 2020, GIVEDIRECTLY had reached 19,000 people in three districts (Gasabo, Kicukiro and Nyarygenge) in Kigali and was seeking to expand to the Western Province (Rusizi and Rubavu). Targeting was done based on the data of affected families gathered by local village leaders and compiled by LODA. From these lists, GIVEDIRECTLY targeted those households with family heads under 40 years. Local staff then conducted enrolment surveys via phone to verify eligibility, after which the cash was transferred via mobile money. Each beneficiary received two transfers of 153.21 k RWF (or $150).[15]

Equity Assessment

In the following short-term equity assessment, we will shed light on the impact of Covid-19 and related responses on the vulnerable groups we have identified across four dimensions of well-being, i.e. material,

---

[15] Interview with GIVEDIRECTLY local officer.

relational, subjective well-being and collective. Material well-being is associated with income and patterns of consumption. At the same time, relational well-being is associated with individual interactions with their kin, clients and those around them. Cognitive well-being is about mindset positivity and satisfaction with one's life. Finally, we examine how the pandemic has created windows of opportunity for political participation and mobilisation of the poor, which relates to the notion of collective well-being (Kingdon, 1984; Sen, 1984).

SHORT-TERM EQUITY ASSESSMENT

Impact on Material Well-being

All the vulnerable people included in this study have been severely affected by the government's response to Covid-19. Taxi-moto drivers approximately 32, 230 drivers in 2018 according to RURA (2018)) and taxi-velo riders form a significant section of people informally employed. They have been vulnerable as many of the adopted Covid-19 containment measures such as mobility restriction ones limited their services. During the lockdown, motorcycle and bicycle-taxi drivers were only allowed to carry goods resulting in income losses for the transporters. The majority (80%) of these are youth. Some have their incomes halved. As a taxi-velo rider in Kigali said, "*my living condition has changed a lot, to the extent that I do not have basic needs like food and shelter*" (taxi-Velo rider, Kigali).

Out of the ten taxi-velo and taxi-moto drivers interviewed, only two reported having received some food support from the government. However, one stated he received some support from the association in terms of payment of his savings. In addition, some received support from their relations.

The market women were also affected economically in various ways. First, all non-essential businesses were closed during the lockdown leaving only those that sell foodstuff to open their shop, but even for these women, business was slow due to a decline in customers and an increase in prices, which made their profit decrease because the government fixed prices of some seventeen items. Also, on August 28, markets started operating at 50% capacity via a rotation system. This has had a severe impact on the incomes of the traders. Nevertheless, they continued to pay the same amount of taxes. Since market women generally fall outside the lowest Ubudehe category, they were not eligible for government support such as food supply.

Similarly, the elderly also lost the support they receive from relations because of economic hardship. *"Before COVID-19, I had something to eat from the supporters and other donors. But now in this period of the pandemic, most people who have supported me are not working as before"* (elderly man in Western Province). While poor older adults fall under the lowest Ubudehe category and are thus received cash transfers from the state, transfers have not been extended in amount or coverage despite an increase in poverty. Consequently, those just above the poverty line now fell below it. The amount for cash transfers are about 8000Frw per household, which is not enough for a dignified condition of living considering the cost of food (1 kg of sweet potatoes is 300Frw and a kilo of beans is 1000frw, e.g.).[16] Furthermore, the cash transfers are given at the household level, without considering the number of members. Due to unemployment, many people returned to the rural areas. As a result, rural households had more members to feed. Development partners have also changed their service provisions due to new priorities and regulations in line with Covid-19.

Impact on Relational Well-Being

In terms of the relational well-being of poor and vulnerable people, low-income families survive through mutual support with family members helping one another. However, Covid-19 induced financial insecurity strained these support networks and consequently affected social relations. The social effects dimensions were highlighted in this statement by a taxi-moto driver in Kigali *"My relationship with my friends and colleagues has been very negatively affected because I have no money to help them"*.

It is customary to borrow money between colleagues, but the economic hardships have made this complicated and stressful. This issue of credit is also significant for market women, who were buying goods on credit as a normal practice. Some women defaulted their credit obligations thereby creating social conflicts. The competition over fewer clients also raised tensions among market women. The relations between clients have

---

[16] Interview with a member of civil society in Western Province.

also been affected as the Covid-19 protocols have made all human inter-actions less spontaneous. Another impact is the pandemic effect on the social character of markets. For the elderly, the restrictions on mobility seemed to have affected them. Some stated that nobody came to visit them, highlighting their loneliness.

Impact on Subjective Well-Being

The pandemic has also influenced the way people felt about their lives and the future. However, only one respondent, a taxi-moto driver from Kigali, mentioned that the pandemic had positively impacted on his life:

> It has made the most significant change in my life, so I must work hard, and saving must be my culture. Therefore, I would say that my life has improved; it made me think that I can do different things and save (taxi-moto driver, Kigali).

In general, people expressed extreme difficulties with the pandemic's impacts on them and their family's future. Some blamed themselves for their misfortunes. This individualism and the belief that one is respon-sible for one's life resonates with the RPF political discourse of moving forward by working hard (Chemouni, 2014). This mindset helps people from getting bitter with the government measures.

Impact on Collective Well-Being

With collective well-being, we refer to the position of the specific vulner-able group within society and their political power and voice. Taxi-moto and taxi-velo drivers were met with public prejudices when the lock-down started, and their businesses were banned as many feared they would resort to theft and other illegal practices to substitute for their loss of income. Interestingly, this negative sentiment spurred public opinion to join the taxi-moto associations in pushing the government to lift the restrictions on their service provision. After a media campaign in which the associations appeared on a popular radio programme and high-lighted their concerns, the government decided to lift the ban on June 1. However, the bicycle-taxi drivers were excluded from this policy change, and their livelihoods remained halted until October. To a certain extent, the government has recognised the importance of their services for urban transport and has incorporated mobile money paying systems, providing loans to them so that they can buy helmets which are now a requirement for both taxi-velo and taxi-moto drivers.

Regarding the market women, it was unclear if the associations were involved in the policy formulation processes. The government has in recent years come a long way in formalising the markets and its vendors, but this process does not seem to have increase the bargaining power of the women decisions take centrally are imposed on them.

The elderly in the study have shown no sign of collective action. Although they are aware their group was more vulnerable to the virus, there has been no collective organisation as their expectations for support were not expressed in citizen-state relations but in family-community or development partner-ties terms.

Long-Term Equity Assessment

Besides the direct impact on people's well-being, Covid-19 and the related responses will also have long-term effects on the other structural inequalities in Rwanda.

Rural Versus Urban

One of the most apparent inequalities within Rwanda is geographical which is between urban and rural communities and between Kigali and the other provinces. Poverty is three times higher in rural areas than in urban ones, and Kigali has, on average, a poverty rate which is half of those in the other provinces. Nonetheless, socioeconomic impact mitigation measures were urban-biased due to the assumption that urban people were more affected by Covid-19. This approach overlooks the (in) direct impact on poor rural people. For example, an Oxfam survey indicated significant job losses in rural areas (Oxfam 2020).

Furthermore, while the direct economic impact might be slightly lower than in Kigali, the indirect impact is very high. As mentioned above, the elderly peoples living in the villages often rely on family in the city. But, with the loss of jobs, remittances to the village decreased, pushing poor older adults and households deeper into poverty. Although people in rural areas might have been hit less, the high poverty rates imply that they are also less resilient and that the impact of a shock will be higher for them.

Furthermore, rural areas present fewer opportunities to find alternative income-generating activities. For example, the VUP public works program, which provides jobs for rural citizens in the second Ubudehe category, was halted during the lockdown. Although in some districts, advances were paid to beneficiaries of the VUP public works program, this was not the case everywhere.[17] According to trade union representatives, the food distribution programme could have been complemented with agricultural productivity support such as hoes, pangas and seeds.

Another inequality with geographical characteristics is the digital divide and the implications on school children to continue learning despite school closures. Despite the efforts of development partners such as UNICEF to address this challenge, more school children in rural areas did not have access to online or television school programmes.

Gender

According to the UNDP (2020a, 2020b, p. XV): *the current crisis threatens to push back the limited gains made on gender equality and exacerbate the feminisation of poverty, vulnerability to violence, and women's equal participation in the labour force. As a result, female-headed households are at a greater risk of being impacted by the adverse effects of the COVID19 crisis; in fact, they could fall into deeper poverty levels and even face extreme poverty.*

Women are overly represented in the daily wage labourers and operators or SMEs, two categories which have been badly affected by Covid-19 and related policies (UNDP, 2020a, 2020b, p. XV).

Income

Income inequality will likely increase in Rwanda as many measures favour formal businesses over informal SMEs. While market women received tax exemptions, companies have benefited from tax relief. Urban bias policies would exacerbate income inequality between and within provinces. There have been no measures targeting informal workers, although they represent most of Rwanda's workforce. Most of them were left to fend for themselves by depleting their savings or diversifying their income. A

---

[17] Interview with CSOs representative.

moto-taxi driver said, *"even though we lived badly, we never missed a meal because I looked for another income-generating activity"*.

Furthermore, due to informal housing situations and regular movements between Kigali and rural areas, day labourers have been left out of food distribution.

EFFECT OF COVID-19 ON STRUCTURES AND SYSTEMS OF POWER

> Whether the people trust or fear their government, Rwandans listen to it and have been following the order regarding masks, washing hands, and staying home (Beaubien, 2020).

Based on our findings, Covid-19 has strengthened existing power systems and reaffirmed state-citizen relations in Rwanda rather than changed them. The centralised response implemented through decentralised government institutions, punitive measures against non-compliance with regulations and control over media is known characteristics of Rwanda's governance system. The high level of compliance by citizens to Covid-19 regulations is embedded in the country's political culture, which is wary of publicly showing discontent and has been infused by the values of togetherness and joint-responsibility because of the post-genocide nation-building discourse. As a result, among respondents from vulnerable groups, there was a high responsibility to follow the restrictions.

The socio-economic policy choices made by the government in response to Covid-19 are embedded in Rwanda's neoliberal growth. A trade union representing the "doing business" model once again prevailed, with huge jobless and related increase in poverty as a result. Moreover, the rush to flatten the curve undermined human rights and civil liberties. The detainment of people for education in stadiums, for instance, was an excessive use of force. The strict control over information, research, and reporting on the impact of Covid-19, which has also had consequences on this research, raises red flags regarding freedom of speech and press.

Another system of power that has been highlighted through Covid-19 has been that between the Rwandan government and international donors. Local CSOS have not been engaged in the policy formulation processes of Covid-19 prevention measure. But they were consulted posterior to share ideas on reactivating specific sectors in a Covid-19-safe way. International donors such as UNDP have, on the other hand, played an essential role in developing the government's response throughout. Unfortunately, this reinforces existing tendencies towards upward accountability rather than accountability towards Rwandan citizens.

From a donor perspective, Rwanda can be seen as a successful case in its fight against Covid-19 as it has flattened the curve relatively quickly. However, the cost of the adopted approach to the poorest and vulnerable has been very high. The civil society and broader population have little political space to voice their concerns, and the media has indicated that while the government has been relatively open about Covid-19 data, they have been much more careful in sharing information about the socioeconomic impact of adopted measures.[18] Critical, independent media trying to dig below the surface have been met with oppression. All the above fall in line with existing systems of power and how Kagame's regime, which is defined as developmental and, for others, authoritarian, sustains power.

One positive development has been how the pandemic has spurred political activism via social media and its influence over political decision-making. An example is the crimes committed by security officers at the beginning of the lockdown in Kangondo II, an informal settlement in Kigali. On March 26, 2020, security officers raped various women and severely beat several men. Independent YouTube journalists who reported on the event were later arrested for not respecting the Covid-19 regulations. Human Rights Watch has, in response, criticised the government in this statement:

> It is unacceptable for Rwanda to use authoritarian tactics to enforce public health measures to contain Covid-19's spread," Lewis Mudge (HRW director for Central Africa) said. "The media crackdown sends a deliberately chilling message at a time when scrutiny of security forces' behaviour is critical.

The government officials including the president were forced to condemn the atrocities following public outrage on social media about the police brutalities. Five police officers related to the crime.[19]

---

[18] Interview with a representative of the media.

[19] Interview with Amnesty International representative.

Conclusion and Recommendations

The Rwandan government activated its robust health management structures, building on its experience with Ebola and long-term support of development partners. The decentralised governance approach, backed by a strong state, allowed for efficient implementation of mitigation measures. The use of village leaders *"who know the vulnerable people"* made it possible to coordinate and implement food distribution relatively rapidly and in an orderly fashion. In addition, the government prioritised "flattening the curve" over other socio-economic considerations. The initial nationwide lockdown was eventually eased and replaced by targeted quarantine measures in "transmission hot spots". The transport of goods, including medicines and agricultural produce, was waivered from restrictions on mobility and essential services. Research respondents largely approved of the measures and primarily complied with them. However, the socioeconomic support provided by the government was disproportionate in terms of the needs of the extremely poor and biased towards formal sector industries and workers, thereby exacerbating existing inequalities.

Food aid distributed by local government officials was insufficient compensation for the loss of income, and the targeting was untransparent. Similarly, an economic stimulus such as loans was not accessible to SMEs in the informal sector. As a result, most poor people were left to fend for themselves and depleted their savings, while others reduced their food consumption to cope with the hardship.

The strict way in which regulations were enforced and the instrumentalisation of local CSOs as implementers and watchdogs of Covid-19 prevention measures highlighted and, at the same time, exacerbated the country's authoritarian governance style. "Unfortunately, this same governance style also allowed for a quick flattening of the curve" during the first wave, which could be used as a legitimation for restricting human rights and civil liberties in the name of efficient service delivery and development.

The following policy recommendations could be considered.

- Social protection for rural citizens should include agricultural inputs to farmers to increase food security.

- Development partners should also engage with the government to include—on equal footing—local CSOs when designing and implementing crisis responses.
- Targeting by village leaders should be more transparent. While monopolisation increases efficiency; it creates challenges to inclusiveness.
- Pandemic responses should also centre on enhancing human rights, press freedom and transparency.
- Appropriate support measures should be fashioned out for various sectors and social groups.

REFERENCES

Africa CCVI. (2020). Rwanda in perspective. *Precision for Covid.* Retrieved from https://precisionforcovid.org/africa

Amnesty International. (2019). *Rwanda: Decades of attacks, repression and killings set the scene for next month's election.* Retrieved from https://www.amnesty.org/en/latest/news/2017/07/rwanda-decades-of-attacks-repression-and-killings-set-the-scene-for-next-months-election/

Ansoms, A. (2020). *Expanding the Space for Criticism in Rwanda.* Retrieved from https://roape.net/2019/03/12/the-green-revolution-in-rwanda-an-expanding-space-for-criticism/

Ansoms, A., Marijnen, E., Cioffo, G., & Murison, J. (2017). Statistics versus livelihoods: Questioning Rwanda's pathway out of poverty. *Review of African Political Economy, 44*(151), 47–65. https://doi.org/10.1080/03056244.2016.1214119

Asala, I. (2020). *Rwanda's extreme Covid-19 prevention tactics.* Africa News. Retrieved from https://www.africanews.com/2020/08/07/rwanda-s-extreme-covid-19-prevention-tactics/

Beaubien, J. (2020). *Why Rwanda is Doing Better Than Ohio When it Comes to Controlling COVID-19.* Retrieved from https://www.npr.org/sections/goatsandsoda/2020/07/15/889802561/a-covid-19-success-story-in-rwanda-free-testing-robot-caregivers

Bizoza, A., & Sibomana, S. (2020). Indicative socioeconomic impacts of the novel coronavirus (Covid-19) outbreak in Eastern Africa: Case of Rwanda. Available at SSRN 3586622.

Bourguignon, F. (2015). *The globalisation of inequality.* Princeton University Press. ISBN: 9780691160528

Bower, J. Apell, D., Twum, A., Adia, U. (2020). Rwanda's response to COVID-19 and future challenges. *International Growth Centre, Kigali.*

Retrieved from https://www.theigc.org/blog/rwandas-response-to-covid-19-and-future-challenges/

BPN and UoR (2020). Measuring the Impact of COVID-19 on Rwandan Entrepreneurs. *Professionals Network (BPN) and the University of Rwanda (UoR), Kigali.* Retrieved from https://bpn.rw/application/files/9615/9047/8175/Impact_of_COVID-19_on_Rwandan_Businesses._Eng.PDF

Broulard, L. (2020). *Coronavirus: au Rwanda, Félix organise la solidarité officielle de quartier.* Le Monde Diplomatique. Retrieved from https://www.lemonde.fr/afrique/article/2020/04/10/coronavirus-au-rwanda-felix-org anise-la-solidarite-officielle-de-quartier_6036269_3212.html

Broulard, L. (2021). *Covid-19: Malgré un contrôle strict, le Rwanda commence à se faire déborder.* Le Monde Diplomatique. Retrieved from https://www.lem onde.fr/afrique/article/2021/01/30/covid-19-malgre-un-controle-strict-le-rwanda-commence-a-se-faire-deborder_6068188_3212.html

Byishimo, B. (2020) COVID-19 cases confirmed in 43% of Rwanda's districts. Retrieved from https://www.newtimes.co.rw/news/covid-19-cases-confirmed-43-rwandas-districts

CDC. (2019). *CDC in Rwanda.* Centers for Disease Control and Prevention (CDC), Atlanta.

Chaplin, D. Twigg J., & Lovell, E. (2017). *Intersectional approaches to vulnerability reduction and resilience-building.* Resilience Intel, 12. BRACED.

Chemouni, B. (2014). Explaining the design of the Rwandan decentralisation: Elite vulnerability and the territorial repartition of power. *Journal of Eastern African Studies, 8*(2), 246–262. https://doi.org/10.1080/17531055.2014.891800

Chemouni, B. (2018). The political path to universal health coverage: Power, ideas and community-based health insurance in Rwanda. *World Development, 106,* 87–98. https://doi.org/10.1016/j.worlddev.2018.01.023

Crisafulli, P., & Redmond, A. (2012). *Rwanda Inc: How a devastated nation became an economic model for the developing world.* Palgrave Macmillan.

Dawson, N. M. (2018). Leaving no-one behind? Social inequalities and contrasting development impacts in rural Rwanda. *Development Studies Research, 5*(1), 1–14. https://doi.org/10.1080/21665095.2018.1441039

Debenedetti, L., Kirke-Smith, D., & Mfura, J., L,.H. (2020). *The Reach of the COVID-19 Crisis in Rwanda: Lessons from the RECOVR Survey.* Retrieved from https://www.poverty-action.org/blog/reach-covid-19-crisis-rwanda-les sons-recovr-survey (Accessed January 2021)

Edwards, N. (2020). *Rwanda's successes and challenges in response to COVID-19.* Retrieved from https://www.atlanticcouncil.org/blogs/africasource/rwa ndas-successes-and-challenges-in-response-to-covid-19/

Gatzinsi, J., Hartwig, R. S., Mossman, L. S., Francoise, U. M., Roberte, I., & Rawlings, L. B. (2019). *How household characteristics shape program access* and asset accumulation: A mixed method analysis of the vision 2020 umurenge programme in Rwanda. The World Bank Group

Gaynor, N. (2015). 'A nation in a hurry': The costs of local governance reforms in Rwanda. *Review of African Political Economy, 41*(1), S49–S63. https://doi.org/10.1080/03056244.2014.976190

Government of Rwanda. (2020). *Covid 19 Corona Virus 17 07 2020.* Retrieved from https://www.rbc.gov.rw/fileadmin/user_upload/annoucement/Update-on-COVID-19-17-07-2020-eng.jpg

Government of Rwanda. (2021). *Covid 19 Corona Virus 19 01 2021.* Retrieved from https://www.africanews.com/2021/01/20/coronavirus-rwanda-covid-19-update-19-january-2021/

HRW. (2017). *Rwanda: Politically Closed Elections: A Chronology of Violations.* Retrieved from https://www.hrw.org/news/2017/08/18/rwanda-politically-closed-elections

HRW. (2020a). *As Long as We Live on the Streets, They Will Beat Us" Rwanda's Abusive Detention of Children.* Retrieved from https://www.hrw.org/report/2020/01/27/long-we-live-streets-they-will-beat-us/rwandas-abusive-detention-children

HRW. (2020b). *Rwanda: Lockdown Arrests, Abuses Surge. End Media Crackdown, Mass Arbitrary Arrests.* Retrieved from https://www.hrw.org/news/2020/04/24/rwanda-lockdown-arrests-abuses-surge

ILO. (2018). *Women and men in the informal economy: A statistical picture.* ILO.

IPA. (2020). *Research for Effective COVID-19 Responses (RECOVR) Survey Analysis Rwanda.* Retrieved from https://www.poverty-action.org/recovr

ISHR. (2016). Rwanda: Participation and protection of civil society is crucial to development. Retrieved from https://www.ishr.ch/news/rwanda-participation-and-protection-civil-society-crucial-development

Kingdon, J. W. (1984). *Agendas, alternatives and public policies.* Little, Brown and Company.

Klopp J., Krueger, A., & Trimble, M. (2020). *COVID-19 impacts cross border traders in East Africa.* Retrieved from https://ace.globalintegrity.org/smallscaletraders/

Laterite. (2017). *Understanding Dropout and Repetition in Rwanda.* Kigali, Rwanda: MINEDUC and UNICEF

LODA. (2018). *Ubudehe Program.* Retrieved from https://loda.gov.rw/programs/ubudehe/

Matengo, D. (2020). *Unemployment rate in Rwanda has increased to 22 percent.* Retrieved from https://africa.cgtn.com/2020/08/20/unemployment-rate-in-rwanda-increases-to-22-percent/

Mcgregor, J. (2004). Researching well-being. *Global Social Policy, 4,* 337–358. https://doi.org/10.1177/1468018104047491

Mcgregor, J. A., & Pouw, N. (2017). Towards an economics of well-being. *Cambridge Journal of Economics, 41*, 1123–1142. https://doi.org/10.1093/cje/bew044

Ministry of Local Government. (2016) Revised Ubudehe categories are out. Available at http://197.243.22.137/minaloc/index.php?id=469&tx_news_pi1%5Bnews%5D=376&tx_news_pi1%5Bday%5D=28&tx_news_pi1%5Bmonth%5D=4&tx_news_pi1%5Byear%5D=2016&cHash=4e719b950f3caa512a3d35b1bda7fc7f (Accessed June 2020)

MoH. (2017) Private Health Facilities in Rwanda Health Service Packages, Ministry of Health.

MoH. (2018). Fourth health sector Strategic plan July 2018–June 2024, Ministry of Health.

MoH. (2019). *Rwanda Health Sector Performance Report 2017–2019*. MoH

Munu, M. L. (2019) *Research on informal workers and social dialogue; Rwanda case study*. FNV Mondiaal. Retrieved from https://www.fnv.nl/getmedia/0fd031da-d864-46f4-910d-12985ad78acf/Mondiaal-FNV-Case-study-Rwanda-final-aug-2019.pdf

Mwai, C. (June 19 2020). *Central bank reinstates mobile money charges*. The New Times. Retrieved from https://www.newtimes.co.rw/news/central-bank-reinstates-mobile-money-charges

Mwasa, F. (2020). *Running Dry: Booming Informal Trade of Cross-border Water Sellers in Rwanda, DR Congo Hit by Border Closure*. Pulitzer center. Retrieved from https://pulitzercenter.org/stories/running-dry-booming-informal-trade-cross-border-water-sellers-rwanda-dr-congo-hit-border

NISR. ((2015). *Rwanda Poverty Profile Report - Results of EICV 4*. Retrieved from https://www.statistics.gov.rw/publication/rwanda-poverty-profile-report-results-eicv-4

NISR. (2016). *Rwanda Poverty Profile Report - Results of EICV 5*. Retrieved from Retrieved from https://www.statistics.gov.rw/publication/rwanda-poverty-profile-report-results-eicv-5

NISR. (2018). *The Fifth Integrated Household Living Conditions Survey. Thematic Report: Rwanda Multidimensional Poverty Report*. NISR. https://www.mppn.org/wp-content/uploads/2018/12/EICV5_Thematic-Report_Multidimensional-Poverty-Index_MPI.pdf

NISR. (2020a). *Labour Force Survey Trends-May 2020(Q2)*. NISR

NISR. (2020b). *COVID-19 and its impact on Labour force in Rwanda*. Retrieved from https://www.statistics.gov.rw/publication/covid-19-and-its-impact-labour-force-rwanda

Nkurunziza, M. (October 21 2020). Teen pregnancy: Activists call for way forward before schools resume. *The New Times*. Retrieved from https://www.newtimes.co.rw/lifestyle/teen-pregnancy-activists-call-way-forward-schools-resume

NODEA. (2020). *The Economic Context of Rwanda*, July 2020, retrieved from https://www.nordeatrade.com/en/explore-new-market/rwanda/econom ical-context

OECD. (2014). *Focus on Inequality and Growth - December 2014*. Paris, France: OECD. Retrieved from www.oecd.org/social/inequality-and-poverty.htm

OECD. (2018). Graph 5.7—Gini coefficients and difference in income share in East African countries. In *Africa's Development Dynamics 2018: Growth, Jobs and Inequalities*, OECD Publishing. https://doi.org/10.1787/978926430 2501-graph74-en.

O'Reilly, P., & Vaughan, C. (2020). East African integration is alive—even though leaders haven't been united over COVID-19. *The Conversation*. Retrieved from https://theconversation.com/east-african-integration-is-alive-even-though-leaders-havent-been-united-over-covid-19-142419

Our World in Data. (2020). *Rwanda: Coronavirus Pandemic Country Profile*. Retrieved from https://ourworldindata.org/coronavirus/country/rwanda?country=~RWA

Piketty, T. (2014). *Capital in the twenty-first century*. Belknap Press. ISBN 9780674430006

Republic of Rwanda (2020). RWANDA DEVELOPMENT PARTNERS. Maximising aid effectiveness in Rwanda. Retrieved from http://www.devpar tners.gov.rw/index.php?id=45

Reyntjens, F. (2015). Reduction of poverty and inequality, the Rwandan way. And the aid community loves it, *IOB Analyses and Policy Briefs, 16*. Universiteit Antwerpen, Institute of Development Policy (IOB).

Reyntjens, F. (2015). Lies, damned lies and statistics: Poverty reduction Rwandan-style and how the aid community loves it. Available at

RURA. (2018) Statistics in Transport Sector as of March 2018. RURA. Retrieved from https://rura.rw/fileadmin/Documents/transport/statistics/Transport_Statistics_Report_as_of_March_2018.pdf

Sabiiti, D. (2020). Rwanda Sets A Covid-19 Economic Recovery Plan. Available at https://www.ktpress.rw/2020/05/rwanda-sets-a-covid-19-eco nomic-recovery-plan/ (Accessed August 2020)

EAC Secretariat. (2020). East African community COVID-19 response plan. EAC.

Sen, A. (1984, Apr). Well-being, agency and freedom: The dewey lectures, *The Journal of Philosophy*, *82*(4), 169–221

Stuart, J. (2020). *Informal Cross Border Trade in Africa in a Time of Pandemic*. Tarlac Blog. Retrieved from https://www.tralac.org/blog.html

The East African. (2020). Rwanda revises policy to meet Covid-19 bills. Available at

UNDP (2020a). *The Socioeconomic Impact of COVID-19 in Rwanda*. UNDP.

UNDP (2020b). *UNDP Rwanda Support to the National Response to Contain the Impact of COVID-19.* UNDP.

University of Oxford (2020). *Relationship between number of COVID-19 cases and government response.* Retrieved from https://covidtracker.bsg.ox.ac.uk/stringency-scatter.

Verpoorten, M. (2014). *Growth, Poverty and Inequality in Rwanda: A Broad Perspective.* WIDER Working Paper 2014/138. UNU-WIDER.

Vlaminck, Z., Dekker, M., Leliveld, A.H.M., Oberst, U. (2014). *Rome wasn't built in a day: the accessibility of social protection for informal workers: a mapping of 5 West African countries.* CNV Internationaal.

WHO (2019). WHO Country Cooperation Strategy (2014–2018) Rwanda. World Health Organisation Resource Office for Africa.

WHO (2020b). *COVID-19 in Rwanda: A country's response, July 20 2020.* Retrieved from https://www.afro.who.int/pt/node/13056

WHO (2020a). *First Case of COVID-19 confirmed in Rwanda.* Retrieved from https://www.afro.who.int/news/first-case-covid-19-confirmed-rwanda

World Bank (2020). *The World Bank In Rwanda, Overview.* Retrieved from https://www.worldbank.org/en/country/rwanda/overview

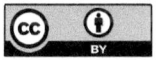

CHAPTER 12

Uganda

Shiphrah Kuria, Miles Lambert-Peck, Tonny Kapsandui, and Laura Ferguson

INTRODUCTION

The Covid-19 pandemic in Uganda exposed pre-existing structural inequalities and their impacts on social groups. Its health system and multiple disease burdens contributed to shaping the pandemic responses and their impacts. In terms of its population structure, the country has a large youthful population, with 72% under 24 years old. Only 2% are 65 years and above. Ordinarily, this should be an advantage since the

M. Lambert-Peck · L. Ferguson
Institute On Inequalities in Global Health, University of Southern California, Los Angeles, CA, USA
e-mail: Laura.Ferguson@med.usc.edu

T. Kapsandui
Reproductive, Maternal Child and Adolescent Health Programme, Amref Health Africa, Kampala, Uganda
e-mail: Tonny.Kapsandui@Amref.org

S. Kuria (✉)
Corporate Programmes' Department, Amref Health Africa Headquarters, Nairobi, Kenya
e-mail: Shiphrah.Kuria@amref.org

© The Author(s) 2024   291
A. Altaf et al. (eds.), *EQUITY IN COVID-19*, EADI Global Development Series, https://doi.org/10.1007/978-3-031-58588-3_12

Covid-19 infection rate for youth is lower than that of older people. However, other critical structural factors are important to note. Due to rapid urbanization, 25% of the population lives in densely populated urban areas. Uganda also has a large refugee population[1] which has tripled since 2016 and adds an essential dimension to the demographic dynamics that are critical for an effective Covid-19 response. The country's social services are under stress because of these demographic dynamics.[2]

Ranked 159 out of 189 countries in the Human Development Index, Uganda is categorized as a lower-middle-income country by the World Bank due to its high poverty levels and other developmental indicators. Economic vulnerability to external shocks is high, with two out of every three people living around the poverty line or falling back below it. In 2016, 42% of the population lived on less than $1.90 per day.[3] Despite the high incidence of poverty, only 3% of the population has access to social protection programmes.[4] Regarding social services, only 38% of households have access to electricity, and around 40% have access to improved sanitation.

Agriculture employs more than 70% of Ugandans. Also, 29% of children under the age of five are stunted, a measure of chronic malnutrition that highlights the need for attention to food security. In Uganda, even before the pandemic, the health system was overstretched, with relatively low ratios of health professionals to population, little intensive care capacity and shortages of medical equipment, including ventilators.[5] The health system throughout the country is chronically underfunded and fragmented. The doctor-patient ratio is one to 24,000 and nurse-patient ratio is one to 11,000. Only 55 ICU beds are available in-country, of which 20 lack ventilatory capacity, only one-third are part of the public health system, and all are in major urban hubs.[6] The disparities in the health infrastructure are stark in rural areas. Though communicable diseases are a considerable burden in Uganda, non-communicable diseases such as hypertension and diabetes, which pose a significant risk

---

[1] World Bank (2021).

[2] Mejia-Mantilla et al. (n.d.).

[3] Thinkwell (2020).

[4] World Bank (2021).

[5] Murthy et al. (2015).

[6] O'Donovan et al. (2020).

to those who contract Covid-19, are rising. Though there is limited data, the available evidence points to rising cases not only in the urban areas but also in the rural areas.[7] The 2014 NCD survey attributed 33% of annual deaths to NCDs. In addition, hypertension and high blood sugar were reported, with many of those affected not being on medication.[8]

The constraints in the health sector and system raise concerns about the country's capacity to mount an effective biomedical response to the pandemic alongside the fear that necessary public health measures such as physical distancing, handwashing, and wearing facemasks might also be challenging to implement, particularly among some social groups such as the poor.

The chapter is guided by a social-ecological framework whereby individuals' experiences are shaped by a range of nested, interrelated factors around them, from seemingly "distant" factors such as laws and policies down to more "proximal" factors such as their immediate living situation. We explored the interplay of these factors, mainly the range of laws, policies, and regulations relevant to Covid-19 and their impact on different social groups.

Methodology

This mixed-methods study includes policy, quantitative and qualitative research, and a joint analysis to combine all these different data types. We reviewed web-based search engines such as Google and Google Scholar for the legal and policy analysis. Searches, carried out in October 2020, were limited by the date range of publication and were restricted to the year 2020. Searches included "Uganda + COVID + policy," "Uganda + COVID + law," "international + COVID + policy + tracker," and "Uganda + COVID + legal + response." Data were assessed for relevance and systematically extracted based on their direct or indirect implications for vulnerable communities.

Searches were conducted on Pubmed, Google Scholar, and Scopus using the search terms "Uganda" AND "covid". Pubmed searches were inclusive of the abstract and article, while Google Scholar and Scopus searches were only inclusive of the title. The Pubmed search yielded

---

[7] Mondo et al. (2013).

[8] The Republic of Uganda Ministry of Health (2014).

90 results, with 30 articles deemed relevant after a title and abstract review and 15 articles included in the final review. The Google Scholar search yielded 67 results, of which 46 were unique to Google Scholar and deemed relevant after a title and abstract review. Twenty-one articles were included in the final review. The Scopus search did not yield any impressive results. Thus, a total of 36 articles were included for a full review.

We also conducted media analysis of major local and international media channels. Reports from influential organizations actively engaged in the Covid-19 response in Uganda were identified from the media analysis, including UN organizations such as the WHO, UNDP, UNICEF, WFP, FAO, UN Women, as well as civil society organizations including Amref Health Africa, the Red Cross, World Vision, Save the Children, Akina Mama Wa Afrika, and the White Ribbon Alliance. Their latest reports on areas of interest were reviewed, and data relevant to answering the study's research questions were systematically extracted.

Nine key informant interviews were conducted with various participants across different sectors at the national level and in the Lango region in northern Uganda. Participants at the national level included heads of departments, programme managers, and principal medical officers at the Ministry of Health. At the regional/district level, these included medical superintendents, hospital administrators, Residence District Commissioners (RDCs), Chief Administrative Officers (CAO) of districts, and District Health Officers (DHO). Interviews were recorded and transcribed verbatim for analysis. Ethical approvals were secured through the MILDMAY Uganda Ethics Review Committee and the USC Institutional Review Board.

Overview of the Timeline of the Legal and Policy Response

In the first year of the pandemic, Uganda was widely lauded by the World Health Organization and the Africa Centres for Disease Control and Prevention (Africa CDC) for its strong response to Covid-19. The government put in place a range of legal and policy measures, each covering different aspects of their response. The pre-existing Public Health Act provided the overall legal framework for designing and implementing the Covid-19 response. The Minister of Health invoked powers under this Act to issue rules and orders aimed at combating Covid-19.

In the Public Health (Notification of Covid-19) Order, 2020, Covid-19 was declared a notifiable disease to which the provisions on prevention and suppression of infectious diseases under the Public Health Act (Cap. 281) apply. This includes the Minister of Health's power to make rules for control of the spread of the disease, order the quarantine of infected persons or those suspected to be infected, inspect premises of persons believed to be infected with the disease, and disinfect premises and buildings which have been covered under these rules and orders. Local government authorities are empowered to enforce such regulations and may make their own.

The national *Covid-19 Preparedness and Response Plan* was developed based on model guidance for countries published by the WHO. The Ugandan plan includes eight pillars: Leadership, Stewardship, Coordination, and Oversight; Surveillance and Laboratory; Case Management; Strategic Information, Research, and Innovation; Risk Communication and Social Mobilization; Community Engagement and Social Protection; Logistics and Operations; and Continuity of Essential Services. This plan was designed to guide the overall national response. It is supplemented by the additional legal and policy measures that have been instituted throughout the pandemic period.

The Ministry of Gender, Labour and Social Development issued Covid-19 guidelines in which it called on employers to retain employees who are paid monthly (regardless of whether they are essential or non-essential staff) and to agree with workers on who may stay home. Casual employees paid hourly or daily were most affected under these arrangements. The guidelines do not, however, have the force of law.

Figure 12.1 provides an overview of the national response until November 2020. A critical characteristic of the government response is the phased re-opening: rather than immediate removal of all restrictions. The government gradually loosened restrictions, continuously tracking their impact on the epidemic.

Covid-19 Response Measures

Further information on these measures is provided below, organized by the different sectors they are designed to impact. The section ends with an analysis of how these measures may have influenced the spread of Covid-19 throughout 2020. The actual impact of the measures will be explored in the subsequent sections. For example, in November (after the

UGANDA'S COVID-19 RESPONSE TIMELINE

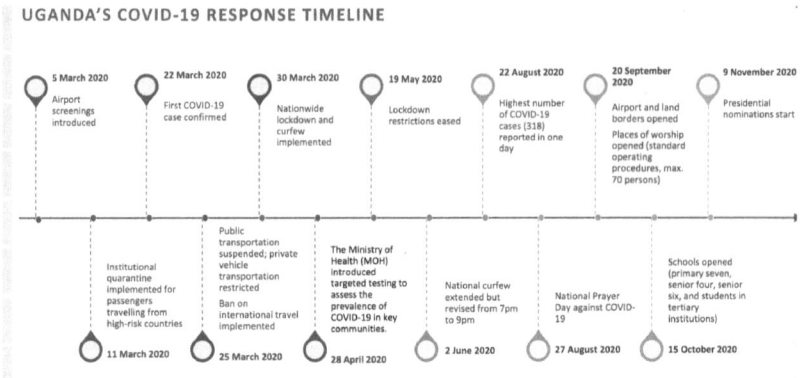

Fig. 12.1 Uganda's Covid-19 response timeline[9] (*Source* https://thinkwell. global/wp-content/uploads/2020/05/COVID-19-Uganda_August-2020-Updates-final.pdf)

period covered in the timeline above), it was reported that a new national strategy had been launched in which community health workers (CHWs) were to be paid a monthly allowance to fight Covid-19 at the community level.[10]

President Museveni imposed various restrictions on different types of mobility. For example, on March 25, airports and land borders were closed. This included banning new refugee arrivals, a significant change from the usual "open door" policy for refugees.[11] A fourteen-day lockdown was imposed on March 30, 2020 and reviewed. In addition, a 7 p.m. to 6:30 a.m. curfew was effected. Apart from transporting food and essential goods, private transportation was also restricted. Some measures were eased sequentially with locational variations.

The government of Uganda decided to open its borders to Ugandan nationals who had been stranded abroad in neighbouring East African Community (EAC) countries. On September 20, land borders and

[9] The Uganda SP4PHC Team (n.d.).

[10] "Donated PPE Protects Health Workers in Africa during Polio Vaccination Campaign, Covid-19 Response." 2020. Direct Relief. November 12, 2020. https://www.directrelief.org/2020/11/caf-africa-ppe-supporting-drc-polio-campaign-uganda-covid-19-response/.

[11] Reuters (2020).

airports were opened, and tourists and citizens who were stranded abroad were allowed to enter the country. As of October 1, Uganda's borders opened, and international flights resumed. Passengers arriving in the country required a negative PCR test certificate within 72 hours of arrival in Uganda.

On April 1, President Museveni ordered the closure of all non-food shops. However, shops that sold food, agricultural products, veterinary products, detergents, and pharmaceuticals were allowed to remain open. Closure of schools and public places was also enforced. These measures were accompanied by hygiene and sanitation protocols such as handwashing, face-mask-wearing, and social distancing mandates.

MITIGATION MEASURES

To mitigate the impact of school closures, the government developed a response plan focusing on continuity of learning during the closure of schools. According to UNHCR, nearly 500,000 children accessed distance learning programmes across Uganda while schools were closed, and 1,127 children with disabilities received support. However, there was some apprehension about e-learning because access was impossible for some social groups.[12]

Regarding fiscal measures, Uganda secured US$491.5 million in emergency financing from the IMF under the Rapid Credit Facility programme, which was intended to boost international reserves and improve health spending on vulnerable populations. In June 2020, Finance Minister Matia Kasaija announced that the Uganda budget for the fiscal year 2020/21 would focus on improving the well-being of Ugandans, boosting economic transformation, and improving peace, security, and good governance.

Tax cuts were announced in June 2020 as part of the stimulus package. In addition, the budget included an economic stimulus and growth strategy, including introducing tax relief to businesses, expanding social protection for the vulnerable, improving household incomes through work programmes and credit facilities, and reduction of mobile transaction costs to prevent the spread of the pandemic.[13] On June 29, the

[12] Tumwesige (2020).

[13] United Nations Agenda (2020).

Uganda Covid-19 Economic Crisis and Recovery Development Policy Financing received $300 million in budget support from the World Bank to support reforms to provide immediate relief to businesses and individuals hit hardest by the pandemic.

NON-STATE ACTORS' INCLUSION IN THE NATIONAL COVID RESPONSE

Within the government, there was cross-sectoral involvement in designing the Covid-19 response. However, evidence suggests that the government acted unilaterally in designing the response, restricting consultation and contributions to decision-making. While the chosen strategies were quickly deemed successful, with few reported Covid-19 cases, this came at a cost. Nevertheless, some key informants felt this approach was justified given the need for the quick action and reported that even community engagement came in much later.[14] It has fuelled growing demands from civil society and the private sector for greater involvement and accountability. There were calls for community involvement in Covid-19 management, including strengthening community structures such as political, religious, and cultural leaders to mobilize their constituencies to improve response measures.[15] Key informants suggested that civil society involvement in the national response increased over time. However, their primary function was often described as support to the government in terms of providing financing and supplies and sensitizing communities rather than playing an active role in designing the Covid-19 response.[16] A national-level official justified this by explaining that "the government response framework is science-based, so there is no need to involve [civil society]."[17] Another key informant, however, thought that civil society could be more effectively involved in policy-making, implementation and monitoring.[18] Some inclusion of religious and cultural leaders was reported to ensure acceptability of and compliance with restrictions

[14] Key Informant Interview 2.
[15] World Health Organization (n.d.).
[16] Key Informant Interviews 2; 3; 6; 9.
[17] Key Informant Interview 2.
[18] Key Informant Interview 7.

on mass gatherings rather than as a matter of inclusive participation of Covid-19 management.

INCLUSIVITY OF MITIGATION MEASURES AND POLICY RESPONSES

Some key informants, especially government representatives at the national level, emphasized that laws and policies apply equally to everyone in the country, which, in their view, meant that it was unnecessary to accord additional attention to any sub-population.[19] While others stated that vulnerable populations were targeted in mitigation measures, there was an acknowledgement that when the government first designed the response, it was based on biomedical criteria without due attention to social factors, such as poverty, that might put some people at greater risk.[20] Finally, some noted that attention was given to vulnerable groups at the intervention level rather than within laws and policies. Food relief, for example, was targeted the urban poor and provisions were made to allow special permission for pregnant women to travel outside curfew to reach health facilities.[21] But, the government's mitigation measures and policy responses have disproportionately affected specific populations, including women, the urban poor, children, people with disabilities, and people living with HIV and other chronic health conditions. For example, the impact on women is reflected by an increase in reported domestic violence, a loss of jobs across sectors dominated by women, a rise in abortion cases, and the limitation of travel for essential health services.[22,23,24]

Overall, it seems that there was little consideration for vulnerable populations. For example, people with disabilities such as people with hearing, speech, or sight impairments were left out, yet they needed communication.[25] Even when vulnerabilities were considered, more health-related

[19] Critical Informant Interview 2; Key Informant Interview 6.

[20] Key Informant Interviews 1; 3; 4.

[21] Critical Informant Interview 1; Key Informant Interview 6.

[22] Akina Mama wa Afrika (2020a).

[23] New Vision (2020c).

[24] New Vision (n.d.-b).

[25] Key Informant Interview 6.

challenges were at the fore, leaving the socioeconomically disadvantaged inadequately covered. Policy responses mainly focused on combating the spread of the infection and protecting those at high risk of Covid-19 but did not consider the effects on the poor.[26]

IMMEDIATE IMPACTS OF THE RESPONSE ON COVID-19-RELATED OUTCOMES

Overall, many interview respondents argued that the legal and policy measures implemented intended to affect Covid-19-related outcomes, including keeping mortality low, shielding the elderly from infection, and improving health infrastructure. While some government officials reported that the response had its intended impact on Covid-19 outcomes, many challenges remained. In the first six months of the pandemic, Uganda was internationally lauded for a successful response, but that changed with fast community transmission. In addition, the level of risk of exposure to the coronavirus was not equally distributed among population groups. Figure 12.2 shows the distribution of risk among different populations based on household exposure to seven risk factors:

    i. levels of overcrowding
    ii. population living with an older person (aged 60+)
    iii. population with no access to water in their dwelling or on their premises (yard/plot)
    iv. population who reports having to collect their water
    v. population sharing sanitation facilities with others or who lack any toilet facilities
    vi. population who reports not having handwashing facilities near their toilets
    vii. population who must collect fuel for cooking.[27]

At the national level, almost 67% of the population has a high risk of exposure to more than four risk factors, while rural areas have a higher risk exposure than urban areas (73% and 46%, respectively). People living

---

[26] Key informant Interview 4.
[27] United Nations Agenda (2020).

HH-EXPOSURE TO COVID19 RISK FACTORS

		NONE		1-3 RISK FACTORS		4+ RISK FACTORS	
		COUNT	ROW N (%)	COUNT	ROW N %	COUNT	ROW N (%)
Uganda	National	869	2	13,012	31	27,587	67
Place of Residence	Rural	130	0	8,104	26	22,823	73
	Urban	739	7	4,888	47	4,764	46
Sub-region	Kampala	160	9	884	49	752	42
	Central1	374	7	2,727	50	2,324	43
	Central2	105	2	1,744	39	2,590	58
	Busoga	23	1	974	23	3,203	76
	Bukedi	19	1	322	15	1,842	84
	Bugishu	11	1	520	25	1,536	74
	Teso	2	0	381	18	1,784	82
	Karamoja	-	0	74	6	1,086	94
	Lango	27	1	619	24	1,891	75
	Acholi	-	0	256	14	1,536	86
	West Nile	12	0	539	18	2,523	82
	Bunyoro	35	1	794	32	1,677	67
	Toro	37	1	1,046	34	1,994	65
	Ankole	59	2	1,591	46	1,818	52
	Kigezi	7	0	523	34	1,030	66
Poverty status (UBOS)	Non-poor	868	3	11,902	36	20,099	61
	Poor	-	0	952	11	7,462	89
Poverty Group	Poor	4	0	3,027	16	16,433	84
	Rising	37	4	371	44	434	52
	Vulnerable	10	0	1,387	33	2,749	66
	Not poor	819	5	8,226	48	7,972	47

Source: UNHS 2016/17 (UBOS, 2018)

Fig. 12.2 Number of risk factors to which people are exposed (*Note* Red indicates higher risk, yellow indicates moderate risk, and green indicates lower risk)

in poverty are also at higher risk than the non-poor, and specific sub-regions such as Karamoja, Acholi, Bukedi, and West Nile are particularly affected.

The socioeconomic features of the country show that the lockdown was unfeasible for the poor. Reliance on a daily wage to meet basic needs is incompatible with lockdown measures. Half of the residents in the Greater Kampala Metropolitan Area live in informal settlements, comprising only 16% of total land, presenting challenges to compliance with measures such as physical distancing and self-isolation.[28] Lockdowns

[28] World Health Organization (2020).

also limited job opportunities for sex workers, which led them to engage in riskier behaviours that could contribute to community transmission.[29]

The costs of food, medicine, and transportation increased, making life unbearable for the poor. Health workers were also affected by mobility challenges. Rural people could no longer travel to access health care in urban areas.

IMPLICATIONS OF MEASURES FOR THE HEALTH SECTOR

By November 10, 2020, at least 1,070 health workers in Uganda were confirmed to have contracted Covid-19.[30] At least 17 frontline health workers had lost their lives to the pandemic.[31] Although some district hospitals and lower-level facilities received personal protective equipment (PPE) and infection prevention and control commodities that had been centrally procured, there were widespread reports of shortages and deficiencies in PPE supply, with some reports indicating that some health workers did not have access to basic PPE such as face masks and gloves.[32,33] Our media analysis showed that health workers were exposed to unsafe working conditions, low pay, long working hours, and violence.[34] Healthcare workers reported being anxious and panicked and had avoided patients with COVID-like symptoms due to concerns of being infected.[35,36,37] One study found that workers in non-Covid-19 designated hospital departments were more at risk because infection prevention and control measures were inadequate.[38] In some places, UNICEF supplied health facilities with PPE, detergents, handwashing stations, and soap for infection prevention and control.[39] Healthcare

---

[29] Kawala et al. (2020b).

[30] New Vision (2020d).

[31] Ssemugabo (2021).

[32] Well (2020).

[33] Key Informant Interview 1; Key Informant Interview 9.

[34] New Vision (2020d).

[35] Semaan et al. (2020).

[36] Olum et al. (2020).

[37] Madinah (2020).

[38] Amanya et al. (2020).

[39] UNICEF (2020b).

workers, particularly midwives, reported increased workloads, frequent schedule changes, and exhaustion[40] which had implications for their mental and physical health.

Mental health has also been affected for some peer support workers due to their inability to meet in person because of the restrictions. Peer support workers in mental health are not salaried employees and therefore have to resort to meal and transport allowances and other small income-generating activities to survive. In addition, while some peer support workers were able to participate in weekly conference calls, mobile phones and cellular data were not affordable for others, meaning that they could not keep in touch with co-workers, leaving them socially isolated.[41]

Although guidance for non-severe Covid-19 was home-based care, there was no provision of PPE for caregivers, which, while understandable in the context of nationwide shortages, presents challenges, particularly in crowded households where true self-isolation might not be possible.

Impacts of Measures on Social Groups

The first issue to note is that managing the Covid-19 crisis created additional problems for the health of non-COVID patients. Due to the ban on public transportation, some pregnant women died because they had to walk long distances to get to hospitals.[42] Regarding livelihoods, many people working in the industries most affected by shutdowns, including tourism, hospitality, horticulture, infant educators, petty trade, markets, and cleaning, are dominated by women.[43,44]

Many women who are over-represented in the informal sector, sex workers, market vendors, hawkers, and caterers, among others, most of whom live hand to mouth and are the only breadwinners of their families, lost their only sources of income because they were forced to stop working indefinitely.[45] Forty-six per cent of workers employed in the informal sector are reported to have been pushed below the poverty

---

[40] Madinah (2020).

[41] Mpango et al. (2020).

[42] Lamony (2020).

[43] Ssali (2020).

[44] Akina Mama wa Afrika (2020a).

[45] Akina Mama wa Afrika (2020a).

line in the first months of the pandemic, with similar trends seen in the hospitality industry (43%) and trading and services (41%), all of which disproportionately affected women.[46] The number of households with no income earner rose by 41% in the first three weeks of the lockdown, with female-headed households, people living with disabilities and older adults most affected.[47] The closure of Kalerwe market resulted in lost livelihood for 10,000 vendors, 80% of whom were women and the vast majority of whom had no access to social safety nets.[48]

The government stated that food markets could only remain operational if workers socially distanced themselves and slept in the markets. Female vendors have an extra burden due to childcare responsibilities and some resorted to either sleeping with their children in the market or leaving them home for days.[49] Some poor women were unable to afford to pay fees to sell in the market and had to resort to hawking and roadside trading.[50] With school closures and isolation in homes, many women who already bore the brunt of unpaid domestic care work had attend to it as a full-time job.[51] Some of these chores also fell to girls as they were not attending school, limiting their opportunities to study. Female refugees were also particularly affected by the additional burden of domestic responsibilities.[52] Many interview participants recognized the impact of movement restrictions on pregnant women's access to health services, but no one mentioned any of these gender-related factors exacerbating the pandemic's impact on women. One participant noted that women might have been left out of livelihood support programmes.[53]

According to the Bureau of Labour Statistics, in Greater Kampala, over 87% of total employment is informal sector workers who experienced a high risk of loss of income and livelihood and Covid-19 infection due to trading with close person-to-person contact.[54] In addition, a survey in

---

[46] United Nations Agenda (2020).

[47] World Food Programme (2020).

[48] United Nations Agenda (2020).

[49] Ssali (2020).

[50] Ssali (2020).

[51] Akina Mama wa Afrika (2020a).

[52] Ssali (2020).

[53] Key Informant Interview 6.

[54] World Food Programme (2020).

April found that approximately 84% of the small- and medium-scale businesses in Kampala had reduced their workforce by more than half since the start of the pandemic.[55] Additional layoffs, pay cuts, and terminations occurred because of cash flow shortages stemming from the lockdown.[56] The layoffs were due to the ban on internal travel, which mainly affected small and medium-sized businesses.

HEALTH: BIOMEDICAL AND PUBLIC HEALTH RESPONSE

Covid-19 also increased gender-based violence (GBV). Between March 30 and April 28, 2020, alone, 3,280 cases of gender-based violence cases were reported to the police. In addition, anger and frustration due to loss of income increased strain on relationships and aggravated emotional and physical violence.[57,58] Due to the isolation regulations being enforced and widespread loss of employment, people spent more time at home, and some women, particularly those who lacked financial independence, may have been unable to escape abusive partners, leaving them at risk of being severely harmed.[59,60,61] Certain districts, including Wakiso, were more impacted than others.[62]

Other dimensions of GBV were the risks posed by curfew, the ban on public transport and its attendant walking to work necessities.[63] Furthermore, sex workers experienced increased violence and were forced to engage in more risky behaviours because of the pandemic.[64] Informal trade closures have led to female refugees engaging in transactional sex

---

[55] Lakuma and Sunday (n.d.).

[56] Madinah (2020).

[57] Parkes et al. (2020).

[58] Bukuluki et al. (2020).

[59] Bukuluki et al. (2020).

[60] Ssali (2020).

[61] JohnBosco and Ggoobi (2020).

[62] JohnBosco and Ggoobi (2020).

[63] Ssali (2020).

[64] Kawala et al. (2020b).

to support their families.[65] This same trend has been reported generally among younger people.[66]

In the five months of lockdown, Uganda registered more than 21,000 cases of child abuse.[67] A recent survey found that 60% of people have observed an increase in sexual violence against children since the lockdown began, and 80% reported that parents used violence against children.[68] Increased child poverty and hunger, child marriage and labour were reported as some of the additional dimensions of violence.[69] Girls from families of low socioeconomic status—pushed further into poverty during lockdown—resorted to trading sex for money, food, and even sanitary towels.[70] Child marriage and teenage pregnancy also increased[71] which led to high school dropout rates. A study indicated that half of street children surveyed had been exposed to violence. In addition, the challenges associated with being on the streets during the pandemic forced some street children to return to their abusive families.[72]

The measures also affected mental health. The inability to attend social gatherings caused fear, uncertainty, and stress, particularly for salaried workers.[73] The suicide rate among men, including a disproportionate number of male teachers, increased during the pandemic, likely due to school closures leading to monthly payment suspension.[74] The lack of social interaction disproportionately affected girls, who were less likely than boys to maintain social contact because of boys' greater access to mobile phones and the ability to meet in person at community gatherings.[75]

---

[65] Bukuluki et al. (2020).

[66] Bukuluki et al. (2020).

[67] New Vision (2020a).

[68] Save the Children (2020).

[69] Childfund Alliance (n.d.).

[70] Childfund Alliance (n.d.).

[71] Ssali (2020).

[72] Kawala et al. (2020a).

[73] Kansiime et al. (2021).

[74] Ssali (2020).

[75] Parkes et al. (2020).

People with disabilities were heavily impacted by barriers to health access and were often met with violence by authorities.[76] They faced challenges accessing health centres and markets to seek medical attention and essential items for their families. Without support from the government or others, people with disabilities were left behind at a time when they needed access to services and support more than ever.[77] The inclusion of representatives from the National Union for Disabled Persons Uganda in district-level meetings in Lira is a good example of inclusivity within the pandemic response.[78]

The high food insecurity experienced by many was due to the many restrictions and measures. In addition, the lockdown amplified the food crisis.[79] It affected the food supply chain at all stages, and income shocks further amplified food insecurity with increased prices, food shortages, and the inability of supply chains to adapt.[80] These changes disproportionately impacted socioeconomically vulnerable households, particularly those not growing their food.[81]

One survey found that compared to a "normal period," there were significant increases in the number of respondents who reduced the amount of food eaten (30 percentage points), were unable to eat healthy and nutritious food (35 percentage points), consumed less diverse diets (45 percentage points), or worried about not having enough food (50 percentage points).[82] Another survey found that 17% of Ugandans living in Kampala faced acute food insecurity, with six in ten families selling productive assets such as land and livestock and begging or turning to illegal activities to find food and two in ten urban households not having enough food to eat.[83] Some young people borrowed money, going into debt, to buy food and other essentials.[84] A decrease in the amount and

---

[76] New Vision (2020b).

[77] New Vision (2020b).

[78] Key Informant Interview 8.

[79] Wemesa et al. (2020).

[80] Trotter et al. (2020).

[81] Kansiime et al. (2021).

[82] EurekAlert! (2020).

[83] New Vision (n.d.-a).

[84] Save the Children (n.d.).

variety of food consumed in urban slums was also documented.[85] Millions of children were no longer receiving school meals due to the schools' closure.[86,87]

Ugandans were worried about insufficient food, were unable to eat healthy food, were eating reduced portions, and consumed limited food varieties.[88] Groups noted to have experienced increased food insecurity include street children, indigenous communities, people with disabilities, the elderly, sex workers, and people with pre-existing chronic health conditions such as HIV or diabetes.[89,90,91,92] The government provided targeted food donations for sex workers in one district, but these efforts were limited in impact and did not entirely address their challenges.[93] Diabetes associations provided food and other support to families that have a child with Type 1 Diabetes in some areas.[94]

In March 2020, the government recognized the severe negative impacts of the lockdown on household earnings, especially the urban poor, and requested US$15 million to provide food for two million poor people living in urban centres.[95] Interview participants widely cited this intervention as a pro-poor and essential response to the unforeseen impact on food security caused by Covid-19-related restrictions.[96] The Uganda Coronavirus Response Team directed food distribution to the urban poor but only targeted major urban groups living in and near Kampala.[97,98,99]

[85] Trotter et al. (2020).

[86] Trotter et al. (2020).

[87] Zavaleta-Cortijo et al. (2020).

[88] Kansiime et al. (2021).

[89] Kawala et al. (2020a).

[90] Kawala et al. (2020b).

[91] Klatman et al. (2020).

[92] United Nations Agenda (2020).

[93] Kawala et al. (2020b).

[94] Klatman et al. (2020).

[95] Thinkwell (2020).

[96] Key Informant Interview 1; 4; 6; 8.

[97] Nathan and Benon (2020).

[98] Haider et al. (2020).

[99] Ssali (2020).

This move benefited women, lactating mothers, the elderly, the sick, and small business owners.[100] However, urban refugees were left out because food distribution programmes required individuals to present national identification cards that refugees do not possess.[101,102] Due to movement restrictions, rural populations were also excluded from food distribution programmes and could no longer access their gardens.[103]

Food aid was insufficient in amount and variety to address the food insecurity crisis.[104] It was reported that about 1.5 million people needed food assistance.[105] Yet, early in the pandemic, the World Food Programme (WFP) cut rations for refugees in the settlements by 30% due to funding shortfalls.[106] The government stated that they would provide food relief to vulnerable workers who were the most impacted by the lockdown, but this was yet to be seen at the time of writing.[107]

Farmers' logistical challenges also contributed to food insecurity. Although the government expressly permitted farm workers to travel, they were often denied access to their farms by security personnel. They also struggled to transport their produce to markets, and many markets closed due to social distancing protocols.[108,109] The risk was that primary rural production, food deliveries, exports, employment, and incomes would be affected. The subsequent agricultural season production would also be affected due to the disruptions. Local businesses and supply chains were more likely to be affected than international ones.[110] Disruptions to food supply chains, caused primarily by travel restrictions and social distancing rules that disrupted food flows, were likely to have a sustained impact on the availability of farm inputs and labour, post-harvest losses, and thus

---

100 Nathan and Benon (2020).

101 Ssali (2020).

102 Bukuluki et al. (2020).

103 Ssali (2020).

104 Trotter et al. (2020).

105 Nathan and Benon (2020).

106 World Food Programme (2020).

107 Kansiime et al. (2021).

108 Madinah (2020).

109 Save the Children (n.d.).

110 Donovan (2020).

farmers' ability to purchase inputs for the following year.[111] The poultry, cattle, and fishing industries were similarly affected as well.

IMPACT ON ACCESS TO OTHER SERVICES

Access to health care for non-Covid-19 patients decreased due to the response measures. For example, between February and March 2020, there was a decline in individuals testing for HIV (16%), linkage to HIV care (20%), antenatal care (ANC) visits (14%), and facility-based deliveries (6%), and increases in deliveries by caesarean section (4%), neonatal deaths (7%), perinatal deaths (9%), maternal deaths (43%), and GBV cases (6%).[112] Routine health system data confirm that most maternal health indicators (e.g. pregnant women with at least 1 ANC visit, pregnant women with 4 ANC visits, health facility deliveries) worsened in the first two or three months of the pandemic but also show that they had recovered by August 2020 (the most recent data available at the time of writing). In addition, the number of women newly diagnosed with HIV during pregnancy and the number then linked to care were lower than in previous years.[113]

Vitamin A supplementation to children under five suffered because biannual campaigns are run in April and October every year, but the April 2020 campaign could not be carried out. Sexual and reproductive health services were initially not listed as essential, impeding access for women of reproductive age seeking services such as contraception or abortion.[114] Patients with chronic illnesses such as diabetes, HIV, heart conditions, cancer and prostate issues were advised to wait or consult online.[115] In addition, certain conditions (diabetic patients, people living with HIV, sickle cell anaemia patients, and patients with cardiac conditions) were not designated as an emergency, negatively impacting access to services.[116,117] No HPV vaccinations were given to adolescents and

---

[111] United Nations Agenda (2020).

[112] UNICEF (2020a).

[113] Violence and Newborn (n.d.).

[114] Akina Mama wa Afrika (2020a).

[115] Ssali (2020).

[116] Ssali (2020).

[117] Barugahare et al. (2020).

women during the lockdown. While the Family Health Days programme had previously increased access to vaccine immunizations, this programme was stopped due to the pandemic.[118]

In April 2020, a coordination mechanism was established, cognizant of the disruption to routine health services and the heavy disease burden attributed to conditions other than Covid-19. In addition, the Ministry of Health published the *Guidelines for Continuity of Essential Services during the Covid-19 Outbreak.*[119,120] These guidelines outline which health services could be continued or discontinued depending on three transmission scenarios. While these guidelines were welcome, health resources, including infrastructure, health workers, and financing, continued to be reallocated from regular services to accommodate the COVID response. For example, at the Hoima Referral Hospital, a coronavirus treatment unit displaced a mental health department and its patients.[121]

SOCIAL PROTECTION PROGRAMMES

Before Covid-19, only 3% of the Ugandan population accessed direct income support.[122] The Social Assistance Grants for Empowerment (SAGE) cash transfer programme for senior citizens pre-dated Covid-19. However, it was expanded, but restrictions on mobility affected access to beneficiaries. This Senior Citizen Grant of UGX 25,000 per month was paid in advance to mitigate the negative impacts of the pandemic on beneficiaries.[123] People had to present a national identification document to access these grants, which was challenging for some.[124]

The GirlsEmpoweringGirls Programme, implemented by Kampala City Council Authority (KCCA), has three components: empowering girls through a network of peer mentors; engaging them through education, training, and referrals to support services; and enabling them to pursue

---

[118] Kajungu et al. (2020).

[119] Key Informant Interview 4.

[120] MOH Uganda (2020).

[121] Isingoma (2020).

[122] The Independent (2020).

[123] Akina Mama Wa Afrika (2020b).

[124] Unwanted Witness (2020).

better opportunities for their future through a small cash transfer.[125] While the programme continued through the pandemic, its reach and impact were unclear.

During the lockdown, the government began distributing food to vulnerable people affected by the pandemic in the Kampala, Wakiso, and Mukono districts. Within the first 37 days of the lockdown, the government distributed food to 1,385,000 people in 372,397 households. The programme was, however, discontinued.[126] Questions have been raised about the decision to provide food relief rather than cash transfers to the urban poor, which many global agencies and countries have promoted as the most effective mechanism to expand access to health and other social services.[127] In another effort to support food security, the government reported that farmers would be supported to access high-quality agricultural inputs, seeds, and fertilizers using e-vouchers. However, its implementation was unclear.

Another scheme that pre-dates the pandemic is the Ministry of Gender Labour and Social Development's National Special Grant for Persons with Disabilities. Although the amounts disbursed were unclear, the Ministry decided to make payments during the pandemic. That said, one study found that social protection programmes were not accessible for people with disabilities because they fall into a category that requires special emotional, financial, and social assistance, and they depend on a third person to access benefits, which may have impeded access during this time.[128]

Conclusion and Recommendations

The pre-existing epidemic response structures were an essential foundation for the national response to Covid-19. They allowed the government to act quickly and decisively, which undoubtedly helped slow the spread of the disease. Initially, health funding focused on case management in high-level facilities. However, more significant investment in community structures and primary health care is also paramount. This includes

---

[125] Akina Mama Wa Afrika (2020b).

[126] Akina Mama Wa Afrika (2020b).

[127] Thinkwell (2020).

[128] Kajungu et al. (2020).

not only investments in infrastructure but also expansion of the health workforce, strengthening of supply chains, and upgrading of health management information systems to efficiently capture and link data at all levels from the community to the national. This will help improve access to a wide range of other services which will better meet community needs and assist the country to reach its universal health coverage targets.

The fact that most resources were invested in Covid-19 management exacerbated the health conditions of other non-COVID patients. Efficient decentralization and allocation of resources in the health sector is needed to prevent the reoccurrence of the fallouts of the Covid-19 management problems. In the longer-term, alternative guidelines for budget and staff allocation during infectious disease outbreaks might be developed to provide a framework within which this could be done.

It is important to note that given the economy's structure, lockdown measures were not viable given the reliance on daily wages for meeting basic needs unless a cash transfer programme could be instituted to reach all those who needed assistance very quickly. It will be essential to consider what policy options might exist in the context of a future pandemic that might be viable across all the different contexts of Uganda and to put in place structures to facilitate this as soon as possible. Instituting targeted social protection programmes could help mitigate the impact of the pandemic on livelihoods. These were very effective in other locations and could be equally valuable in this context. For example, payments to households whose income is derived solely from everyday work would allow greater compliance with any future movement restrictions or lockdown measures allowing families to survive with dignity. However, this will require a complete social protection plan to support vulnerable and marginalized populations.

Early engagement with communities and the private sector is critical to effective disease response. Even in an emergency where time pressure is immense, involving these partners from the outset will help promote trust in government and cohesive response to which all stakeholders can commit. The importance of public trust in the government during an infectious disease outbreak cannot be overestimated: it is critical to comply with government directives and willingness to collaborate in the disease response. Establishing protocols and mechanisms for how this should be done and where responsibility lies might help facilitate this for future disease outbreaks. In addition, civil society has demonstrated that its advocacy can influence the government response. Capacity building of civil society organizations will expand their ability to engage in and advocate for appropriate responses to future pandemics. They can also play a beneficial watchdog role, helping to hold duty bearers to account.

The need for investment in the food supply chain has also been highlighted. Investment in infrastructure to create resilience in domestic food production, storage, and distribution can help mitigate food insecurity and ensure a timely government response if food distribution is needed.[129] In addition, creating a strategic food reserve could facilitate a rapid government response to sudden shocks to food and nutrition security among vulnerable and marginalized households. During future disease outbreaks, if schools are closed again, alternative mechanisms would be helpful to sustain school feeding programmes in place.

REFERENCES

Akina Mama Wa Afrika. (2020a). *The gendered implications of COVID-19*. https://www.akinamamawaafrika.org/the-gendered-implications-of-cov id-19/. Accessed February 15, 16, and 17, 2021.

Akina Mama Wa Afrika. (2020b, June). *The state of social protection in Uganda in response to Covid-19*. https://www.akinamamawaafrika.org/wp-content/uploads/2020/10/akina_The-state-of-social-protection-in-Uganda-in-res ponse-to-Covid-19.pdf. Accessed February 24, 2021.

Amanya, S. B., et al. (2020). Knowledge and compliance with Covid-19 infection prevention and control measures among health workers in regional referral hospitals in Northern Uganda: A cross-sectional online survey. *Research Square*. https://doi.org/10.21203/rs.3.rs-63627/v1

Barugahare, J., et al. (2020). Ethical and human rights considerations in public health in low and middle-income countries: An assessment using the case of Uganda's responses to COVID-19 pandemic. *BMC Medical Ethics, 21*(1), 91.

Bukuluki, P., et al. (2020). The socio-economic and psychosocial impact of Covid-19 pandemic on urban refugees in Uganda. *Social Sciences & Humanities Open, 2*(1), 100045.

Childfund Alliance. (n.d.). *Keeping children safe in Uganda's COVID-19 response (May 2020)—Uganda*. https://reliefweb.int/report/uganda/kee ping-children-safe-uganda-s-covid-19-response-may-2020. Accessed February 23, 2021.

Donovan, M. (2020). *Do not forget about the impact of COVID-19 on the rural poor and food security*. https://www.cimmyt.org/blogs/dont-forget-about-the-impact-of-covid-19-on-the-rural-poor-and-on-food-security/. Accessed February 23, 2021.

---

[129] Trotter et al. (2020).

EurekAlert! (2020). *New research highlights the impact of COVID-19 on food security in Kenya and Uganda*. https://www.eurekalert.org/pub_releases/2020-09/c-nrh092120.php. Accessed February 23 2021.

Haider, N., et al. (2020). Lockdown measures in response to COVID-19 in nine sub-Saharan African countries. *BMJ Global Health, 5*(10). https://doi.org/10.1136/bmjgh-2020-003319

Isingoma, T. (2020). How COVID-19 health responses impact displaced fishing communities in Uganda. *Africa at LSE*, 6.

JohnBosco, L., & Ggoobi, N. S. (2020). *COVID-19 and the rising levels of domestic violence in Uganda*. https://www.africaportal.org/documents/20473/COVID-19-THE-RISING-LEVELS-OF-DOMESTIC-VIOLENCE-IN-UGANDA-SEPTEMBER-2020-1.pdf

Kajungu, D., et al. (2020). *Catch-up vaccination drives may mitigate the effects of COVID-19 response measures on routine immunisation services in rural Uganda—use of real-world data*. Preprints. https://search.proquest.com/openview/99f4a6452cd2e3bfbc54d901d9119e00/1?pq-origsite=gscholar&cbl=4361587

Kansiime, M. K., et al. (2021). COVID-19 implications on household income and food security in Kenya and Uganda: Findings from a rapid assessment. *World Development, 137*, 105199.

Kawala, B. A., Kirui, B. K., & Cumber, S. N. (2020a). Effect of COVID-19 response in Uganda on street children. *The Pan African Medical Journal, 35*(Suppl. 2). https://doi.org/10.11604/pamj.supp.2020.35.2.23545

Kawala, B. A., Kirui, B. K., & Cumber, S. N. (2020b). Why policy action should focus on the vulnerable commercial sex workers in Uganda during COVID-19 fight. *The Pan African Medical Journal, 35*(Suppl. 2), 102.

Klatman, E. L., et al. (2020). COVID-19 and type 1 diabetes: Challenges and actions. *Diabetes Research and Clinical Practice*, 108275.

Lakuma, C. P., & Sunday, N. (n.d.). *Impact of COVID-19 on micro, small, and medium businesses in Uganda*. https://www.brookings.edu/blog/africa-in-focus/2020/05/19/impact-of-covid-19-on-micro-small-and-medium-businesses-in-uganda/. Accessed February 16, 2021.

Lamony, S. A. (2020). *A comparative analysis of COVID-19 responses and their effects on human rights protections in East Africa*. http://opiniojuris.org/2020/06/09/a-comparative-analysis-of-covid-19-responses-and-their-effects-on-human-rights-protections-in-east-africa/. Accessed February 16, 2021.

Madinah, N. (2020). *The COVID-19 pandemic: Economic effects and government measures in Uganda*. University of Malaya.

Mejia-Mantilla, C., et al. (n.d.). *Impact of fiscal policy on poverty and inequality in Uganda: Fiscal incidence analysis using the UNHS 2016/17*. https://elibrary.worldbank.org/doi/abs/10.1596/1813-9450-9051. Accessed February 15, 2021.

MOH Uganda. (2020, April). *Guidance on continuity of essential health services.* http://www.c19hub.io/wp-content/uploads/2020/05/MoH-Uganda_Gui dance-on-Continuity-of-Essential-Health-Services-during-the-COVID-19-out break_April-2020.docx

Mondo, C. K., Otim, M. A., Akol, G., Musoke, R., & Orem, J. (2013). The prevalence and distribution of non-communicable diseases and their risk factors in Kasese district, Uganda. *Cardiovascular Journal of Africa, 24*(3), 52–57. https://doi.org/10.5830/CVJA-2012-081

Mpango, R., et al. (2020). Challenges to peer support in low- and middle-income countries during COVID-19. *Globalization and Health,* 90.

Murthy, S., Leligdowicz, A., & Adhikari, N. K. J. (2015). Intensive care unit capacity in low-income countries: A systematic review. *PLoS ONE, 10*(1), e0116949.

Nathan, I., & Benon, M. (2020). COVID-19 relief food distribution: impact and lessons for Uganda. *The Pan African Medical Journal,* 35. https://doi.org/10.11604/pamj.supp.2020.35.2.24214

New Vision. (2020a). *COVID-19 Hand Washing.* https://www.newvision.co.ug/news/1529578/covid-19-hand-washing-increase-61

New Vision. (2020b). *Persons living with disability suffering effects of pandemic.* https://www.newvision.co.ug/news/1522442/covid-19-persons-living-disability-suffering-effects-pandemic

New Vision. (2020c). *Spike in unplanned pregnancies and abortions.* https://www.newvision.co.ug/news/1528596/spike-unplanned-pregnancies-abo rtions

New Vision. (2020d, November). *Counting the cost of COVID-19 on health.* https://www.newvision.co.ug/news/1532238/counting-cost-covid-19-health

New Vision. (n.d.-a). *Kampala residents facing acute food insecurity.* https://www.newvision.co.ug/news/1529425/kampala-residents-facing-acute-food-insecurity

New Vision. (n.d.-b). *Police warn of ridiculing pregnant students.* https://www.newvision.co.ug/news/1530387/covid-19-police-warn-ridiculing-pregnant-students

O'Donovan, J., Carr, D., Welch, H. G., Peterson, A., Karlawish, J., Largent, E., Warraich, H. J., Shell, M., Monach, P., & Branch-Elliman, W. (2020, March 28). *Community health workers must lead the Covid-19 fight in Uganda—STAT.* https://www.statnews.com/2020/03/28/community-health-workers-lead-covid-19-fight-uganda/

Olum, R., et al. (2020). Coronavirus disease-2019: Knowledge, attitude, and practices of health care workers at Makerere University Teaching Hospitals, Uganda. *Frontiers in Public Health, 8,* 181.

Parkes, J., et al. (2020). Young people, inequality and violence during the COVID-19 lockdown in Uganda. https://doi.org/10.31235/osf.io/2p6hx

Reuters. (2020, March 25). *Uganda, usually welcoming to refugees, bars all new arrivals to contain coronavirus.* U.S. News & World Report. https://www.usnews.com/news/world/articles/2020-03-25/uganda-usually-welcoming-to-refugees-bars-all-new-arrivals-to-contain-coronavirus

Save the Children. (2020). *Save the children protection assessment on the impact of COVID-19 in Uganda.* https://resourcecentre.savethechildren.net/library/save-children-protection-assessment-impact-covid-19-uganda. Accessed February 23, 2021.

Save the Children. (n.d.). *Ugandan youth speak out on the impact of Covid-19—Uganda.* https://reliefweb.int/report/uganda/ugandan-youth-speak-out-impact-covid-19. Accessed February 23, 2021.

Semaan, A., et al. (2020). Voices from the frontline: Findings from a thematic analysis of a rapid online global survey of maternal and newborn health professionals facing the COVID-19 pandemic. *BMJ global health, 5*(6). https://doi.org/10.1136/bmjgh-2020-002967

Ssali, S. N. (2020). Gender, economic precarity and Uganda Government's COVID-19 response. *African Journal of Governance & Development, 9*(1.1), 287–308.

Ssemugabo, C. (2021). *How workplaces are fuelling the COVID-19 pandemic in sub-Saharan Africa.* https://www.internationalhealthpolicies.org/featured-article/how-workplaces-are-fuelling-the-covid-19-pandemic-in-sub-saharan-africa/. Accessed February 16, 2021.

The Independent. (2020). *World Bank economic report urges Uganda to increase social protection.* https://www.independent.co.ug/world-bank-economic-report-urges-uganda-to-step-up-social-protection/. Accessed February 24, 2021.

The Republic of Uganda Ministry of Health. (2014). *Non-communicable disease risk factor baseline survey.* https://www.who.int/ncds/surveillance/steps/Uganda_2014_STEPS_Report.pdf

The Uganda SP4PHC Team. (n.d.). *COVID-19 summary update for Uganda.* https://thinkwell.global/wp-content/uploads/2020/05/COVID-19-Uganda_August-2020-Updates-final.pdf. Accessed February 15, 2021.

Thinkwell. (2020). *Uganda's emergency response to the COVID-19 pandemic: A case study.* https://thinkwell.global/wp-content/uploads/2020/09/Uganda-COVID-19-Case-Study-_18-Sept-20201.pdf. Accessed February 16, 2021.

Thinkwell. (2020). *Uganda-indicators-fact-sheet-final.* https://thinkwell.global/wp-content/uploads/2020/09/Uganda-Indicators-Fact-Sheet-Final.pdf

Trotter, P., et al. (2020). *Between collapse and resilience: Emerging empirical evidence of COVID-19 impact on food security in Uganda and Zimbabwe.* https://doi.org/10.2139/ssrn.3657484

Tumwesige, J. (2020). *COVID-19 educational disruption and response: Rethinking e-learning in Uganda*. The University of Cambridge. https://www.kas.de/documents/280229/8800435/COVID-19+Educational+Disruption+and+Response+-+Rethinking+e-Learning+in+Uganda.pdf/6573f7b3-b885-b0b3-8792-04aa4c9e14b7?version=1.0&t=1589283963112

UNICEF. (2020a). *Retrospective Analysis of DHIS 2 Non-COVID Services, February–March 2020*. UNICEF, Kampala.

UNICEF. (2020b). *UNICEF helps to keep health workers safe during the COVID-19 pandemic*. https://www.unicef.org/uganda/stories/unicef-helps-keep-health-workers-safe-during-covid-19-pandemic. Accessed February 16, 2021.

United Nations Agenda. (2020). *Leaving no one behind: From the COVID-19 response to recovery and resilience building. Analyses of the socioeconomic impact of COVID-19 in Uganda.*

Unwanted Witness. (2020). *Uganda's National ID system; an access hindrance to the Social Assistance Grants for Empowerment (SAGE)*. https://www.unwantedwitness.org/ugandas-national-id-system-an-access-hindrance-to-the-social-assistance-grants-for-empowerment-sage/. Accessed February 24, 2021.

Violence, G.-B., & Newborn, M. (n.d.). *The effects of the COVID-pandemic on the continuity of essential health services delivery, access, and uptake in Uganda*. http://library.health.go.ug/sites/default/files/resources/CEHS%20Monthly%20Report%20-%20August-1.pdf

Well, T. (2020). *Uganda's emergency response to the COVID-19 pandemic: A case study*. https://thinkwell.global/wp-content/uploads/2020/09/Uganda-COVID-19-Case-Study-_18-Sept-20201.pdf. Accessed February 16, 2021.

Wemesa, R., et al. (2020). The economic impact of the lockdown due to COVID-19 pandemic on low income households of the five divisions of Kampala district in Uganda. *Open Journal of Business and Management, 8*(4), 1560–1566.

World Bank. (2021). *Uganda Overview*. https://www.worldbank.org/en/country/uganda/overview

World Food Programme. (2020). *WFP Uganda country brief*. https://reliefweb.int/sites/reliefweb.int/files/resources/WFP-0000119279.pdf. Accessed February 16, 2021.

World Health Organization. (2020). *Kampala turns data into action against COVID-19 inequalities*. https://www.who.int/news-room/feature-stories/detail/kampala-turns-data-into-action-against-covid-19-inequalities. Accessed February 16, 2021.

World Health Organization. (n.d.). *Easing COVID-19 impacts critical health services*. https://www.afro.who.int/news/easing-covid-19-impact-key-health-services. Accessed February 15, 2021.

Zavaleta-Cortijo, C., et al. (2020). Climate change and COVID-19: Reinforcing indigenous food systems. *The Lancet. Planetary Health, 4*(9), e381–e382.

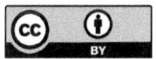

PART III

North Africa

CHAPTER 13

Tunisia

Majdi Hassen, Mohamed Ali Marouani, and Emilie Wojcieszynski

INTRODUCTION

Tunisia, like every other country in the world, was hard hit by Covid-19 and suffered social and economic consequences (Hasell, 2020). Indeed, the crisis began in a situation of relative instability in which the development model was losing momentum and in which there were also distinct inequalities in labour markets relating to location, sex, and differences in levels of education (Assaad et al., 2018; World Bank, 2015). The existence and the post-revolutionary extension of social protection in the form of cash transfers (PNAFN) and free access to health care (AMGII) for the poorest made it possible to mitigate the social consequences of sluggish growth for families most in need (CRES, 2017; Krafft et al., 2020).

M. Hassen
University of Tunis, ESSECT, Tunis, Tunisia

M. A. Marouani (✉)
UMR Développement Et Sociétés, Université Paris 1 Panthéon-Sorbonne, Paris, France
e-mail: marouani@univ-paris1.fr

E. Wojcieszynski
School of Economics, Utrecht University, Utrecht, Nederland

© The Author(s) 2024   323
A. Altaf et al. (eds.), *EQUITY IN COVID-19*, EADI Global
Development Series, https://doi.org/10.1007/978-3-031-58588-3_13

Tunisia went into this crisis with few financial resources and against a background of government instability since 2019. Nevertheless, it had the advantage of well-trained medical staff (many of whom have been emigrating to Europe for a decade) and health institutions, such as the National Observatory for New and Emerging Diseases (ONMNE) or the Pasteur Institute that were mobilized immediately to manage the crisis. Psychological support units were also established quickly by civil society.[1]

To contain the spread of the pandemic and mitigate its likely impacts, the Tunisian authorities opted for a proactive strategy that emphasized protecting lives and supporting vulnerable families and people in precarious employment (Krafft et al., 2021). The government adopted a battery of staged preventive measures, with a total lockdown preceding a phase of gradual relaxation. The action taken by the authorities also focused on introducing a set of measures to support affected businesses and people, in addition to the additional spending on managing the pandemic's effect on health. The budgetary cost of these interventions exceeded 7.2%[2] of G.D.P. in 2020.

This unprecedented crisis and the total lockdown have had severe effects on the economic and social fabrics (I.N.S., 2020; Krafft et al., 2021) due to the specific features of the economic structure prior to the crisis, viz. a high level of openness and structural fragilities (World Bank, 2015). Sectors vulnerable to the crisis, such as tourism, employ large numbers of people, with implications for the economic activities in the sectors (Marouani & Minh, 2020); Krafft et al., 2021). Socially, low-income households and those who lost their jobs were particularly hard hit. Despite the large-scale government intervention, the crisis accentuated social inequalities (I.N.S., 2020; Krafft et al., 2021; I.N.S./World Bank, 2020).

In this chapter, we combined an objective analysis of all the data sources available to date with the assessment including interviews with stakeholders. First, we examined the impact of the pandemic on various socioeconomic groups. We also showed that the households' pre-Covid-19 situation conditioned how this shock affected them. Second, the interviews highlighted the contribution of non-State actors and the limits they faced while trying to support the vulnerable.

---

[1] According to our interviews.

[2] Authors' calculations are based on data from the complementary 2020 Finance Act.

The Pandemic and Crises

The focus here is on managing the first wave of the pandemic, although we also analysed restrictions and impacts during the second wave. The management of the second wave was radically different, as in many countries of the world, due to economic constraints and social considerations. The analyses will be backed up by interviews with governmental and non-governmental actors.[3]

The first case of Covid-19 in Tunisia was recorded on 2 March 2020. At the Scientific Committee's recommendation, the Tunisian authorities adopted staged preventive measures (e.g.: installation of thermal cameras in airports, cancellation of congresses and cultural events, prohibition of gatherings, curfews, etc.). A total lockdown was decreed from 20 March to 4 May 2020 before the country entered a phase of gradual relaxation between 5 May and 14 June of the same year.[4]

In addition, strict health protocols were put in place for people entering the country, including a mandatory quarantine in hotels. This seems to have been the most effective measure of stopping infections from outside the country. At the same time, a screening strategy was put in place to identify clusters and to help establish a clear picture of the spread of the pandemic. The measure made it possible to contain the pandemic reasonably during the first wave. However, these measures proved inadequate and relatively ineffective in managing the second wave. Indeed, infections rose to 220,000 and deaths to more than 7000 in early February 2021, as opposed to 4679 cases and 96 deaths in early August 2020.

The economic cost of the measures implemented to parry the impact of the pandemic and the lockdown was relatively high for the Tunisian economy, which was faced with a dual crisis of an unprecedented supply

---

[3] The leading agencies surveyed were the World Bank, UNICEF, the Ministry of Finance, the Ministry of Health, the Ministry of Women, the Family and the Elderly, the Tunisian Institute for Competitiveness and Quantitative Studies, the Tunisian Institute for Strategic Studies, the Tunisian League for Human Rights, the Tunisian Association for the Defence of Children's Rights, the Tunisian Association for the Right to Health, Enda Tamweel and Enda Inter-Arab, the Center for Arab Women for Training and Research and the non-governmental organization BADR.

[4] Without the measures taken by the authorities, in particular the lockdown, the number of cases for 22 April would have been 26,246 and the number of deaths 4000, as opposed to the actual numbers of 726 cases and 34 deaths. Study—Estimation of Tunisia COVID-19 infected cases based on mortality rates—April 2020.

crisis due to production shut down and a demand crisis due to the fall in individual consumption caused by lower household demand and a breakdown in investment due to global uncertainty.

The impact of the pandemic was first felt in sectors focusing on the external market and then, in a second round and after the lockdown, in sectors focusing on the internal market. Remote working as an appropriate way of safeguarding the continuity of business operations affected only one in ten workers and one in three for the richest quintile.[5]

The Covid-19 crisis also accentuated social inequalities and highlighted the problems of inclusiveness in the Tunisian economy and society. Before the pandemic, the resources allocated to the poorest households were relatively low compared to the actual needs of this population. In the context of a sanitary emergency, the needs in terms of liquidities, goods, and services increased while the resources available to manage the crisis were even scarcer compared to the pre-pandemic situation. Moreover, informal workers who had access to fewer benefits before Covid-19 suffered a double burden with dwindling employment opportunities and social protection (except those benefiting from PNAFN cash transfers).

MEASURES TO MITIGATE COVID-19 IMPACTS

In addition to the health, economic, and social issues, this crisis required the implementation of article 70 of the Constitution, which empowers the head of the government to issue decrees to address the consequences of Covid-19. This is an exceptional extension of regulatory power in the legislative domain. The laws support businesses and preserve jobs and relate primarily to the temporary suspension of specific provisions of the Labour Code. They were also in relation to the execution of employment contracts following an enforcement order (hours lost because of a collective work stoppage, etc.) and support for companies and employees affected by the total lockdown and exceptional measures (Fig. 13.1).

The efficient management of the first wave in Tunisia originated from the government's prompt and strict responsibility to manage the first cases of Covid-19 within the territory. However, the economic crisis was at the core of the government's preoccupations and social policy as restrictions eased at summertime (27 June). Two months later, the second wave

---

[5] First wave of the socioeconomic impact of COVID-19 on households (I.N.S.).

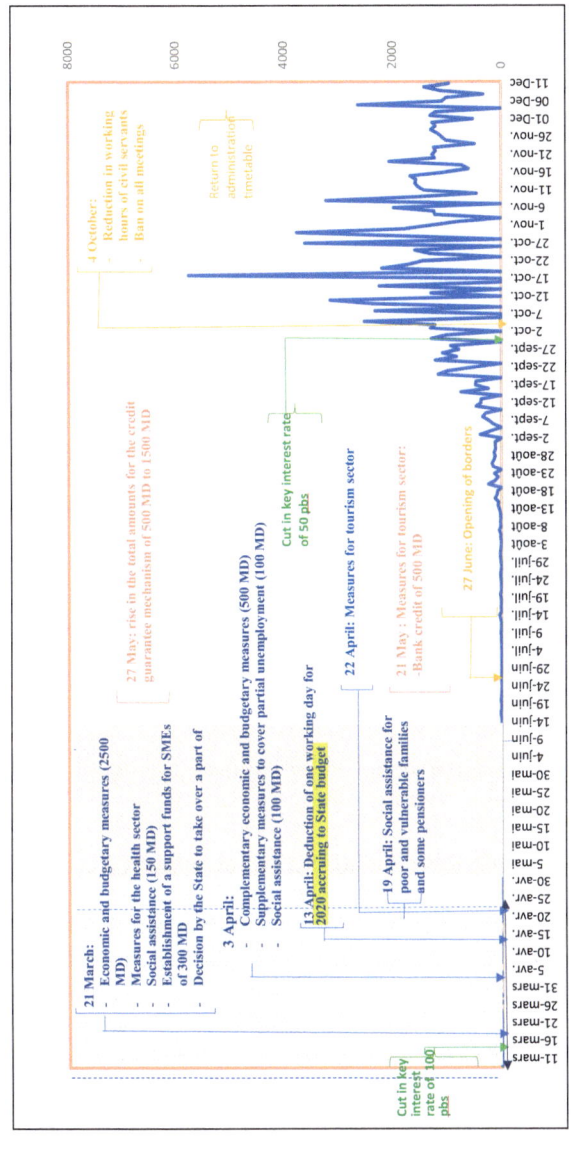

Fig. 13.1 Government policies and measures to mitigate the impact of the crisis ( ) *Source* Compilation by authors

started to hit the country, leading to stricter restrictions (4 October). The case count was about 200 cases per day at the beginning of September, while in mid-October, the country was witnessing 3000 cases per day (first peak).

Access to health services was almost exclusively limited to cases of Covid-19 and very urgent cases. The Ministry of Health prepared a strategic reserve of medicines (amounting to 150 million dinars) at the Central Pharmacy and guaranteed minimum staffing of public establishments by medical professionals. Schools were also shut down as a Covid-19 prevention measure.

Approximately 332 million dinars were allocated to vulnerable groups[6]. The allocation was to be used to help the poor and groups with specific needs during the total lockdown. This consisted of support for the families in need programme in the form of direct aid to be paid to the vulnerable groups directly affected by the crisis. The Ministry of Social Affairs managed this support. Direct cash transfers were granted to:

(i) 260,000 families in need (50 dinars in addition to the initial monthly aid of 180 dinars);
(ii) 464,000 families with limited incomes (200 dinars per family);
(iii) 382 families caring for children without support (200 dinars per family), 121 families caring for the elderly (200 dinars per family), 286 families caring for persons with special needs (200 dinars per family), 120 foreign families and students (200 dinars per family).

An exceptional welfare payment of 100 dinars was made to 140,000 retired persons receiving a pension of less than 180 dinars (a total of 60 million dinars).

Electricity and water subsidies were also introduced for a short term. In addition, the government postponed the introduction of measures to rationalize the subsidies for essential commodities and raised the volume of grain subsidies by 616 million dinars to cover additional food needs. At the same time, exemptions and financial support were granted, such as the deferral of repayments of bank loans for 6 months for employees with a salary of less than 1000 dinars a month and three months for employees with a salary of more than 1000 dinars.

---

[6] One dinar is the approximate equivalent of 0.3 euros.

In parallel with the cut in the central bank's key interest rate by 100 pbs, the authorities introduced a package of measures[7] to shore up companies affected by the crisis and cushion the harmful effects of the lockdown. The package announced by the government amounted to 2500 million dinars (see Box 13.1 in the Annex).

Special assistance in the form of a bonus of 200 dinars per employee was paid to 12,250 companies (which were identified in the "Help Enterprise" procedure[8] launched by the Ministry of Social Affairs) employing about 247 thousand workers who were laid off temporarily. The payment of the remainder of the remuneration remains the responsibility of the employer.[9]

In addition, approximately 34,000 self-employed workers affected by the lockdown measures and registered on the Batinda platform received a provisional exceptional allowance of 200 dinars. The global package was 100 million dinars. These allowances were charged to the budget of the Ministry of Social Affairs.

At the same time, the government provided financial support packages to businesses amounting to 1700 million dinars in total, consisting of bank guarantees and investment funds (see Box 13.1). Other financial support has been granted to the business. It includes the deferral of repayments on bank loans for six months for companies affected by the crisis.

---

[7] Websites of the Tunisian Investment Authority and MEFAI.

[8] The government proposed a platform through the Ministry of Social Affairs to help businesses: "Help Enterprise" provided businesses with assistance to cope with the consequences of the total lockdown and to help the employees concerned. The conditions for eligibility are (i) affiliation to the CNSS by 15 May 2020 at the latest, (ii) declaration of salaries to the CNSS for the fourth quarter of 2019 or the first quarter of 2020, (iii) regularisation of the situation of employees not registered with the CNSS by 15 May 2020 at the latest and (iv) documentation showing financial difficulties or a downturn in activity or cash flow difficulties resulting from the total lockdown.

The temporary cessation of activity must be confirmed by the competent department of the labour and conciliation inspectorate or by the directorate-general of the labour inspectorate

The solutions proposed to address the effects of the general lockdown: settlement of all annual leave days and early leave, and the total or partial payment of salaries by the employer during the temporary cessation of activities, with the possibility of recoupment during the six months after the lockdown

[9] Provided that the amount of the amount granted and that of the part of the salary paid by the employer does not exceed the amount of the salary registered with the National Social Security Fund.

A deduction of one working day for 2020 accruing to the State budget[10] was decreed by the government. This contribution was deducted for the month of April 2020 and paid to the Treasury based on the same terms and time limits as those applicable to the deduction of tax at source.

At the same time, the government took austerity measures to address the impact of Covid-19. These include freezing civil service recruitment, except for priority specialization of an urgent nature, and the rationalization of the performance bonus awarded to employees so that it did not exceed an average of 80%. In addition, promotions for 2020 were to come into effect only in 2021 and those for 2021 were postponed to 2022, and the packages of bonuses and overtime will be reduced by 50% for all departments except for Defence, the Interior, Health, and the Presidency of the Republic. Although these measures helped to control the spread of the pandemic, they were inadequate to compensate for the effects of the lockdown, particularly on working-class people and inland regions.

IMPACT AND PERCEPTION OF PANDEMIC SUPPORT AND MITIGATION STRATEGIES

Surveys were conducted by various institutions since the lockdown phase (I.N.S./World Bank, IACE, ERF, ANRS etc.).[11] They made it possible to compensate for the lack of regular surveys of household living condition in Tunisia.[12] These surveys made it possible to conduct a regular evaluation of the effects of the pandemic and the views of the various actors and beneficiaries of the measures adopted.

First, the I.N.S. collaborated with the World Bank on a telephone survey of a panel of 1339 households to study and monitor the impact of Covid-19 on the daily lives of Tunisians. Five rounds were completed successfully between late April and early October. Second, The Arab Institute of Business Managers (IACE) conducted two surveys, one in April (with 600 businesses) and a second one in December 2020 (950 businesses with 10 employees or more, 200 businesses in creation and 1000 individuals of 18–35 years old) to assess the socioeconomic consequences

---

[10] MEFAI site

[11] Using C.A.T.I method.

[12] The budget-consumption survey takes place every five years.

of Covid-19 on employment. Third, the Economic Research Forum, with the support of the I.L.O., conducted four waves of household (2000) and firms surveys (500), starting in October 2020 (Covid-19 MENA Monitor)[13]. The CORES project survey[14] was conducted in July/August 2020 to assess the economic consequences of the lockdown on 1200 SMEs in April/May 2020. All the surveys employed the C.A.T.I method, except the ANRS survey where face-to-face interviews were conducted with the enterprises.

To complement the analysis of the available data delivered by the above surveys, we conducted semi-directive interviews with the above-mentioned set of governmental and non-governmental organizations based on a questionnaire adapted to the needs of this report.

The results of these surveys were backed up by interviews with numerous institutions about the views of government actors, civil society, and international cooperation agencies relating to the management of, and responses to Covid-19. The main findings show that 44.1% of these institutions maintained their activities at a distance and that 29.4% have cut back on their activities. In addition, 50% of the associations continued their activities with a total workforce.

THE ECONOMIC AND BUDGETARY IMPACT OF THE CRISIS

The negative growth rate expected in 2020 (-7% according to the I.M.F.) can be primarily explained by the direct and indirect repercussions of the pandemic but also by the structural problems, which were accentuated by the crisis in some economic sectors.

The results of the econometric analysis[15] (conducted based on the difference between the growth forecasts made in February 2020 and the growth update in October[16]) to distinguish between the impact of Covid-19 and the structural impact shows that the effect of the pandemic exceeded 70% in 2020 (Table 13.1).

---

[13] Krafft et al. (2020).

[14] The project launched by the I.R.D. and ESSEC and financed by the French ANRS.

[15] Double exponential smoothing based on the quarterly series of added values (STATA).

[16] Economic Budget 2021—MEFAI.

Table 13.1 Structural impacts of Covid-19 on economy

(Added values, Accr yoy)	Share	Feb 2020	October 2020	Structural impact (%)	Impact of Covid-19 (%)
Manufacturing industries	**16.2**	**1.0**	**−11.5**	**2.6**	**97.4**
Textiles	2.8	−1.0	−22.0	8.5	91.5
IMCCV	1.4	1.0	−12.0	8.9	91.1
IME	5.8	−0.5	−19.0	3.2	96.8
Non-manufacturing industries	**8.5**	**3.4**	**−9.2**	**20.5**	**79.5**
Mines	0.5	10.0	0.5	28.3	71.7
Construction	4.2	0.8	−18.0	7.4	92.6
Trade services	**46.1**	**1.0**	**−10.6**	**8.4**	**91.6**
Commerce	10.1	0.9	−7.0	16.3	83.7
Tourism	3.6	1.8	−37.0	6.0	94.0
Transport	7.6	−2.0	−21.0	5.7	94.3
Non-trading production	**22.0**	**1.6**	**−1.9**	**41.8**	**58.2**
GDP	**100**	**1.6**	**−7.3**	**22.2**	**77.8**

Source Ministry of economy, finance and investment support—authors' calculations

Impact on the State Budget

The urgency that characterized the government's response to this unprecedented crisis, particularly in the first wave, led to exceptional interventions and spending in three areas: safeguarding the continuity of public services, the procurement of essential materials and equipment, and support for groups in difficulty. Against a backdrop of falling tax revenues and little budgetary room for manoeuvre, decisions must be made, particularly in prioritizing crisis management spending and social transfers.

The measures announced by the government, which were not budgeted for, and the reallocation of some spending to the health sector, had an impact on public finances and required the adoption of the complementary Finance Act for 2020. The sharp decline in economic activity combined with the fall in private consumption had a substantial impact on tax revenues (direct and indirect). The shortfall in the State's revenue was estimated to have been nearly 5600 million dinars,[17]

---

[17] Complementary Finance Act 2020—MEFAI.

in 2020, the equivalent of 5.1% of G.D.P. At the same time, state expenditure increased because of additional interventions in response to the crisis (social transfers, support for affected businesses, procurement of medical equipment, strategic stockpiling of medicines at the central pharmacy, etc.). The total budgetary cost of the pandemic in 2020 was approximately 7.2% of G.D.P., requiring more significant levels of additional financing.

Impact on Household Living Standards

The crisis has highlighted the absence of detailed statistics for regularly monitoring household living conditions. Many households have seen their living conditions deteriorate because of the lockdown. The various post-lockdown surveys found a relative improvement in the situation with the gradual lifting of restrictions prior to October when the socioeconomic situation began to deteriorate again.

Indeed, in the survey conducted by the I.N.S. of household living conditions during the first wave, 60% said they had been affected in one way or another by the pandemic. This number fell to 38% during the second wave. During June, 40.8% of households experienced a deterioration in their standard of living, with 10.2% being more seriously affected.[18] Of the poorest 20% of households, 58% suffered a deterioration in their living conditions. The suspension of work was one of the main factors where 57% of respondents reported being laid off before the lockdown. This number was 41% in the second round, and 5% for October. After the termination of the lockdown, 5.9% of workers lost their jobs, and 29,000 unemployed people did not return to work, even when their employers resumed their activities.[19] Sixty per cent of the respondents could not obtain their salary. This number rose to 80% in the poorest groups (see Fig. 13.2).

The inter-quintile difference is a persisted where according to the results of the fourth round, 70% of households in the first quintile were able to obtain their salary, and 17% of them were unable to do so. The figures were 92% and 4% respectively in the richest quintile. During

[18] The 4th round of the survey of household living standards was 22-28 June 2020.

[19] Indicators of employment and unemployment, Third quarter 2020—I.N.S.

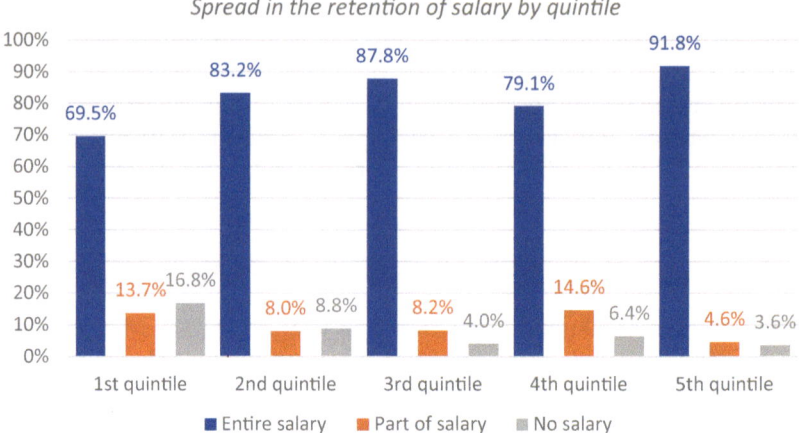

Fig. 13.2 Spread in retention of salary in Tunisia *Source* I.N.S. 4th round of the household living standards survey

October, the vast majority were able, ultimately, to obtain their salaries in full.

It is interesting to note, however, that the sectors developed differently from one period to the next. For example, industry and agriculture were most affected in the first round. After that, many service sector workers were most likely to be unpaid (73% as opposed to approximately one-third for both agriculture and industry). This is because industry and agriculture were no longer subjected to the restrictions imposed on the service sector.

This deterioration was mainly seen in the incapacity to pay fixed charges, as 28% of the households surveyed were unable to do so. However, this improved since this proportion was previously more than half in the two quintiles (40%) with the poorest respondents. Therefore, these results show that the distribution of financial aid to families in need or households that lost some or all their income during the suspension of economic activity was not adequate to cover the needs of those households (Fig. 13.3).

The survey results show that the poorest people found it more difficult to pay expenses associated with education (33%) or health (34%). Despite these fluctuations, the number of households able to find a sum of 200

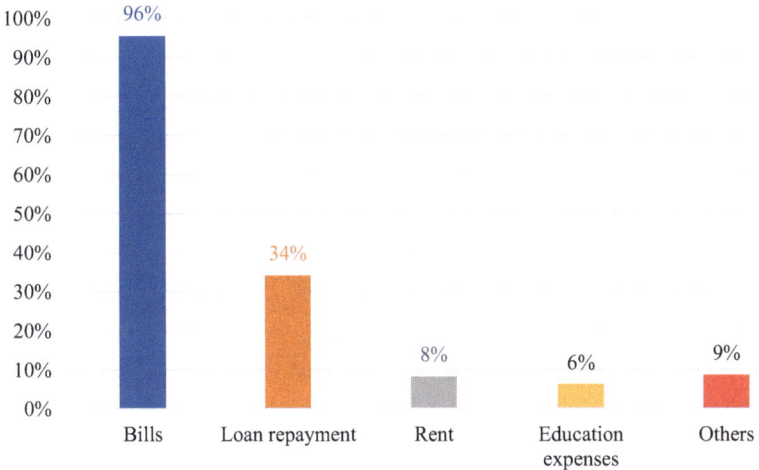

Fig. 13.3 Rate of failure to pay fixed charges by type (*Source* I.N.S. Survey—fourth round of the household living standards survey)

dinars in an emergency rose from 44% in the first round to 55% in the second and 62% in October.

Nevertheless, the ERF survey shows that, when restrictions were reintroduced, 51% of households experienced a drop in income relative to February (of more than 25% in 38% of households and less than 25% in 13%). More specifically, the socio-professional categories most affected were farmers, of whom 61% experienced a loss of income, the self-employed (69%), regular informal workers (63%), irregular informal workers (61%),[20] and the unemployed (60%).[21]

Vulnerable people do not only belong to the first wealth quintile. According to Krafft et al. (2021), the second and third quartiles have experienced the most significant losses (49%) while at the same time, the richest have experienced an increase in their income (13%). In addition, a small share of the population is getting richer while the losses are consistent in time for a large part of the population (it is important to note

---

[20] Regular workers have a permanent jobs, while irregular ones do not work permanently.

[21] November 2020 COVID-19 MENA Monitor (ERF).

that data on the richest people in Tunisia are not included in this survey) (Krafft et al., 2021).

In addition, it should be mentioned that these realities were experienced differently depending on gender. The pandemic has been experienced as a "double lockdown" for many Tunisian women, which can sometimes lead to parental burnout. At first, we can still note the large share of women in the public sector in Tunisia, which was also one of the most protected sectors during the pandemic. In addition, many women work in the informal sector, particularly in domestic and agricultural work, and, on the one hand, they are over-represented in frontline jobs, those related to the hospital environment. Also, the pre-pandemic trends were catalysed by the pandemic. It should be noted that women tend to leave the labour market for family reasons relatively earlier compared to men (Selwaness & Krafft, 2020). This is even more true due to Covid-19-related issues (Krafft et al., 2021). Thus, women are present in many essential sectors for the proper functioning of society and, paradoxically, are subject to insecurities related to working conditions and employment.

In summary, the various surveys show a relative improvement in the situation with the gradual lifting of restrictions until October, when the socioeconomic situation began to deteriorate again. Indeed, nearly 44% of respondents stated that their finances were worse in early October than before the crisis.

Impact on Employment

Since employment is the primary determinant of income, our analysis will begin with the social impact of this variable. As stated above, the most acute effects were seen during the lockdown phase, but the subsequent improvement was patchy given the restrictions and social distancing measures. To complete and refine the analysis of the impact of employment, we draw on rounds 2 and 3 of the I.N.S. National Population and Employment Survey and the ERF survey. The ERF survey focused on a more recent period which allows for a more concrete analysis of the consequences of the pandemic in late 2020 (Table 13.2).

The health crisis led to a rise in the unemployment rate to 18% in the second quarter of 2020 compared with 15% in the first quarter and a loss of 161,000 jobs, 132,000 of which involved salaried employee. The unemployment rate fell to 16.2%, with an increase in the number of people employed of 107,000 by comparison with the second quarter

Table 13.2 Pandemic effects on employment indicators

Indicator	T1 (2020)[22]	T2 (2020)	T3 (2020)
Minimum wage (hourly)		1.984 dinars	
Minimum wage (daily)		15.504 dinars	
Unemployment rate	15%	18%	16.2%
Unemployment rate (male)	12.3%	15.2%	13.5%
Unemployment rate (women)	22%	25%	
Unemployment rate (youth)			
Workers in Employment	28%	36.5%	22.8%
Workers in employment (male)	48%	−4.5%*	35.7%
Workers in employment (female)		−3.92%	30.2%
Unemployed graduates		−6.14%	47.7%
Active labour force		31.2%	
Participation rate		−1.17%	
		47.4%	

Source Compilation of the results of the ENPE 2020 survey, National Institute of Statistics

of the year. According to the ERF survey, the unemployment rate in November was 3 percentage points higher than before Covid-19. This increase was seen primarily among men, particularly those who had completed primary education. Indeed, working women are generally better educated and prefer public service when they can.

Secondly, there is the impact on salaries. According to the ERF survey,[23] the employment situation in November was still affected even though it had improved by comparison with the situation during the total lockdown. Thirty-two per cent were laid off temporarily, and 13% made redundant. In terms of the number of hours worked, 29% of workers were working for fewer hours. In addition, the wages of 21% of the respondents declined, and there was a delay in the payment of wages for 36%. The tourism sector was the most affected sector.

Moreover, the consequences were more manifest in specific socio-professional categories. Farmers were most affected where 8% employed before the pandemic were no longer engaged in active employment.

[22] It should be noted that data collection for the National Population and Employment Survey had to be suspended when the lockdown began. According to the I.N.S., 78% of the sample was surveyed.

[23] "Assessing the impact of Covid-19 on Households, Firms and Farmers—Tunisia—ERF—November 2020." The survey took place from 25 October to 30 November 2020.

In addition, 16% of private sector workers who were still employed in February were unemployed (6% of informal workers and 2% of farmers).

During the previous 60 days, 32% of employees were laid off temporarily, and 13% were made redundant; 36% were experiencing delays in payment, 29% were working fewer hours, and 21% were being paid less. The survey found that irregular and regular informal workers were most affected during this period.

The trends were consistent over time, but we can still note a less significant integration into the labour market for women according to the results of the surveys conducted by the Economic Research Forum. For example, between November 2020 and February 2021, the labour force participation (standard) increased significantly more for men (79 to 87%) than women (47% to 46%). It is also the case for the employment rate. Men (69 to 77%) were more employed than women (27–28%).

These results indicate that precarious employment was most affected. That type of employment is most common in small and medium-sized enterprises.[24] An understanding of supply-side effects and the coping strategies of business is needed for a better analysis of the results described here.

According to the first round of the I.N.S./World Bank survey, private sector businesses made limited changes during April 2020.[25] About half (50.1%) of businesses reported making no changes, 18.7% reported giving paid holidays and 9.6% unpaid holidays. Another 11.5% of businesses reported wage cuts. Only 4.5% of enterprises said they had implemented redundancies in April, and 1.2% said they took on new employees. In particular, the construction sector and the mechanical and electronic industries made most employment-related changes.

According to the I.N.S. survey,[26] 59.0% of businesses made employment-related changes in July: 17.7% of them implemented redundancies, 18.2% granted paid leave and 7.2% unpaid leave, 10.9% cut wages and 27.1% cut the number of hours worked, while 4.8% took on new staff.

---

[24] Inequalities, vulnerabilities to poverty and unemployment—Tunisian Forum for Economic and Social Rights.

[25] Socio-Economic Impact Study of the private sector—an IFC/INS partnership—1st phase.

[26] Socio-Economic Impact Study of the private sector—an IFC/INS partnership—2nd phase.

According to the ERF survey, 38% of domestic businesses implemented temporary layoffs, and 28% implemented redundancies.

According to the ANRS survey, more than half of the companies declared they had not received government assistance. The measures that have benefited most companies are the postponement of the payment of contributions from the CNSS for the second quarter for three months (22%) and the postponement of tax payments for three months from April 1 (16%). Employment remained stable for April (77% and 81% of companies declare stability in terms of employment) despite a decrease that remains to be considered (20% in April and 16% in May). Full payment in April and May remains the minority and represents around 1/3 of the companies surveyed. During June, no reductions were known within the companies.

Paradoxically, the businesses that needed assistance most were not those which submitted most applications to the authorities. Only a quarter of them applied for assistance or are in the process of receiving it.[27] During the crisis, the financial assistance granted to companies under the "Help Enterprise" platform or in the Batinda context has not been adequate to preserve jobs, particularly during the lockdown.

Overall, according to the four rounds of the Household Living Standards Survey, only 5% of respondents who had been employed before the lockdown had not yet returned to work by early October. The vast majority of those who returned to work did so with the same employer (90%), and they received their full salary (85%).[28]

Impact on Informal Employment and Social Protection

The formal sector recorded a decline of 86,000 jobs, in comparison with an increase in the number of jobs in the informal sector of 31,300. According to the third round of the 2020 Employment Survey, the agriculture and construction sectors were in first and second place in terms of the proportion of informal jobs (85% and 72%, respectively), followed by the commercial sector (66.2%). Income losses for workers in the informal sector were quite significant, particularly during the lockdown. Indeed,

[27] "Assessing the impact of Covid-19 on Households, Firms and Farmers".

[28] INS Survey.

the hardest-hit sectors were those with a high proportion of workers in informal employment.

Otherwise, 44.9%[29] households surveyed by the I.N.S. during the month of June reported that they could not find paid work. After deducting the proportion of households that lost wages as reported by their employers (5.9%)[30] during the same period, we can conclude that 39%[31] of workers in the informal sector lost their jobs.

Vulnerable groups face multiple situations reflecting combinations of factors that exacerbate their vulnerability. Examples include the situation of workers in the construction industry.[32] Sixty-eight per cent of workers in the construction sector are employed informally. The condition of workers in the context of the pandemic reflects three main factors namely, transport, wage system and delivery assistance crises. They are two categories affected namely administrative poverty (holders of cards for free health or a "white book") and the category of persons with free health insurance (AMG II), commonly known as the "yellow book," which are not covered by any health protection scheme. In addition, workers in this sector report a sense of injustice and indifference towards the government, mainly because of the perceived inconsistency in the conditions for obtaining assistance. Moreover, obtaining a "white book" is controversial because the list of legal beneficiaries has not been updated. In addition, a successful application process sometimes requires a bribe.[33]

The circumstances of workers in the agricultural sector have been affected due to knock-on effects and the position of their sector in the value chain.[34] For example, the shutdown of the tourism sector has significantly impacted the demand for agricultural products because of the border closures. Although demand has been high during the lockdown

---

[29] Data from the fourth round of the I.N.S./World Bank household survey.

[30] Data from the INS/IFC survey.

[31] This figure is for information purposes only since the data come from two different surveys.

[32] Tunisia: consequences of the pandemic for construction workers: the lockdown between government action and lived reality—Maddouri Haythem.

[33] According to the FTDES report on the impact of the COVID-19 pandemic on farmers.

[34] Agriculture in the context of a health crisis linked to COVID-19: reducing inequalities in the olive-oil value chain in Tunisia.

for essential commodities,[35] many farmers have been faced with the interruption of supplies of inputs such as imported feed materials or plant protection products. According to an ERF survey, 58% of the farmers surveyed used fewer inputs due to this reason.

On top of mobility restrictions, this specific situation has been conducive to speculation and monopolization in some food supply contexts. The National Anti-Corruption Authority also stated that 300 reports were received daily from the public about speculative practices. Moreover, the authorities seized basic food products such as semolina, subsidized flour, and vegetable oil. The same applied to large quantities of sanitary products. For example, delegates were dismissed, including the delegation of Kalaat Sinan on the Algerian border were arrested for having concealed a large quantity of semolina to resell it in Algeria.[36]

Like construction workers, farmers are also exposed to the risk of having no social security cover. Initially, the circumstances led to an actual and expected fall in harvests for three-quarters of the farmers surveyed.[37] This issue has already been targeted by civil society action, particularly concerning women working in agriculture through the Ehmini project, which involves identifying women working in agriculture to benefit from social security.

Ultimately, informal sector workers were excluded from the scope of the measures implemented for households and businesses, except for some types of assistance granted to families in need, and they were therefore affected more by a loss of income. More specifically, there is an important share of women working in the informal sector (domestic workers, agricultural and textile-related workers). Furthermore, workers' challenges might differ depending on the sector or the region. For instance, businesses in some regions tend to operate less than nine years due to fiscal advantages permitted by the law investment, who must proceed by the mean of delocalization to re-operate after that. Workers are then left in difficult situation, especially older people.[38]

---

[35] At the beginning of the pandemic, 65% of respondents had difficulty obtaining flour and semolina. According to the I.N.S. survey, this figure fell to 40% at the end of May.

[36] La Tunisie face au Covid-19 pp. 59–60.

[37] According to the ERF survey of households and farmers in Tunisia.

[38] https://inkyfada.com/fr/2021/03/25/ouvrieres-textile-monastir-covid-tunisie/.

Their proportion increased significantly after the crisis since the proportion of informal workers reached 46.4% in the third quarter of 2020, by comparison with 44.8% in the previous year (fourth quarter of 2019), as did the proportion of precarious jobs. This exacerbates the severity of the impact of possible major crises on employment, poverty, and household living standards.

Concerning social assistance, only 14.2% of households surveyed by the National Institute of Statistics in May reported receiving social assistance in cash. It is important to point out that the share of public transfers in the assistance granted during the lockdown (transfers of money, food or other assistance) amounted to 88.1%,[39] which reflects the importance of the social role of the State in times of crisis.

On the poverty scale, it emerged that there were targeting errors in the distribution of households receiving money transfers by quintile. Only 27.9% of the poorest households received cash assistance. In other words, fewer than 6% of the households that most deserve social benefits received cash assistance. It should be noted that the PNAFN currently covers nearly 9% of the Tunisian households that automatically qualify for exceptional assistance. Paradoxically, the survey results showed that 6.5% of the richest 20% of households received financial assistance.

According to ERF MENA Covid-19 Monitor (Krafft et al., 2021), the percentage of this population benefiting from regular social assistance (PNAFN/AGMII) or recent Covid-19 related programmes decreased from 22% in November 2020 to 20% in February 2021. Nevertheless, a considerable share of beneficiaries belonging to the fourth quintile (9%) of income was receiving this support from the State (Krafft et al., 2021).

In summary, the allocation of financial assistance suffered from a major targeting problem that has limited the expected impact in terms of mitigating negative effects on the living standards of households. Moreover, during the lockdown, only 4000 families were covered by the PNAFN programme[40] (Fig. 13.4).

According to the ERF survey, 18% of respondents were able to obtain government assistance. The socio-professional categories[41] more likely to receive government assistance were regular informal workers (35%), the

---

[39] The second round of the household living standards surveys during the period 15–21 May 2020.

[40] According to an internal CRES source.

[41] As of February 2020.

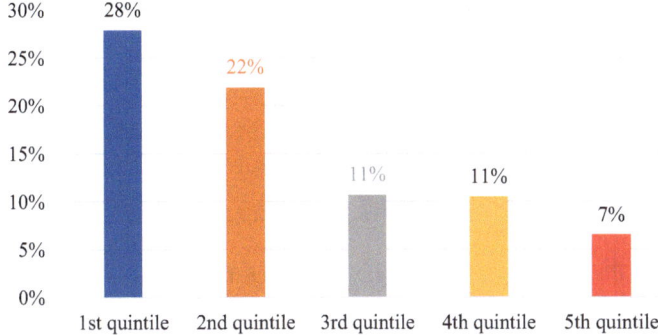

Fig. 13.4 Households receiving financial aid by wealth status () *Source* I.N.S. 2nd round of the household living standards survey

self-employed (23%), the unemployed (22%), people not included in the labour force (21%), irregular workers (20%), farmers (12%), and regular formal workers (12%).[42]

Nevertheless, with the return of restrictions, the ERF survey shows that 51% of households experienced a drop in income in February (more than 25% for 38% and less than 25% for 13%). More specifically, the socio-professional categories most affected were farmers, of whom 61% experienced a loss of income, the self-employed (69%), regular informal workers (63%), irregular, informal workers (61%), and the unemployed (60%).

The spatial distribution of households receiving assistance favours non-urban households, where poverty is more highly concentrated than urban households. Moreover, the targeting of financial assistance was better at this level (Fig. 13.5).

Regarding service delivery, the I.N.S./World Bank survey showed that 14.7% of governmental and non-governmental institutions offer services that strongly emphasize the most vulnerable groups. This proportion is higher for governmental institutions with a social or health focus (28.6%) and national associations (37.5%). During the spread of the first wave of Covid-19, the overall demand for the services offered increased for

---

[42] The Impact of COVID-19 on Middle Eastern and North African Labor Markets: Vulnerable Workers, Small Entrepreneurs, and Farmers Bear the Brunt of the Pandemic in Morocco and Tunisia.

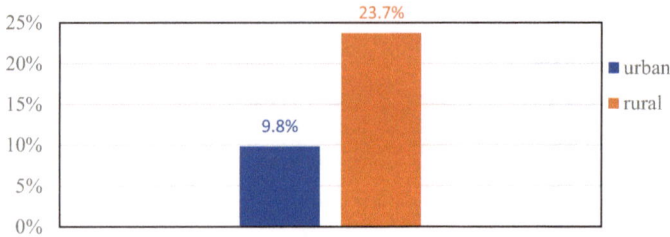

Fig. 13.5 Percentage of households receiving financial assistance () *Source* I.N.S. 2nd round of the household living standards survey

41.2% of the institutions surveyed. This increase was more pronounced for government social and health institutions (71.4%) and national associations (75%). The interviews revealed the lack of monitoring of the most vulnerable households by almost all the institutions interviewed. About 85.3% of the organizations interviewed are dissatisfied with the level of government assistance delivered to businesses and households. Moreover, 61.8% of the organizations believe this assistance falls short of the actual need (Fig. 13.6).

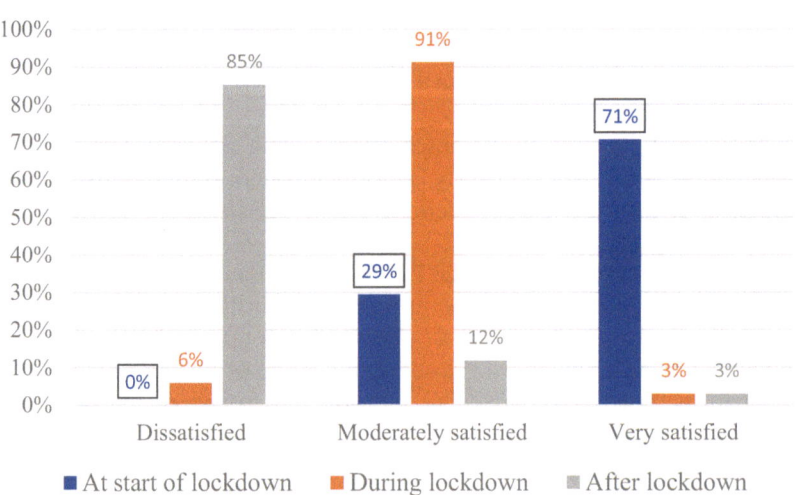

Fig. 13.6 Satisfaction with assistance allocated to businesses and households

Most actors said that they believed government assistance was not adequate for the most vulnerable groups. In addition, those most in need have not been able to obtain assistance because of problems with organization and resources. A failure to identify vulnerable persons was also noted. The difficulties of finalizing the response devised to process applications and the follow-up to those applications are more problematic. In addition, a series of interviews with agricultural workers[43] confirms this. The distribution of the assistance is thought to have been uncoordinated because the assistance was not covered by the circulars issued by the State due to infrastructural problems.

IMPACT ON POVERTY

Overall, the pandemic undoubtedly weakened population groups that were not necessarily vulnerable previously, resulting in the emergence of a category of "new poor".[44] This category represents all the new poor, and the marginal population thought to have left the poverty category in 2020.[45] This definition is particularly relevant in administrative poverty and the problems with targeting government assistance. To some extent, it is consistent with the categorization on lines of perceived poverty, recorded poverty, and poverty as assessed by the Ministry of Social Affairs.[46]

The results of the simulations proposed by UNDP must be presented in a context where survey data were not available at this level of disaggregation. The rate of monetary poverty worsened during the two months of lockdown following the spread of the pandemic, primarily because of falling consumer spending and rising prices for basic foodstuffs. In fact, according to UNDP simulations, 457,500 individuals fell below the poverty line. Moreover, the monetary poverty rate reached 19.2%[47] as opposed to 15.2% before the Covid-19 crisis. This can be explained by

---

[43] FTDES report on farmers.

[44] "Profiles of the new poor due to the COVID-19 pandemic" 6 August 2020, World Bank.

[45] According to projections.

[46] These categories were formulated in the report "Pandémie Covid-19 en Tunisie: Les inégalités, les vulnérables à la pauvreté et au chômage" Mahjoub Azzam - FTDES.

[47] Study on the economic impact of COVID-19 in Tunisia - UNDP.

the decline in consumer spending by household groups and the increase in the price of basic foodstuffs. The categories most affected by Covid-19 were unemployed and inactive workers, who have experienced a more considerable fall in their income than other household categories. As far as the last two of these categories are concerned, although inactive people do not receive any direct income, they receive assistance from their families and relatives. Inactive people and the unemployed were among those most affected by the health crisis. This is because, in addition to rising prices, they suffered from the effect of the fall in the incomes of their relatives. In addition, the economic recession caused by the coronavirus has affected multidimensional poverty. Indeed, the multidimensional poverty index[48] exceeded 15.6%, compared with 13.2%, due to the difficulties encountered by poor households in terms of food and health expenses (Box 13.1).

Box 13.1: Principal findings relating to the impact of the pandemic on poverty according to UNDP.

– Multidimensional poverty rose from 13.2% to 15.6%
– Food expenditure rose from 14.4% to 21.3%
– Healthcare spending rose from 44.5% to 49.1%
– The proportion of the poor increased in the category of agricultural workers (45.1% as opposed to a 38.3% before the health crisis), in the category of non-agricultural workers (27.3% as opposed to 21.8% before the health crisis), in the category of farmers (26.8% as opposed to 21.4% before the health crisis), in the category of the unemployed (41.7% as opposed to 35.6% before the health crisis) and in the category of other inactive persons (24.5% as opposed to 19.5% before the health crisis)
– According to the multidimensional approach, the poorest Tunisian households were poorer after the crisis. Indeed, the

---

[48] Multidimensional poverty is based on calculating an index (M.P.I.) that identifies privation in terms of education, health and income. This index is based on 10 indicators covering (i) education (duration of schooling, children in school), (ii) health (infant mortality, nutrition), and (iii) standard of living (electricity, sanitation, drinking water, land, cooking fuel, equipment).

> poverty rate rose in the category of agricultural workers (23.4% as opposed to 20.7% before the health crisis), in the category of non-agricultural workers (15.7% as opposed to 13.1% before the health crisis), in the category of farmers (19.6% as opposed to 16.8% before the health crisis), in the category of the unemployed (24.3% as opposed to 21.5% before the health crisis) and in the category of other inactive persons (24% as opposed to 17.7% before the health crisis)

Source UNDP (2020)

THE IMPACT OF THE LOCKDOWN ON ACCESS TO BASIC SERVICES

The total lockdown in response to the pandemic included the closure of all schools and academic institutions. The options for online education in the public sector were limited due to the shortages of connection options, equipment, and distance learning materials.

More specifically, most pupils and students were not able to maintain educational continuity, and after the lockdown, only 39% of school children were able to participate in a learning activity.[49] These activities consisted of completing homework (48%), following educational programmes (40%) and using digital platforms (37%). In addition, only 26% of households were able to contact a teacher. This proportion was 53% for the richest quintile and 11% for the poorest quintile. It should be noted, however, that the authorities, with assistance from civil society, produced educational television programmes to safeguard the continuity of distance learning for a large population of pupils, particularly in rural areas with less internet connection. However, the impact of those programmes remains uncertain.

Education is, therefore, not exempt from the stark reality of greater inequality because of the crisis. Indeed, the proportion of students who

---

[49] The second round of the household living standards survey for the period 15-21 May 2020.

have had contact with teachers is five times higher in richer households than in poorer ones. Furthermore, children whose parents come from modest families or who have poorly educated parents would face more difficulties when they return to school. The main reasons for the educational shortfall are the lack of remote options (33%), a lack of interest (22.5%), lack of communications with teachers (18%), and lack of equipment and educational materials at home (11% of households).[50]

The poor performance of remote education can be explained, in part, by the lack of digital resources and equipment in the education system, which is even more serious in the era of digital transformation, but also by the modest digital resources produced as a matter of urgency in combination with the lack and inadequacy of teacher training and the poor mastery of digital tools. Moreover, it is important to note that two-thirds of respondents in the four rounds of the household living standards survey believed that the health measures taken in schools were inadequate to protect students and teachers and that priority should be given to improving infrastructure and equipment in schools.

The considerations set out here about the educational options available in Tunisia should also be seen in conjunction with the circumstances of children, which the pandemic has severely impacted. In addition, it has also been noted[51] that there was an increase in insomnia, violence, and depression among children in 34%, 33% and 18% of households respectively. More specifically, impaired concentration was seen in one-third of the children. Housing conditions may also influence their psychological condition. According to the 2014 national census, 27.6% of dwellings consist of fewer than two rooms, and about 54% of dwellings in non-municipal areas are "*dar/houch arbi*" (traditional houses). These living conditions can be particularly affected by the family context: according to the Ministry for Women, the Family, Children and Seniors, violence against women has increased seven times during the lockdown. Calls to dedicated numbers increased drastically during the lockdown (multiplied

[50] The first round of the Household Living Standards Survey for the period 29 April-8 May 2020.

[51] The 2nd round of the household living standards survey during the period 15 May-21 May 2020.

by 7).[52] In other words, the problems associated with delivering education are catalysed by the living conditions of children and the family circle in the context of uncertainty associated with the pandemic.

The short-term consequences referred to here should be viewed in the context of the situation prior to the pandemic. Indeed, this "missed year" for young Tunisians will exacerbate cumulative under-achievement at whatever level of education.

In summary, education is unquestionably one of the sectors most affected by the crisis, mainly because of the disruption of educational continuity, and the repercussions are irremediable, particularly for the most vulnerable. The inequalities in educational infrastructure access should be of a concern to government going forward.

IMPACT ON ACCESS TO THE HEALTH SERVICES

Access to medical assistance has gradually improved after the difficulties during the total lockdown. Household access to medical care after the lockdown has returned to almost the same level as before the spread of the pandemic, according to the I.N.S. survey conducted during June. Indeed, 5.3% of the households surveyed could access health services during the total lockdown, and 25.5% reported being able to access health services during the progressive relaxation of restrictions. However, of the poorest 20% of households, only 7% had access to medical assistance during the total lockdown, and 18.8% had access during the targeted lockdown (Fig. 13.7).

Turning to the quality of health services, 30.4% of the households surveyed reported dissatisfaction with the quality of care obtained. In addition, 44.3% of the poorest 20% of households reported being dissatisfied. The main reasons are the financial charges involved (22% overall and 20.4% of the 20% of poorest households) and the distance from health facilities (10.9% overall and 21.8% of the 20% of poorest households).

Moreover, the pandemic has had a negative impact on the public health sector[53] in the light of the following listed in the Box 13.2:

---

[52] https://lapresse.tn/59099/retombees-sociales-du-confinement-total-la-femme-tunisienne-doublement-sanctionnee/

[53] Economic budget for 2021.

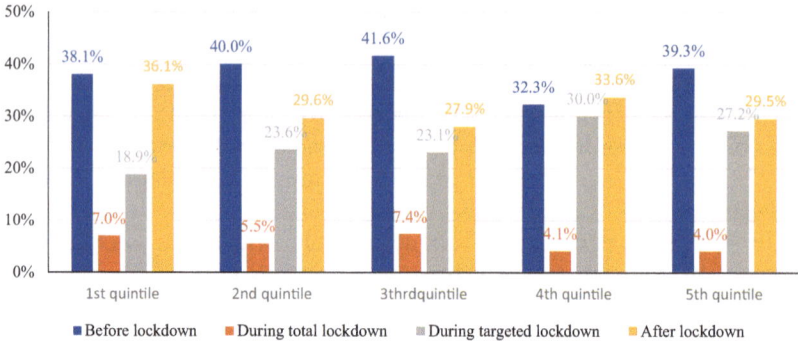

Fig. 13.7 Spread of households access to medical care by quintile (*Source* I.N.S. 4th round of the household living standards survey)

Box 13.2: Pandemic Impact on Health Sector

- The fall in the level of activity of the public health structures and, consequently, the decline in their revenue
- The worsening health status of patients with chronic diseases
- An urgent need for additional beds in the intensive care units (the available number of beds with oxygen facilities is 450 and the number of intensive care beds is just 240)[54]
- The depletion of stocks of medicines and shortages of medical equipment[55]. Particularly for people from the lower categories
- The poor management of medical staff and medical specialists. In addition, the reduction and restriction of medical assistance during the lockdown have had an impact on health services
- The increasing need for medical organizations to protect themselves against the pandemic[56]
- The delay in the establishment of some twenty hospital units

[54] Emergency Response Project—Environmental and Social Management Framework—Ministry of Health—September 2020.

[55] "Appeal to the public authorities to safeguard supplies of medicines in the public health structures and to provide one million chronically ill people with the right to medication"—Civil society collective for the defence of the public health sector.

[56] "Frontline health service contribution to the continuity of services and the fight against the COVID-19 pandemic" Tunisian Association for the Right to Health.

In addition, the cost of the PCR test represents a significant proportion of the household budget in the context of private clinics, given that most of them were not able to find 210 dinars in emergencies.

Moreover, the crisis has shown that the lack of means of transport and the minimum service requirements for medical assistance, both public and private, have negatively affected the quality of health services, particularly during the total lockdown. While the government's proactive strategy to contain the spread of the virus did succeed in limiting the number of deaths and infections during the first wave, the acuity of the sector's shortcomings and problems, and the lack of a coherent crisis management plan involving all stakeholders after the period of the progressive relaxation of the lockdown, was strongly felt. The worsening of the health situation and the exponential increase in the number of cases, both infections and mortalities, bear witness to this.

CONCLUSION

Tunisia was particularly successful in managing the first wave of the pandemic from a health perspective due to the early and strong response. However, this response had a very high economic cost and a disproportionate social impact that the State was able to mitigate in part only. Indeed, the economic difficulties of the previous decade left the Tunisian State with no room to manoeuvre in response to major crises. In addition, the presence of a large informal sector and the delay in the implementation of the unique identifier did not make the task any easier for the government, which had to respond exceptionally quickly.

In addition to the cost of jobs and income, the education of working- and middle-class children have been the big loser: public education, unlike private education, has not made any provisions for remote schooling.

After the lockdown phase, Tunisia went through a partial recovery during the summer and early autumn due to the lifting of restrictions. However, the second wave had a more dramatic health impact because of the need to work with socioeconomic constraints. The State no longer had the resources to compensate households or businesses. The most vulnerable therefore had to pay the price for this crisis.

The pandemic has once again highlighted malfunctions in monitoring, continuity, and quality of services, especially for those who need them most. It has deepened inequalities and revealed the presence of a two-speed Tunisia. This pandemic is, therefore, not only a reflection of stark structural and social needs but also a window of opportunity to precipitate structural reforms. The ordeal of the pandemic has also highlighted the resilience of the Tunisian social fabric, particularly the capacity for adaptation of civil society and the public.

One of the few positive aspects of this exceptional Covid-19 crisis is that it has helped accelerate certain structural reforms, particularly the digitalization of the administration of the economy. In addition, the completion of the Amen Social programme and of the unique identifier, the minimization of inclusion and exclusion errors in the allocation of assistance, and the strengthening of financial inclusion are now seen as absolute priorities.

The success of these reforms will depend on the ability of leaders to forge consensus and compromise by organizing a dialogue about reforms that can remedy structural difficulties along the lines of the dialogue that anchored the democratic transition.

In line with the findings, the Tunisian government needs to mainstream social inclusion in the fight against the pandemic as it did for the first wave. Given the low availability of financial resources, it should envisage all the possibilities of mobilizing more resources locally, including coordinating better between the different stakeholders. It should also present a clear plan to international donors to guarantee more external support and simplify any cumbersome procedures impeding the funds from reaching the final beneficiaries. In the longer run, the country needs to extend social protection to a larger share of the population by inciting informal workers and enterprises to become formal.

References

Ali, N., & Marouani, M. A. (2020). *Household enterprises: The impact of formality on productivity and profits*. Working Papers 1452, Economic Research Forum.

Assaad, R., & Krafft, C. (2016). Labor market dynamics and youth unemployment in the middle East and North Africa: Evidence from Egypt, Jordan and Tunisia. Economic Research Forum Working Paper Series No. 993.

Assaad, R., Ghazouani, S., & Krafft, C. (2018). The composition of labor supply and unemployment in Tunisia. In R. Assaad & M. Boughzala (Eds.), *The Tunisian Labor market in an era of transition* (pp. 1–38). Oxford University Press.

Assaad, R., Rana, H., Moundir, L., & Yassin, S. (2020). Explaining the MENA Paradox: Rising educational attainment, yet stagnant female labor force participation. *Demographic Research, 43*(28), 817–850.

Association tunisienne de la défense du droit à la santé. (2016). *Le droit à la santé en Tunisie.*

Avocats sans Frontières. (2020). *Deux mois de lutte contre le Covid-19 en Tunisie. Analyse en matière d'État de droit.*

Centre de recherches et d'études sociales. (2017). *Note d'orientation des pistes de réformes pour l'instauration d'un Socle de Protection Sociale.*

Centre de recherches et d'études sociales. (2017). *Évaluation de la performance des programmes d'assistance sociale en Tunisie.*

Forum tunisien des droits économiques et sociaux (2014). *L'abandon scolaire volontaire : le phénomène et les causes.*

Forum tunisien des droits économiques et sociaux (2020). *L'agriculture en contexte de crise sanitaire liée au Covid-19 : Réduire les inégalités dans la chaîne de valeur de l'huile d'olive en Tunisie.*

Forum tunisien des droits économiques et sociaux (2020). *Rapport mensuel des mouvements sociaux, suicides et violences.*

Institut national de la statistique. (2018). *Enquête nationale sur la consommation et le niveau de vie des ménages pour l'année 2015.*

Institut national de la statistique (2019). *Tunisie en chiffres 2018.*

Institut national de la statistique (2020). *Suivi de l'impact socio-économique du Covid-19 sur les ménages tunisiens - Résultats de la quatrième vague (22 juin 2020–28 juin 2020).*

Institut national de la statistique (2020). *Suivi de l'impact socio-économique du Covid-19 sur les ménages tunisiens - Résultats de la seconde vague (15 mai 2020–21 mai 2020).*

Institut tunisien des études stratégiques (2020). *La Tunisie face à la COVID-19 à l'horizon 2025 : Fondements d'une stratégie conciliant l'urgence du court-terme et les impératifs du moyen-terme.*

Institut national de la statistique (2020). *Suivi de l'impact socio-économique du Covid-19 sur les ménages tunisiens (Octobre 2020).*

Institut national de la statistique & IFC (2020). *Études d'impact socio-économiques sur le secteur privé—1ère phase.*

Institut arabe des chefs d'entreprises (2020). *Évaluation du dernier gouvernement, impact de l'instabilité politique et les actions à entreprendre par le prochain gouvernement selon les chefs d'entreprises.*

Institut national de la statistique (2020). *Suivi de l'impact socio-économique du Covid-19 sur les ménages tunisiens - Résultats de la première vague (29 avril 2020 - 8 mai 2020).*

Institut national de la statistique & IFC (2020). *Études d'impact socio-économiques sur le secteur privé - 2ème phase.*

Krafft, C., Assad, R., & Marouani M. A. (2021). *The Impact of COVID-19 on Middle Eastern and North African Labor Markets: Vulnerable Workers, Small*

Entrepreneurs, and Farmers Bear the Brunt of the Pandemic in Morocco and Tunisia. ERF Policy Brief No. 55.

Maddouri, H.(2020). *Tunisie : Conséquences de la pandémie sur les ouvriers du bâtiment. Le confinement entre mesure gouvernementale et réalité vécue.* Forum tunisien des droits économiques et sociaux.

Azzam Mahkoub. (2020). *Pandémie COVID-19 en Tunisie: Inégalités, vulnérabilités à la pauvreté et au chômage.* Forum tunisien des droits économiques et sociaux.

Marouani, M. A, & Minh, P. L. (2020). The first victims of Covid-19 in developing countries? The most vulnerable workers to the lockdown of the Tunisian economy, DIAL Working Paper DT 2020/6.

Ministère de l'Économie, des Finances et de l'Appui à l'Investissement (2020a). *Budget du Ministère des Affaires Sociales pour l'année 2020.*

Ministère de l'Économie, des Finances et de l'Appui à l'Investissement (2020b). *Budget économique de l'année 2021.*

Ministère de l'Économie, des Finances et de l'Appui à l'Investissement (2020c). *Loi des finances complémentaires 2020.*

Ministère des Affaires Sociales & Bureau international du travail (2020). *Évaluation de l'intervention des communes dans la lutte contre la propagation de la pandémie de Covid-19 en Tunisie.*

Ministère du Commerce de la République Tunisienne (2020). *Présentation de la caisse de compensation.*

Ministère de la Santé (2020). *Projet d'intervention d'urgence - Cadre de gestion environnementale et sociale.*

Ministère de la Santé (2020). *Santé Tunisie en chiffres 2018.* Direction des Études et planification.

Nguyen, M. C., Yoshida, N., Wu, H., & Narayan, A. (2020). *Profiles of the new poor due to the COVID-19 pandemic.* Poverty and Global Equity Practice, Global Unit, World Bank.

OCDE (2016). *Les résultats du PISA 2015 à la loupe.* (PISA à la loupe, n°67, Éditions OCDE).

Programme des Nations Unies pour le Développement (2020). *Impact économique du COVID 19: Analyse en termes de vulnérabilité des ménages et des micros entreprises.*

Redissi, H. (2020). *La Tunisie à l'épreuve du Covid-19.* Observatoire tunisien de la transition démocratique.

UNICEF (2020). *Tunisie : Impact des mesures de confinement associées à la pandémie Covid-19 sur la pauvreté des enfants.*

World Bank. (2015). *The unfinished revolution—bringing opportunity, good jobs and greater wealth to all Tunisians.* The World Bank.

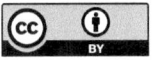

CHAPTER 14

Conclusion

Dzodzi Tsikata and Gertrude Dzifa Torvikey

The chapters in this book have examined the implications of the Covid-19 pandemic and the early containment and support measures by governments to respond to its projected impacts on the fortunes of African economies, societies, and democratic politics. They also consider the implications for the livelihoods of working people, poverty, and inequalities. While the studies were preliminary, they enable us to draw some conclusions on a range of issues. This conclusion discusses a few of the key findings and notes their implications for policy. These include (a) the need to pay attention to pre-existing economic weaknesses and structural inequalities; (b) the importance of policy sovereignty; and c) the need to build stronger and more effective democracies and social policy institutions and infrastructure.

G. D. Torvikey (✉)
Institute of Statistical, Social and Economic Research (ISSER), University of Ghana, Accra, Ghana
e-mail: gdtorvikey@ug.edu.gh

D. Tsikata
Department of Development Studies, SOAS, University of London, London, UK
e-mail: dt48@soas.ac.uk

© The Author(s) 2024
A. Altaf et al. (eds.), *EQUITY IN COVID-19*, EADI Global Development Series, https://doi.org/10.1007/978-3-031-58588-3_14

Pre-existing Economic, Social, and Political Conditions Cast a Long Shadow

As the African Union and other commentators noted, the Covid-19 pandemic was a health crisis with profound socioeconomic consequences for countries and their populations in Africa (African Union, 2020). The twelve studies presented in this book, which have focused on the first year of the pandemic have demonstrated that the degree of the impacts on sectors of the economy and people depends on pre-existing socioeconomic conditions prevalent in a country. Similarly, countries' responses to the crisis also closely derive from their resource base and are contingent on the nature and state of government institutions in these countries. This demonstrated clear interlinkages between structural conditions and responses to pandemic impacts.

Of the twelve countries, only four—Ghana, Tunisia, Kenya, and Nigeria are lower-middle income, while the other eight are low-income countries. Most of the twelve countries, in keeping with the situation in Africa are primary export commodity-dependent and agrarian and therefore have been exposed to the global market turbulence blamed on Covid-19-related trade disruptions. In addition, the services sectors contribute substantially to the GDP of countries such as Ghana, Kenya, Ethiopia, Nigeria, Rwanda, Tunisia, and Uganda. These are also countries with substantial informal economies which concentrate largely precarious forms of work. Thus structural informality is the norm in most study countries, with Tunisia as an outlier which has a bigger formal economy. These economic factors generate social issues which have been exacerbated by the Covid-19 pandemic and policy responses.

On the question of institutional capacity, the studies found that a few countries such as Rwanda and Tunisia had more robust data and targeting systems, while others such as Ghana and Nigeria had deficits in the availability of data. Rwanda's decentralisation structure and robust datasets enhanced social protection targeting. The lack of robust datasets and national social registers had an adverse effect on Covid-19 responses. However, the Rwanda case also demonstrates that data while important, is not sufficient. Although programme delivery has been efficient due to existing robust data used for social protection and the decentralisation of implementation at the village level, the excessive use of preventive measures did not compensate for the heavy impacts on vulnerable social groups.

The state of politics and democracy in a country was also an important dimension of Covid-19 management. Politically, Covid-19 represented a crisis within a crisis with heightened security threats related to Islamic insurgencies of different degrees of severity in countries such as Burkina Faso, Niger, Mali, Mozambique, and Nigeria. Other countries were facing different types of insecurities. Ethiopia was on the brink of civil war while political instability arising from the Arab Spring had unsettled Tunisia. In Ghana's case, elections in 2020 heightened partisan tensions and partisanship and distrust of government. These political challenges affected citizens' engagement and compliance with pandemic containment and support measures.

WHY POLICY SOVEREIGNTY AND DEMOCRATIC POLITICS ARE IMPORTANT

The twelve country studies found that many countries were prompt, proactive, and zealous in some cases in their responses to the Covid-19 outbreak. As well, country responses were quite common across the board in that they consisted of containment measures such as social distancing, face mask-wearing, restrictions on mobility, and sanitary and hygienic practices, among others. The measures were remarkably similar. This was not surprising given the influence of Africa CDC, WHO, and donors on policymaking in Africa. Country lockdowns were on a continuum between severe and long-duration lockdowns such as those experienced in Rwanda and selective and shorter lockdowns in Ghana and Benin.

Given the lack of resilience of economies and institutions, and the poor state of health sector infrastructure across Africa, the Covid-19 containment measures adopted by governments are understandable since the fallouts from high rates of infection could be devastating. However, in their excessive zeal, States paid scant attention to human rights and human dignity, and in some cases, there were serious human rights abuses, particularly concerning curfews in Rwanda, Kenya, Uganda, and Nigeria.

Related to this, citizens in some countries such as Rwanda modelled high levels of compliance with Covid-19 regulations while in Ethiopia and Tunisia, compliance with restrictions was more mixed. Despite the differences in the severity of contaminant measures and mixed levels of citizen compliance, there were no marked differences in levels of infections and success with containment.

The structure of Covid-19 policy decision-making is a common thread in the studies, which found that centralisation and top-down approaches remained the norm. This excluded the voice of the people, CSOs, and other groups from the policy space. The concentration of decision-making power and information asymmetry deepened citizens' mistrust and distrust of the State creating a distance between the people and their government. Given the dire data situation, the lack of consultation with wider segments of society could not have helped the observed lapses in targeting beneficiaries of assistance in several countries. Even when the government used its information systems, as in Rwanda, there have been concerns about patronage and the misuse of local government power to exclude certain categories of persons.

The fact that almost all study countries experienced some form of pandemic-related protests (see Tsikata and Torvikey, 2022) and non-compliance with protocols is an expression of dissatisfaction and disenchantment with the handling of the pandemic by State. The pushback from citizens resulted in some countries such as Niger reconsidering their measures while others such as Nigeria and Rwanda used lethal force to quell resistance and force compliance. These findings point to the importance of paying attention to differences in context and involving citizens in crafting responses to crises in order that government actions do not squander the goodwill of citizens and threaten the democratic dispensation.

Responses to COVID-19 Were Poorly Targeted and Biased in Favour of Certain Social Groups and Spaces

The studies found that pre-existing class, gender, spatial and generational inequalities, weak social protection programmes, and weak social data required for intervention planning and targeting affected the outcomes of responses to the pandemic. There were structural biases in responses that shaped the effects of preventive measures and access to support measures.

In countries such as Ethiopia and Rwanda, Covid-19 prevention-centric measures increased the vulnerability of many people without adequate compensatory support measures. There have been ambiguities, contradictions, and ambivalences of measures and their outcomes for social groups that have widened inequality and worsened the precarious material conditions of certain groups. In Ghana, for example, the authorities intercepted young vulnerable female head porters travelling to their home region to contain the spread of COVID-19 and brought them back to Accra. This exposed them to more vulnerabilities as they were also targets for harassment by city authorities on suspicion that they were vectors in the spread of the virus. Land border closures were common in all countries, and they proved damaging to food security and the livelihoods of small traders.

Furthermore, the public and education authorities adjudged school closures to have been premature, too long and damaging in accentuating inequalities in access to certain kinds of e-learning media and depriving poor children of the benefits of school feeding programmes.

The studies have shown that the pandemic responses in the health sector which included the construction, refurbishment, and conversion of existing health facilities, undermined the capacity of the health sector to undertake non-Covid-19 health interventions. This was the case in Uganda and Kenya where the neglect of equally important health crises increased the vulnerabilities of people who most needed other health care services. In addition, Covid-19 centric health measures did not put measures in place to protect groups with pre-existing health conditions that were most vulnerable to Covid-19 infections.

In sum, preventive protocols failed to take account of the informality of spaces and work and therefore deepened the vulnerability of informal workers. Thus, women, rural dwellers, urban poor, workers in the informal economy and ununionised or unorganised workers were the mostly adversely affected by the pandemic and its containment measures. Paradoxically, these categories of people benefitted less from social support programmes than formal unionised workers. Few countries such as Tunisia and Ethiopia took proactive measures to protect workers' rights with measures such as the suspension of layoffs. Benin implemented measures targeted at artisans. However, these measures targeted formal workers, and not those in the informal economy.

In relation to mitigating and support measures, the country studies highlighted the use of universally applied support measures such as utility subsidies. However, the structural inequalities in the provision of infrastructure that supports these services meant that they benefitted the wealthy instead of the populations most in need. This is because there are existing rural–urban divides and poor and non-poor gaps in access to services. Even support measures, such as business stimuli which target businesses, exclude the very poor and those operating without a modicum of formality such as registration and tax identification number ownership. Many of these sectors are traditionally dominated by women. In addition, during the period, several governments gave tax waivers. As many of these were on consumption, they benefitted the rich more than the poor.

Since the pandemic also had implications for livelihoods and the larger economy, governments instituted mitigation measures such as social support for the poor and the most adversely affected and economic stimulus packages for businesses in many countries. The country studies have shown in many ways how such support measures deepened inequalities since governments policies did not take into account the gaps in the ownership of specific infrastructure such as electricity and water metres, which shape access, and terms of condition and procedures of access.

Several of the research countries expanded social protection programmes numerically or enhanced the social packages. Nigeria for example, increased the eligible numbers on its national social register while Ghana enhanced cash transfer access conditions. However, the overwhelming conclusion was that these programmes were inadequate and so left out many vulnerable social groups. The inadequacy of the support measures has been a common finding of the country studies. Even countries with more robust social protection programmes faced challenges. Tunisia, which was already addressing inequalities through mass social protection programmes before Covid-19, had to confront issues of bureaucratic red tape which restricted access for vulnerable groups, and budgetary pressures which cut short useful programmes. Not surprisingly, Covid-19 has generated many discussions about social protection and the role of the state in social provisioning in health, education, food security, and protecting livelihoods.

In sum, while mitigation and stimulus measures were appropriate, they were poorly targeted and implemented. They showed biases against rural and informal economies and women and therefore exacerbated structural inequalities against those just above the poverty line. For example, in Tunisia and Rwanda, it was itinerant workers had to suffer some of the consequences of the mobility restrictions. In Ghana, it was against certain regions such as the poor north and rural and informal workers.

In conclusion, tackling poverty is different from tackling inequalities. Tackling inequalities requires measures that respond to the structural basis of inequalities, and not to the immediate pandemic effects. The fact that many countries identified urban areas as being the most affected and threw resources at them shows the structural biases and the delinking of urban economies from the rural ones. Apart from the incorrect assumptions about how to reach the poorest of the poor involved in the choice and method of application of these measures, the measures were short-term and ignored pre-existing structural inequalities such as regional, rural–urban, income, and gender, among others. As a result, beneficiaries of both economic and social protection measures were only a minuscule proportion of those suffering dislocation and the opportunity to address inequalities was lost. The pandemic raised new awareness about the need for robust social policies and effective protection programmes for the vulnerable in society which must be part of the systems in place to address structural inequalities and poverty.

References

African Union. (2020). Impact of the Coronavirus (Covid-19) on the African Economy. AU.

Dzodzi, T., & Gertrude, T. D. (2022). COVID-19 in Africa: A synthesis of 12 country studies. INCLUDE.

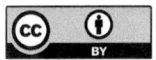

CHAPTER 15

Recommendations and Reflections

Anika Altaf, Dzodzi Tsikata, Gertrude Dzifa Torvikey, and Marleen Dekker

Equity for Future Preparedness: Learning from the Policy and Implementation Gaps During the COVID-19 Pandemic in Africa

Many insightful and valuable recommendations and reflections can be derived from the case studies presented in this book. The unique focus of the case studies on equity within policies and programming at the onset of the COVID-19 pandemic has unveiled serious (future) implications for exacerbating structural inequalities. The health effects of COVID-19 have been limited in Africa; however, the socio-economic consequences of mitigation measures have been substantial. Although the pandemic itself

A. Altaf (✉)
INCLUDE Knowledge Platform for Inclusive Development Policies, African Studies Centre Leiden, Leiden, The Netherlands
e-mail: a.altaf@asc.leidenuniv.nl

D. Tsikata
Department of Development Studies, SOAS, University of London, London, UK
e-mail: dt48@soas.ac.uk

© The Author(s) 2024
A. Altaf et al. (eds.), *EQUITY IN COVID-19*, EADI Global Development Series, https://doi.org/10.1007/978-3-031-58588-3_15

is no longer considered a global threat, the aftermath for the African continent unequivocally is. While some of the studies suggested ways to alleviate part of the harmful remnants of COVID-19, lessons that can be drawn are predominantly warnings for future disruptive changes and crises. During COVID-19, the vision of "*building back better*" was heard loudly within and outside of the development realm. Yet getting back to business as usual quickly overshadowed this aspiration.

Missing Data and Single Registries

If preparedness for future shocks and threats is not commenced soon, slogans such as "*building back better*" will once again remain slogans in a next crisis. For Africa, one of the major constraints in reaching equity and targeting vulnerable and disadvantaged groups with COVID-19 policies and programming was a lack of data and systems. Governments, even with the best intentions of reaching the poorest, generally failed to do so due to outdated population data. Those who required support of the government were not on their radar, despite the fact that they carried the heaviest burden as a result of the containment measures. Moreover, existing data sources were found to be applying systems of patronage (Tsikata & Torvikey, 2022). Countries that had data systems such as single registries in place, e.g. Kenya, Senegal and Mauritius or Togo, where voter registration information and other means to reach a broader population were used, were able to quickly put these to use and scale-up (Swinkels & Altaf, 2022). These types of data were crucial in rolling-out social policies. Especially the single registry system functions well, it is a system that ideally includes all programmes supported by the government, making coordination between social policies possible, such as education, taxes, health care, agricultural livelihoods programmes and other social

G. D. Torvikey
Institute of Statistical, Social and Economic Research (ISSER), University of Ghana, Accra, Ghana

M. Dekker
African Studies Centre Leiden, Leiden, The Netherlands
e-mail: m.dekker@asc.leidenuniv.nl

programmes (Swinkels & Altaf, 2022). Single registries could also function to formalize informal work in order to mitigate the impact of loss of work, which was evident during the COVID-19 pandemic for example during the lock-downs. At the same time, those working in the informal sector may want to stay off the radar. It is crucial that single registries do not cause harm to those who need to be protected, e.g. through misuse of data by governments. Moreover, for single registries to function well, the quality of data and coverage requirements make it a costly affair. Political will and sufficient funding are essential for successful single registries. Global or bilateral funds could play an important role in the set-up of national single registries.

The Shift of Power

While there is no justification for hoarding vaccines and patents, a positive side-effect of these and other exclusionary processes of the global North during the pandemic have pushed the acceleration of the consciousness on the African continent to speeding-up self-reliance (further decreasing dependance on primary commodities), decolonization and regional cooperation and continental unification (e.g., African Union, African Continental Free Trade Agreement). The pandemic offered room to rethink neoliberal development models that had reached their finest hour even before COVID-19. Moreover, possibilities to invest in, develop and promote indigenous and homegrown innovations, research and development sprung up (Kanu, 2020). The global north can learn from the innovations and developments in Africa during the pandemic, for example, the way the private sector in some African countries, such as Ghana, rose to the occasion (e.g., by providing health facilities). This is in stark contrast to for example large companies in the Netherlands profiting from the pandemic while many citizens were in a precarious situation.

Despite the determinedness of African countries to pursue their vision of an independent continent, the global community has a responsibility not to impede these developments, e.g. through the mounting debts crisis and subsidies of countries in the North creating unfair competition within African markets. However "simply" restructuring debts will not be enough, debts and subsidies are part of a financial system based on power imbalances. These imbalances have been magnified during COVID and other events the past years creating a sense of unfairness amongst African countries and a push back on the current system facilitating these imbalances. Hence, the global community has an important task to tackle the inequity within the (financial) system to sustainably address the debt issues and create a level playing field for African countries. Supporting a power balance voluntary will benefit both African countries and the global community, instead of a more forceful and perhaps resentful push from the African continent to restoring balance.

Knowledge Gaps

We already know that inequalities have exacerbated as a consequence of the pandemic and the measures following from that. These measures were developed for the short-term and with the idea that the harm caused by the pandemic would be easily reversible. Thus policies and programming to address structural inequalities are not in place. Moreover, the mid- and long-term consequences of the pandemic are yet to come to light. School closures and related to that drop-out, loss of income and employment of those working in the formal, but particularly informal sector, the impact on political stressors, such as postponement of elections, the role of civil society and civic space, whether and how innovations initiated during the pandemic can be leveraged are some aspects that require further digging.

Using INCLUDE's Equity Lens to Leave No One Behind

The concept of equity, focusing on social and spatial aspects, and the central question in INCLUDE's approach to equity: who gets what, when, where and why, have been crucial in exposing several biases such as gender (more job loss and other disruptions to livelihoods amongst women), as well as a rural and informal economies' bias, revealing poor targeting and implementation of COVID-19 policies and programmes in the case studies. Answering those central questions gives insights into the types of tailor made policies that are necessary to reach the different vulnerable and disadvantaged groups in the context of COVID-19, but also applicable in other crisis and non-crisis contexts. These questions can however only be answered if those who are vulnerable and disadvantaged are heard, directly or through representation. The case studies showed the importance of representation in the design, planning and governance of policy responses (Tsikata & Torvikey, 2022). Trade unions and civil society organizations played a major role in some of the case studies both in representing and in reaching vulnerable and disadvantaged groups, for example, in Ghana and Mozambique.

The intention to do better and not fall back into the way things were is not lost yet and not a utopia either. But it means that in order to do better next time, we start today with a genuine willingness to know who lives in poverty, who lives in a precarious situation and who could potentially fall into such a situation and listen to them. Only then can we safeguard equity in policies and programming and leave no one behind.

REFERENCES

Kanu, I. A. (2020). Covid-19 and the economy: An African perspective. *Journal of African Studies and Sustainable Development, 3*(2), 29–39.

Swinkels, C., & Altaf, A. (2022). Single and ready to mingle: Single registries in social protection. INCLUDE.

Tsikata, D., & Torvikey, D. G. (2022). COVID-19 in Africa: A synthesis of 12 country studies. INCLUDE.

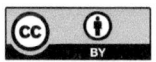